CARDIAC LEAD EXTRACTION

A Case-Based Contemporary Approach

EDITORS

Yong-Mei Cha, MD

Siva K. Mulpuru, MD, MPH

cardiotext

Cardiotext Publishing, LLC
3405 W. 44th Street
Minneapolis, Minnesota 55410
USA
www.cardiotextpublishing.com

Any updates to this book may be found at: www.cardiotextpublishing.com/electrophysiology-heart-rhythm-mgmt/cardiac-lead-extraction

Comments, inquiries, and requests for bulk sales can be directed to the publisher at: info@cardiotextpublishing.com.

Library of Congress Control Number: 2021941855

ISBN: 978-1-942909-54-5
eISBN: 978-1-942909-55-2

Printed in the United States of America

21 22 23 24 25 7 6 5 4 3 2 1

CARDIAC LEAD EXTRACTION

A Case-Based Contemporary Approach

ONLINE ACCESS

The purchase of a new copy of this book entitles the first buyer to free personal access to a digital version of this edition.

Please send a copy of your purchase receipt to info@cardiotext.com with subject LEADS EBOOK, and we will email you a redemption code along with instructions on how to access the digital file.

Dedications

To my loving husband, LeRoy, my son, and his wife (John and Mingjia) for their remarkable support.

To my mentors, colleagues, students, and patients for their encouragement and quest for excellence.

—Yong-Mei Cha

To the three people who lovingly taught me to view the world from a different perspective: P.V. Rama Rao, my grandfather; Balendu C. Vasavada, MD; and Samuel J. Asirvatham, MD.

—Siva K. Mulpuru

Table of Contents

Editors

Yong-Mei Cha, MD
Director of Cardiac Device Practice, Professor of Medicine, Department of Cardiovascular Medicine, Mayo Clinic, Rochester, Minnesota

Siva K. Mulpuru, MD, MPH
Professor of Medicine, Department of Cardiovascular Medicine, Mayo Clinic, Rochester, Minnesota

Contributors

Fatima A. Ali-Ahmed, MD
Fellow, Clinical Cardiac Electrophysiology, Mayo Clinic, Rochester, Minnesota

Arman Arghami, MD
Assistant Professor of Surgery, Department of Cardiovascular Surgery, Mayo Clinic, Rochester, Minnesota

Samuel J. Asirvatham, MD
James M. and Lee S. Vann Professorship in Cardiovascular Medicine; Director, Electrophysiology Laboratories; Director, Cardiac Electrophysiology Training Program, Department of Cardiovascular Diseases, Mayo Clinic, Rochester, Minnesota

Walid M. Barake, FRCPC
Cardiac Electrophysiologist, Kelowna General Hospital, University of British Columbia, Kelowna, British Columbia, Canada

Ulrika Birgersdotter-Green MD
Professor of Medicine; Director, Pacemaker Services, Division of Cardiovascular Diseases, University of California San Diego Health System, San Diego, California

Antonio Maria Canu, MD
Cardiac Electrophysiologist, Second Division of Cardiology, Cardiac Thoracic and Vascular Department, New Santa Chiara Hospital, Azienda Ospedaliero Universitaria Pisana, Pisa, Italy

Gregory A. Cogert, MD
Cardiac Electrophysiologist, Cottage Heart and Vascular Center, Santa Barbara, California

Freddy Del-Carpio Munoz, MD
Associate Professor of Medicine, Department of Cardiovascular Diseases, Mayo Clinic, Rochester, Minnesota

Andrea Di Cori, MD
Cardiac Electrophysiologist, Second Division of Cardiology, Cardiac Thoracic and Vascular Department, New Santa Chiara Hospital, Azienda Ospedaliero Universitaria Pisana, Pisa, Italy

Paul A. Friedman, MD
Norman Blane & Billie Jean Harty Chair, Department of Cardiovascular Medicine, Professor of Medicine, Mayo Clinic, Rochester, Minnesota

Bradley Genovese, MD
Resident, Surgery, Division of Cardiovascular and Thoracic Surgery, University of California San Diego Health System, San Diego, California

Mario Giannotti Santoro, MD
Cardiac Electrophysiologist, Second Division of Cardiology, Cardiac Thoracic and Vascular Department, New Santa Chiara Hospital, Azienda Ospedaliero Universitaria Pisana, Pisa, Italy

Shane M. Gillespie, MS, DO
Assistant Professor of Anesthesiology, Department of Anesthesiology and Critical Care, Mayo Clinic, Rochester, Minnesota

Erik A. Green, MD, MPH
Resident Surgery, Department of Surgery, Tulane University School of Medicine, Tulane, New Orleans, Louisiana

Gordon Ho, MD
Assistant Professor of Medicine, Division of Cardiovascular Diseases, University of California San Diego Health System, San Diego, California

Roshan Karki, MD
Fellow, Clinical Cardiac Electrophysiology, Mayo Clinic, Rochester, Minnesota

Akbar H. Khan, MD
Cardiologist, Minneapolis Heart Institute East, St. Paul, Minnesota

Klitos Konstantinidis, MD
Fellow, Clinical Cardiac Electrophysiology, Johns Hopkins University and Hospital, Baltimore, Maryland

Gurukripa N. Kowlgi, MBBS
Assistant Professor of Medicine, Department of Cardiovascular Medicine, Mayo Clinic, Rochester, Minnesota

Fred M. Kusumoto, MD
Professor of Medicine, Department of Cardiovascular Disease, Mayo Clinic, Jacksonville, Florida

Adetola Ladejobi, MD, MPH
Fellow, Clinical Cardiac Electrophysiology, Mayo Clinic, Rochester, Minnesota

Chin Lee, MD
Fellow, Clinical Cardiac Electrophysiology, University of California San Diego Health System, San Diego, California

Justin Z. Lee, MBBS
Fellow, Clinical Cardiac Electrophysiology, Mayo Clinic, Rochester, Minnesota

Charles J. Love, MD
Professor of Medicine; Director, Cardiac Rhythm Device Services, Johns Hopkins University and Hospital, Baltimore, Maryland

William J. Mauermann, MD
Associate Professor of Anesthesiology, Department of Anesthesiology & Perioperative Medicine, Mayo Clinic, Rochester, Minnesota

Olurotimi Mesubi, MD, MBBS, MPH
Assistant Professor of Medicine, Johns Hopkins University and Hospital, Baltimore, Maryland

Kevin J. Mulligan, RCIS
CVIS Program Coordinator, Mayo Clinic, Rochester, Minnesota

Travis Pollema, DO
Assistant Professor of Surgery, Division of Cardiovascular and Thoracic Surgery, University of California San Diego Health System, San Diego, California

Luca Segreti, MD
Cardiac Electrophysiologist, Second Division of Cardiology, Cardiac Thoracic and Vascular Department, New Santa Chiara Hospital, Azienda Ospedaliero Universitaria Pisana, Pisa, Italy

Samuel A. Shabtaie, MD
Fellow, Cardiovascular Diseases, Mayo Clinic, Rochester, Minnesota

Kunal Shah, MD
Fellow, Clinical Cardiac Electrophysiology, University of California San Diego Health System, San Diego, California

Imran S. Syed, MD
Cardiologist, United Heart & Vascular Clinic, St. Paul, Minnesota

Martin van Zyl, MBBCh
Fellow, Clinical Cardiac Electrophysiology, Mayo Clinic, Rochester, Minnesota

Pierce J. Vatterott, MD
Affiliate Professor of Medicine, University of Minnesota; Cardiac Electrophysiologist, Minneapolis Heart Institute East, St. Paul, Minnesota

Stefano Viani, MD
Cardiac Electrophysiologist, Second Division of Cardiology, Cardiac Thoracic and Vascular Department, New Santa Chiara Hospital, Azienda Ospedaliero Universitaria Pisana, Pisa, Italy

Giulio Zucchelli, PhD, MD
Cardiac Electrophysiologist, Second Division of Cardiology, Cardiac Thoracic and Vascular Department, New Santa Chiara Hospital, Azienda Ospedaliero Universitaria Pisana, Pisa, Italy

Forewords

Joshua M. Cooper, MD

Lead extraction is a somewhat solitary niche within our specialty of cardiac electrophysiology. The high-stakes, unpredictable nature of these procedures whittles down the number of interested trainees. The resource-heavy support system needed for a responsible lead extraction program limits the number of well-equipped and interested medical centers. The optimization of procedural safety and success compels us to concentrate the experience into as few hands as is feasible. Consequently, there tend to be a limited number of lead extractors within a medical institution (often only one) or geographic region. This scarcity results in the performance of lead extraction in a figurative silo, with personal experience being the primary guide for the incremental honing of skills.

Lead extraction is the discipline with the greatest amount of case-to-case variability, requiring the physician to continuously exercise intra-operative judgment, including the leveraging of a great breadth of approaches and tools. The seasoned extractor will invariably innovate and improvise during difficult cases, often relying on the creative application of techniques never originally intended to be used for the freeing and removal of indwelling pacemaker and ICD systems.

So how exactly is a lead extractor in isolation supposed to expand their toolbox and thereby maximize operative success? Personal experience moves at a fixed pace, limited by what that individual has seen before. This mode of learning by self-experience also requires each novel scenario to be encountered more than once for the extractor to directly benefit, assuming there were self-taught innovations during the first struggle that are worth repeating.

The ability to learn from the collective wisdom of the lead extraction community is a game-changer. Dr. Yong-Mei Cha and Dr. Siva Mulpuru fill an essential void with this text by bringing together detailed and practical expert guidance from preoperative planning through all phases and dimensions of the procedure itself, as well as 26 carefully selected case studies that span a wide range of clinical challenges. This compendium showcases a breadth of techniques and expertise that extends far beyond what any individual could achieve. The detailed visual and descriptive presentations provide a virtual "operating theater" to the reader, who is then able to draw from this exposure and apply new methods and insights without having to reinvent the wheel on their own. I wish the editors and contributing authors heartfelt congratulations on the publication of this important work, which will benefit physicians and patients alike.

Joshua M. Cooper, MD, is a Professor of Medicine at Lewis Katz School of Medicine at Temple University, and the Director of Cardiac Electrophysiology for Temple University Health System, Philadelphia, Pennsylvania.

Maria Grazia Bongiorni, MD

It is my pleasure to contribute a foreword to this case-based lead extraction book, which covers a topic often forgotten or not sufficiently explored in electrophysiology and devices books. In the last decades, procedures for lead extractions have soared. Like the authors, I was fortunate to see the birth of these techniques and to have contributed to their growth.

Having a case-based contemporary approach to and explanation of lead extraction is essential. In my experience, I have learned that the lead extraction procedure is not a "routine" procedure, but that each situation needs to be treated individually, on its own merits. Many times, I had to figure out ingenious solutions to overcome challenging situations, such as the use of the internal jugular approach. As described in this book, many solutions have been developed in the last decade to increase the efficacy and the safety of this procedure, making it accessible and workable in many centers.

Lead extraction is one of the medical areas where the need for a solution has led to continued research and resulted in many ingenious ideas. Since that time when the father of the lead extraction, Dr. Charles Byrd, first developed the system of sheaths to make an efficient and safe procedure of transvenous lead extraction, substantial progress has been made in the field. Today, transvenous lead extraction has become a widespread procedure throughout the world.

Lead extraction is a true team procedure. Each participant must keep in mind that all the steps of the lead extraction procedure are intertwined, and by working together to anticipate, manage, and prevent potential complications, the team can achieve the best potential outcome for the patient.

In summary, I highly recommend *Cardiac Lead Extraction: A Case-Based Contemporary Approach* as a superb contribution—one that benefits not only fellows or beginning trainees in the sector, but also experienced colleagues and electrophysiologists. A proper understanding of the challenges of lead extraction should reflect in procedural decisions during device implantation, removal of leads, and overall patient care.

Maria Grazia Bongiorni, MD, is Director of Cardiology and Arrhythmology Division at University Hospital in Pisa, Italy.

Kenneth A. Ellenbogen, MD

Lead extraction has become an increasingly important technique for managing patients with cardiac implantable electronic devices (CIEDs) and leads. It is estimated about 26,000+ procedures are undertaken worldwide. At first glance, this book may seem directed towards the small group of individuals who remove pacemaker and defibrillator leads from the heart. However, after reviewing this book, I think it is far more—and it will appeal to a larger and more diverse group of readers.

In eight chapters and 26 case-based studies, the authors take us from patient evaluation, to lead evaluation and performance, to preprocedural evaluation and risk stratification, to procedural tips and tricks, and finally to postprocedural management and planning. The teaching points are well summarized at the end of each chapter, and in typical Mayo Clinic fashion, the figures and videos are of excellent quality.

I tremendously enjoyed reading this book and extend my congratulations to the outstanding contributors who combined to give us a wide spectrum of cases. It would be impossible to read this monograph and not take away a number of important tips and tricks. For those who do not perform lead extraction, this is a useful book that helps one appreciate lead and device management even more. For those in training or caring for patients with devices, I could not think of a better place to learn about these important techniques for patient management and procedure performance.

This is a comprehensive book that provides everyone—from the learner to the experienced practitioner—with insights into management of the common clinical problems seen with patients with implantable devices, and especially with regard to managing and removing leads. I can highly recommend this lovely monograph.

Kenneth A. Ellenbogen, MD, is the Kimmerling Professor of Cardiology at Virginia Commonwealth University School of Medicine in Richmond, Virginia.

Preface

Modern cardiac electrophysiology procedural training encompasses catheter ablation, appendage occlusion, device implantation, and device extraction procedures. While many articles and books are devoted to device implantation and follow-up, we felt that the comprehensive and up-to-date materials available to trainees and practitioners on device extraction are currently lacking. It is our sincere attempt to provide relevant educational material to the reader in a case-based format.

This collaborative work was possible with contributions from experts from various academic institutions. We are grateful to our patients for not only allowing us to provide clinical care but also permitting us to use their de-identified clinical information to create educational materials. At the Mayo Clinic, our allied health staff (20+ technicians and 30+ device RNs) are the glue that keeps our teams together. Patient care, education, and clinical research would not be possible without their contribution. Our trainees inspire us to better clinicians, often providing us with a fresh perspective on challenging procedural problems. This book would not be possible without our media services support, providing us with high-quality illustrations and video clips. Lastly, we would like to thank our publishers from Cardiotext Publishing for effectively guiding us through the process.

Cardiac Lead Extraction: A Case-Based Contemporary Approach is divided into two main parts. The first section, consisting of eight chapters, provides the reader with the background information to perform lead extraction procedures safely. Anatomical considerations for the proceduralist are presented in Chapter 1. Chapters 2 and 3 provide an overview of clinical evaluation and imaging evaluation before lead extraction procedures. In Chapter 4, we review various tools and equipment used during the extraction procedures. Chapters 5, 6, and 8 provide planning from an anesthesiologist, allied health staff, and a cardiovascular surgeon's perspective, respectively. Chapter 7 reviews the underlying principles of medical decision-making, teamwork, and mental skills training to navigate challenging clinical scenarios.

In the second section, the 26 clinical cases present a variety of unique clinical scenarios and are arranged thematically. Each case starts with a clinical vignette followed by procedural details and a list of key learning points. The videos presented in the electronic version of the book allow the reader to have a realistic clinical scenario experience. We envision that the case-based presentation will allow the operator to quickly study the clinical scenario, review available tools, and take note of potential challenges before their procedures.

Lastly, we want to emphasize that lead extraction is a team sport. Collaborative relationships between the team members are essential for good patient outcomes. We thank you for the interest in our book, and we wish you all success in your lead extraction procedures.

—Yong-Mei Cha, MD
—Siva K. Mulpuru, MD, MPH

Abbreviations

ACT	activated clotting time
AF	atrial fibrillation
AHS	allied health staff
AP	anteroposterior
AT	atrial tachycardia
AV	atrioventricular
BMI	body mass index
bpm	beats per minute
CABG	coronary artery bypass graft
CIED	cardiovascular implantable electronic devices
CITA	continuous, in-situ targeted, ultra-high concentration of antibiotics
CPB	cardiopulmonary bypass
CRT	cardiac resynchronization therapy
CRT-D	CRT with defibrillator
CRTP	CRT with pacemaker
CS	coronary sinus
CT	computed tomography
CV	cardiac vein
CVP	central venous pressure
CXR	chest X-ray
ECG	electrocardiogram
ECMO	extracorporeal membrane oxygenation
EF	ejection fraction
EGM	electrogram
EP	electrophysiology, electrophysiologic
ESRD	end-stage renal disease
FDA	U.S. Food and Drug Administration
ICD	implantable cardioverter-defibrillator
ICE	intracardiac echocardiography
IVC	inferior vena cava
IR	interventional radiology
LA	left atrium/atrial
LAA	left atrial appendage
LAO	left anterior oblique
LV	left ventricle/ventricular
LVOT	left ventricular outflow tract
NICM	nonischemic cardiomyopathy
NYHA	New York Heart Association
OR	operating room
PA	posterior-anterior / posteroanterior
PET	positron emission tomography
PFO	patent foramen ovale
PLSVC	persistent left superior vena cava
PV	pulmonary vein
RA	right atrium/atrial
RAO	right anterior oblique
RIPV	right inferior pulmonary vein
RSPV	right superior pulmonary vein
RV	right ventricle/ventricular
RVA	right ventricular apex
RVOT	RV outflow tract
SVC	superior vena cava
TEE	transesophageal echocardiography/ echocardiogram
TLE	transvenous lead extraction
TPS	transcatheter pacing system
TR	tricuspid valve regurgitation/tricuspid regurgitation
TTE	transthoracic echocardiography/ echocardiogram
VATS	video-assisted thoracoscopy surgery
VF	ventricular fibrillation
VT	ventricular tachycardia

Video Legends

CHAPTERS

Chapter 3: Lead Extraction Imaging

Video 3.1 (A) 2D RV inflow with device lead causing impingement of the septal leaflet of the tricuspid valve. (B) Color Doppler interrogation of the RV inflow view showing severe TR. [00:03]

Video 3.2 Cine venogram demonstrating a patent subclavian vein with scar adherence to SVC coil. Prior traction on the ICD lead entrapped within scar resulted in uncoiling of the SVC coil. [00:12]

Video 3.3 Subclavian venogram from procedure initiation. A medial approach for placement resulted in clavicular crush and bony growth along the lead. [00:04]

Video 3.4 Subclavian venogram from procedure end. At extraction, a Bone Rongeur was used to allow advancement of extraction tool. For comparison, the new system implanted with the more lateral first rib approach. [00:04]

Video 3.5 AP view cine images obtained from a 63-year-old female with pacing leads placed 16 years earlier. Imaging demonstrates very free lead movement, suggesting little lead-to-lead or vascular adherence. [00:03]

Video 3.6 RAO 30-degree cine images obtained from a 63-year-old female with pacing leads placed 16 years earlier. Imaging demonstrates free lead movement, suggesting little lead-to-lead or vascular adherence. [00:03]

Video 3.7 LAO 30-degree cine images obtained from a 63-year-old female with pacing leads placed 16 years earlier. Imaging demonstrates free lead movement, suggesting little lead-to-lead or vascular adherence. [00:02]

Video 3.8 AP view cine images obtained from a 36-year-old female with pacing leads placed 8 years earlier. There is little free lead movement suggestive of a heavy scar burden with lead adherence. [00:03]

Video 3.9 RAO view cine images obtained from a 36-year-old female with pacing leads placed 8 years earlier. There is little free lead movement suggestive of a heavy scar burden with lead adherence. Classic "railroad tracking" is seen in the RAO view demonstrating lead-to-lead adherence from the subclavian to the distal SVC. [00:03]

Video 3.10 LAO view cine images obtained from a 36-year-old female with pacing leads placed 8 years earlier. There is little free lead movement suggestive of a heavy scar burden with lead adherence. LAO cine reveals the distal portion of the ventricular lead adhered to the ventricular septum. [00:03]

Video 3.11 RAO view cine images taken just prior to extraction of a dislodged nonfunctioning LV lead. Note the redundant lead loop extending into the IVC with concerns over possible adherence to the IVC. [00:01]

Video 3.12 LAO view cine images taken just prior to extraction of a dislodged nonfunctioning LV lead. Note the redundant lead loop extending into the IVC with concerns over possible adherence to the IVC. [00:03]

Video 3.13 AP view cine images taken demonstrating calcified scar along pacing leads. The red arrow points out calcium along the lead while the yellow arrow points out a heavy band of calcified scar binding the 2 leads as they exit the innominate into the SVC. These images influence tool selection (please see text). [00:03]

Video 3.14 The corresponding video taken from the patient illustrated in Figure 3.18. This ICE video demonstrates the lack of any lead SVC wall adherence. [00:59]

Video 3.15 In comparison to Video 3.14, this ICE video shows a different patient's pacing leads adhered to the SVC wall within a scar. [02:17]

Video 3.16 Fluoroscopic position of the ICE catheter in the SVC region. [00:02]

Video 3.17 ICE video of pacing leads bound within scar adhered to SVC wall. Wire for possible use of an SVC balloon seen on ICE video but not included on X-ray image. [00:31]

Video 3.18 After both leads were removed, residual scar is seen within the SVC lumen illustrating prior SVC attachment points and lead path. [00:20]

Video 3.19 ICE scan of SVC finds large burden of vegetations (not scar) affecting contrast flow. [00:15]

Video 3.20 ICE images from a patient in whom preprocedure contrast CT scan suggested SVC lead adherence. In this patient, the SVC ICE images illustrate leads encased in a scar adhered to the SVC wall. [00:06]

Video 3.21 ICE images from a patient in whom preprocedure contrast CT scan suggested SVC lead adherence. In this patient, leads are encased in scar and adhered to each other but not to SVC wall. Note the leads move independent of the SVC wall. The scar mass directs the bolus of contrast away from the vessel wall imitating adherence. [00:19]

Chapter 4: Extraction Planning and Preparation

Video 4.1 This video shows the mechanism of Liberator Locking Stylet and its application. (Permission for use granted by Cook Medical, Bloomington, IN.) [00:43]

Video 4.2 The lead (pace-sense) inner lumen is locked, but not the conductance coils. Pulling the lead inner lumen alone results in insulation breach and conductor cable externalization. A multi-lumen ICD lead is used to illustrate the concepts. [00:20]

Video 4.3 Pulling the lead inner lumen and high-voltage conductor cables together (tied by separate sutures), is illustrated in a multi-lumen ICD lead prepared with the locking stylet. Note that as pulling force is not applied to the insulation, bunching can occur. Bunching of the insulation, in turn, leads to difficulty in advancing the extraction sheath. [00:25]

Video 4.4 Uniform force transmission on the components of a multi-lumen ICD lead is illustrated. The pace-sense lumen is locked with a locking stylet. Separate sutures on placed on the high-voltage cables and the outer insulation. All the components are pulled together for more straightforward advancement of the inner extraction sheath and the outer sheath. [00:23]

Video 4.5 Laser sheath with circumferential fiber-optic cables delivering pulses of wavelength 308 nm in the ultraviolet spectrum (green) and photo-ablating the fibrous adhesions. In the animation, we illustrate the use of laser energy to pass through adhesions. When greater lateral forces are noted, the sheaths are pulled back, and only the inner laser sheath is advanced. The combination of inner and our sheaths results in a stiffer system over the lead. It may be easier to advance the outer sheath when the inner sheath is in the low right atrium. Countertraction using the inner sheath is used to free the lead tip. [01:03]

Video 4.6 Laser sheath (blue) is advanced over the lead, separating the lead from the surrounding fibrosis. The outer sheath (orange) is pushed forward for support and countertraction. [00:36]

Video 4.7 When the laser sheath is advancing from innominate vein to SVC, caution is undertaken to align the sheath with the lead in a straight downward force and avoid focusing the energy to the lateral SVC wall. [00:22]

Video 4.8 When lead-to-lead binding is significant, alternating the laser sheath to a different lead helps to free the lead from the binding site. [02:06]

Video 4.9 A pacing lead is captured by the Goose Neck snare, pulled down, and creates a straight line for the mechanical sheath railing down. [00:01]

Video 4.10 The right atrial lead is captured by a Jumbo Jaw biopsy forceps (Boston Scientific) through a deflectable sheath and pulled down towards IVC. The mechanical sheath is railing down close to the Jumbo Jaw. [00:01]

EXTRA VIDEO LEGENDS

Video 4.11 How to use a Bull Dog device (Cook Medical). [03:15]

Video 4.12 How to use a One-Tie device (Cook Medical). [01:47]

Video 4.13 Lead preparation for extraction. [10:14]

Video 4.14 Principles of using a Needle's Eye Snare (Cook Medical). [03:21]

Video 4.15 How to use a fish hook tool to pull a prepared lead through the extraction sheath. [01:26]

CASES

Case 1: Case of Device Extraction from Superior Venous Access

Video 1.1 A locking stylet was placed in the atrial lead. However, the tip of the stylet (yellow arrow) could not be passed to the lead's tip. [00:01]

Video 1.2 Separation of the ring (yellow arrow) and tip electrode (green arrow) can be appreciated when traction was applied on the lead. A conductor cable still connected the 2 electrodes. [00:01]

Video 1.3 An endoscopy biopsy forceps (Radial Jaw 4 biopsy forceps, Boston Scientific) was used to grab the lead proximal to the ring electrode to prevent transection of the lead tip. [00:01]

Video 1.4 A 12-Fr laser sheath was advanced over the lead, and good separation between the ring electrode (yellow arrow) and the tip electrode (green arrow). Note the acute angulation between the long axis of the extraction sheath and the tip electrode's long axis. [00:02]

Video 1.5 The lead was cut in the pocket area. The body of the lead was grabbed using the biopsy forceps (pink arrow), and the proximal end (lead cut in the pocket) was internalized and was pulled down to the level of IVC. Notice the significant separation between the ring (yellow arrow) on the tip electrode (green arrow) connected by the conductor cable. [00:02]

Video 1.6 A Goose Neck snare was placed on the lead's body and was advanced to the ring electrode (yellow arrow). The cut end of the lead was grabbed by the biopsy forceps placed inside a 16-Fr sheath. The green arrow indicates the tip of the femoral sheath. The ring and the tip electrode are still connected by a conductor cable (blue arrows). [00:02]

Video 1.7 3D TEE delineates the conductor cable between the ring and tip electrode. Notice that the tip electrode was attached right below the superior vena cava (SVC)–RA junction. [00:01]

Video 1.8 The femoral sheath (yellow arrow) was slowly advanced until the tip electrode (green arrow). Notice that the angle between the femoral sheath's long axis and the pacemaker lead is favorable for preventing tip transection. The Goose Neck snare (pink arrow) is advanced as distally as possible to apply traction near the tip electrode. [00:01]

Video 1.9 As traction was applied on the lead using the biopsy forceps and countertraction was applied using the tip of the femoral sheath, an echo-free space (yellow arrow) can be appreciated on echocardiography. This echo-free space mimics the presence of a pericardial effusion (pseudo pericardial effusion) and is caused by inversion of the atrial wall. An oval-shaped Goose Neck catheter (green arrow) pulled back on to the shaft of the femoral sheath can be appreciated in the video. [00:02]

Case 2: Extraction of Recalled Riata Lead

Video 2.1 Laser sheath was advanced from subclavian to an innominate vein using laser energy. [00:13]

Video 2.2 Laser sheath was advanced from subclavian to an innominate vein using laser energy. The conductor externalization is shown between the proximal and distal coils. [00:05]

Video 2.3 The laser sheath was moved forward in the SVC and entered the right atrium without lasing. The lead tip was freed from the RV apex by traction. [00:31]

Video 2.4 The laser sheath had difficulty to be advanced further to pass the distal coil. "Snowplowing" (tissue or externalized conductors) was suspected. The outer sheath was then advanced over the laser sheath. The lead was successfully pulling back into the outer sheath. [00:13]

Video 2.5 This video shows a small lateral coronary vein by coronary venogram. [00:02]

Video 2.6 Right atrial, right ventricular, and left ventricular leads placement in LAO view. [00:01]

Case 3: Importance of Lead Countertraction

Video 3.1 Bridge Occlusion Balloon catheter is inflated in the SVC. The RV lead proximal coil is on the lateral wall of SVC (blue arrow) in AP view. [00:01]

Video 3.2 The RV lead proximal coil is now on the medial side of SVC (solid blue arrow). The dashed blue arrow shows the original proximal coil location. [00:02]

Video 3.3 Laser sheath is advancing from the left subclavian to the innominate vein. [00:15]

Video 3.4 TightRail sheath is advanced to RV distal coil but met the resistance and cannot be advanced farther. [00:02]

Video 3.5 Using outer sheath apply for countertraction against RV endocardium where the lead tip was embedded in the myocardium (red arrow). [00:17]

Video 3.6 The RV lead was successfully removed back into the outer sheath. [00:02]

Case 4: Lead Extraction (Right-Sided ICD)

Video 4.1 Transesophageal echocardiography showing a mobile mass attached to the lead in the right atrium (both 2D and 3D). [00:03]

Video 4.2 Another view with TEE showing a mobile mass attached to the lead in the right atrium (both 2D and 3D). [00:05]

Video 4.3 Postextraction intracardiac echocardiography shows no accumulation of pericardial fluid. [00:06]

Videos 4.4 and 4.5 Cardiac MRI after hospital discharge shows normal left ventricular function. [00:02] [00:02]

Case 5: Lead Management (Pocket Pain)

Video 5.1 Intracardiac ultrasound placed in the right atrium before the extraction (9 Mz mechanical, Boston Scientific Ultra Ice Plus). No pericardial effusion is present, and no echogenic masses are identified on the leads. [00:10]

Video 5.2 Gentle traction under fluoroscopy leads to removal of the right ventricular lead without requiring any sheaths. [00:03]

Video 5.3 When the extraction tool reached the distal electrode, traction-countertraction techniques lead to the elongation of the helix. The ultrasound catheter can be seen at the base of the right atrium. In this position, it does not interact with any of the extraction tools, and this location is extremely sensitive for identifying the presence of pericardial effusion. [00:03]

Video 5.4 Removal of the lead with traction and counterclockwise twisting of the lead. Notice that the locking stylet has retracted slightly during this final process (compare the location of the radiopaque tip of the locking stylet in Video 5.3 and Video 5.4). [00:06]

Video 5.5 Postextraction intracardiac echocardiography demonstrates no accumulation of pericardial fluid. [00:05]

Case 6: Case of Superior Vena Cava Obstruction Due to Pacemaker Leads

Video 6.1 Contrast venogram of the SVC was performed through a balloon-tipped catheter in the left anterior oblique (LAO 40) view shows complete occlusion of the SVC with the prominent azygous vein (arrow). [00:06]

Video 6.2 The lead helices were retracted, and the leads were prepared with locking stylets. [00:01]

Video 6.3 A deflectable catheter was used to hook the J portion of the atrial lead and pull the lead down to the IVC (RAO 30). [00:01]

Video 6.4 A 14-Fr laser sheath (GlideLight, Philips Medical) was used to break adhesions around the right ventricular lead. Notice that the other sheath is positioned in the RA, as it may be difficult to navigate additional curves across the tricuspid valve with the outer sheath. [00:05]

Video 6.5 After the 14-Fr laser sheath was advanced over the RA lead to the IVC level, the Amplatz Goose Neck snare (GN 1500, Medtronic) was released from the RA lead. The lead was pulled back into the inner sheath. The inner sheath was then pulled into the outer sheath, which was then used to retain access. [00:30]

Video 6.6 A 16-mm PE-MT low-pressure balloon (Boston Scientific) was used to dilate the region of stenosis. [00:05]

Case 7: Lead Extraction for Superior Vena Cava Occlusion

Video 7.1 Preleadless pacemaker implant. Note the 5 leads (2 from the left and 3 from the right), with the leads in the atrium moving together, suggesting that they are fibrosed to one another. [00:18]

Video 7.2 Leadless pacemaker delivery catheter being advanced to the right ventricle. Note that there was some difficulty crossing the tricuspid valve due to the leads and fibrosis in the right atrium. [00:56]

Video 7.3 Postdelivery of the leadless pacemaker showing that the tines are embedded into the myocardium. [00:04]

Video 7.4 The tether is removed from the pacemaker, and it rests securely in its final position. [00:31]

Video 7.5 Scout cine prior to lead extraction procedure showing the 5 leads once again. Note the superior track of the oldest lead that had been placed via the right internal jugular vein. Note also the leads moving in unison within the right atrium, suggesting they are bound together. [00:12]

Video 7.6 RA Lead part 1: The first lead attempted was the left atrial lead from 2013, using a laser sheath and VisiSheath together in a telescoping fashion. The subclavian vein is entered, remaining coaxial with the lead. [00:35]

Video 7.7 RA Lead part 2: Continuation of the laser/VisiSheath on the left-sided atrial lead, with advancement through the innominate vein. [00:45]

Video 7.8 RA Lead part 3: Further advancement of the laser/VisiSheath down the SVC to the RA. [00:30]

Video 7.9 RA Lead part 4: Final advancement of the sheath to the anode of the RA lead. Due to the acute angle and lack of room in the RA, counter-traction could not be performed. However, by pushing the sheath inferiorly, the RA lead was able to be removed from the myocardium and then extracted. [00:55]

Video 7.10 Once the RA lead was removed while maintaining the extraction sheath through the occluded SVC, a guidewire was advanced (with some difficulty) into the IVC and was maintained for use later in the procedure. [00:56]

Video 7.11 The second lead attempted was the RV lead from 2013. The same sheath system was used. The RV lead pulled free from the myocardium before the sheath was entirely into the RA. [00:49]

Video 7.12 Once the left-sided RV lead was removed, an attempt was made to retain a second guidewire as a backup should we lose the first one. Despite multiple attempts, the wire was not able to be guided into the IVC. [00:56]

Video 7.13 From the right side, the first lead attempted was the RV lead from 1993. The TightRail was used due to its flexible nature and ability to cut through difficult and calcified binding sites. However, the sheath was stopped at the innominate vein and SVC junction, where the 3 remaining leads were bound together. [00:35]

Video 7.14 Working again on the RV lead from 1993, this time with a Cook Evolution RL, further progress through the binding of the 3 leads was not possible. [00:33]

Video 7.15 Using a laser/VisiSheath from the right internal jugular vein, the RV lead from 1978 was attempted next, again with the sheath being unable to pass the same binding site as noted for the RV lead from 1993. [00:53]

Video 7.16 This loop shows the heavy calcification around the electrodes of the RV leads. It also shows calcification in the right atrium just above the tricuspid valve. [00:01]

Video 7.17 Using a snare from the femoral vein, the RV lead from 1998 was captured, but it would not release from the myocardium due to the fibrous and calcified binding sites. [00:08]

Video 7.18 A 13-Fr TightRail was introduced over a snare, and the RV lead from 1998 was again captured. While attempting to bore through the binding site, the lead was severed. The proximal portion of the lead was pulled down from the SVC and removed, leaving the lead's distal end embedded in tissue. [00:56]

Video 7.19 Next, the RV lead from 1978 was captured using a bioptome (we were unable to grasp it with other snares). Though much traction was applied, the lead would not pull out of the RV, nor would it pull through the SVC. [00:27]

Video 7.20 The guidewire retained in the IVC from the left implant site is grasped using a Goose Neck-type snare. [00:06]

Video 7.21 The guidewire is pulled from the femoral vein through the introducer to allow for the introduction of interventional catheters, balloon, and stent. [00:09]

Video 7.22 Contrast injection via a catheter placed superior to the SVC obstruction showing the SVC occlusion extending up to the right internal jugular vein and major collateral flow through the azygous and hemizygous veins. [00:11]

Video 7.23 Deployment of a stent into the SVC. Note that a stent has already been placed in the left innominate vein. [00:10]

Video 7.24 Venogram superior to the SVC showing excellent blood flow down the SVC, with minimal flow via the collateral veins. [00:14]

Case 8: Management of a Patient with Lead Perforation

Video 8.1 2D echo showing perforation of the lead through the RV wall. [00:19]

Video 8.2 3D echo showing perforation of the lead through the RV wall. [00:11]

Video 8.3 The lead in a high position; however, one cannot tell if it is anterior or septal in this projection. [00:02]

Video 8.4 The lead pointing towards the image intensifier and not to the right (i.e., not posterior), suggesting that it is in the RV free wall. [00:05]

Video 8.5 Preextraction access to the pericardium. The access needle is advanced slowly, using a small amount of contrast. The needle is seen at the end of the cine as it enters the pericardial space. [00:56]

Video 8.6 After the pericardial access needle is in the pericardial space, an 0.014-inch guidewire is advanced into the pericardial space. [00:06]

Video 8.7 The 0.014-inch guidewire is then exchanged for a long 0.035-inch guidewire, which is advanced to show that it is not in the right ventricle. [00:08]

Video 8.8 The pericardial drain tube is advanced over the 0.035-inch guidewire. This has been placed prophylactically to be able to both immediately detect a hemopericardium and drain it should it occur. [00:08]

Video 8.9 Initial use of a Cook Byrd telescoping polypropylene extraction sheath. The sheath was easily advanced to the SVC, but a binding site prevented further advancement. [00:52]

Video 8.10 Use of a Philips TightRail extraction sheath. This passed through the biding site and was advanced to an area near where the lead was perforated through the RV free wall. [00:23]

Video 8.11 Further advancement of the TightRail to slowly advance to the myocardium, then use countertraction to extract the lead. The patient remained completely stable at this point, without evidence of pericardial effusion on TEE or blood from the pericardial drain. [00:22]

Video 8.12 Access to the central circulation was retained by placing a guidewire through the TightRail. [00:09]

Video 8.13 Final view of the new leads in the right atrium, right ventricle, and Bundle of His positions. [00:02]

Case 9: The Use of Shockwaves to Facilitate Lead Management (Intravascular Lithotripsy)

Video 9.1 Left axillary venogram cine is depicted. The contrast injection (venogram) suggests severe narrowing and possible occlusion in the left axillary vein as it crosses below the clavicle and becomes subclavian vein. A prominent collateral venous circulation can be also noted. [00:03]

Videos 9.2 and 9.3 Cine clips obtained at maximum inflation (near burst pressure) at the different stenotic lesions. Over-the-wire balloon venoplasty was attempted with a 6-mm noncompliant OPTA Pro, Cordis. Note the inadequate venoplasty results limited by the hard calcification lesions. [00:01] [00:01]

Case 10: Lead Extraction in a Patient with Patent Foramen Ovale and Paradoxical Embolism

Video 10.1 (A) TEE image showing the PFO. Note the device lead in the right atrium. [00:03] (B) PFO shown in Figure 10.1 with color flow Doppler imaging. Note left to right shunting as indicated by the blue color jet. [00:01]

Video 10.2 TEE image showing new mobile echo-densities seen in the right atrium after transvenous lead extraction. The right panel is an orthogonal view of the left one at the level indicated by the white dotted line. [00:06]

Video 10.3 Intracardiac echocardiographic image showing debris attached to the right atrial side of the interatrial septum. The close proximity of the debris to the PFO precluded initial PFO closure, given the high risk of systemic embolization. [00:06]

Video 10.4 Fluoroscopic image showing the SpiderFX embolic protection device in the right and left common carotid arteries. [00:01]

Video 10.5 Fluoroscopic image showing PFO closure with an Amplatzer device. [00:01]

Video 10.6 (A) Fluoroscopic image showing the deployment of an Amplatzer device across a PFO [00:06] (B) Retrieval of the Amplatzer device after use to temporarily close a PFO during transvenous lead removal. [00:04]

Video 10.7 Fluoroscopic image showing temporary patent foramen ovale closure with a balloon occluder (yellow arrow points to dog bone effect on the balloon as it passes through the PFO). [00:06]

Case 11: Large Lead Mass

Video 11.1 TEE showing a 3.2 × 1.9 cm mass attached to the right ventricular and right atrial lead. [00:04]

Video 11.2 TEE showing a free-floating mass in the right atrium. [00:05]

Video 11.3 TEE showing that the mass had embolized. [00:04]

Video 11.4 CT angiogram of the chest showing a large, near-occlusive acute pulmonary embolism in the distal right main pulmonary artery. [00:31]

Case 12: Using AngioVac for Lead Extraction

Video 12.1 TEE shows mobile vegetation attached to the RV lead moving between the right atrium and right ventricle (red arrow), 3 × 2 cm in size. [00:04]

Video 12.2 TEE illustrates TR was present around the device lead and vegetation. [00:01]

Video 12.3 TEE shows that the AngioVac inserted from the right femoral vein cannot reach the vegetation, instead directing into the atrial septum. [00:04]

Video 12.4 Right internal jugular approach to place the AngioVac suction cannula 35-cm DrySeal sheath, which is advanced down to the lower right atrium and tricuspid annulus. [00:01]

Video 12.5 TEE shows AngioVac cannula (red arrow) in contact with vegetation (blue arrow). [00:06]

Video 12.6 Following the AngioVac suction, TEE shows the large vegetation is removed, and no remnant was noted on the lead. [00:04]

Case 14: Early Detection of Superior Vena Cava Tear Using Video-Assisted Thoracoscopy During Lead Extraction

Video 14.1 VATS (right side) shows pericardium and the beating right atrium and its junction to SVC under the pericardium. Right-sided phrenic nerve is seen. The right lung is deflated. [00:25]

Video 14.2 Proximal lead is transected and retracted to the innominate vein (red arrow). The distal lead is snared from below and pulled into IVC (blue arrow). [00:01]

Video 14.3 Snaring proximal RV lead from the subclavian vein was attempted but unsuccessful. [00:01]

Video 14.4 Contrast injection shows subclavian to innominate vein fibrosis with dissection at the broken RV lead area. [00:02]

Video 14.5 All 3 leads are removed by extraction from above and below. [00:01]

Video 14.6 A different patient who underwent a combined VATS procedure and lead extraction for pacemaker pocket infection. The right atrial appendage movement is visualized under the pericardium (yellow arrow). Note that the traction force on the atrial lead is pulling the appendage downward until the lead is removed from the appendage. The blue arrow follows the atrial lead tip, which is pulling back along the SVC lateral wall. [01:11]

Case 15: Percutaneous Management of Superior Vena Cava Tear

Video 15.1 TEE report large mobile echo-density (2.1 × 1.6 cm) consistent with vegetation prolapses into the right atrium and appears to be attached to the ICD lead. [00:04]

Video 15.2 14-Fr Excimer laser sheath is advancing over the RA lead at subclavian vein region. [00:06]

Video 15.3 14-Fr Excimer laser sheath is advancing over the RA lead at SVC. [00:05]

Video 15.4 14-Fr Excimer laser sheath is advancing over the RA lead at SVC and RA region. Outer sheath is supporting the laser sheath, which is in alignment to the lead. [00:37]

Video 15.5 14-Fr Excimer laser sheath is advancing over the LV lead at subclavian vein region. [00:05]

Video 15.6 The laser sheath is at SVC and LV lead is removed by pulling back without laser energy application at this point. [00:05]

Video 15.7 Pericardial effusion was present. Note organized and calcified apical thrombus in the left ventricle. [00:02]

Video 15.8 Pericardial effusion. During pericardiocentesis, agitated saline is injected to confirm the needle in the pericardial space (red arrow). Note left ventricular systolic function is severely reduced. [00:02]

Video 15.9 Contrast injection through the pigtail catheter, which is located at innominate vein (A) and SVC [00:06]. (B) shows that contrast flows into right atrium without apparent extravasation into the pericardium. [00:05]

Video 15.10 SVC Bridge Occlusion Balloon inflation to control the bleeding after all leads are removed. [00:01]

Case 16: Tools and Techniques for the Extraction of Leadless Pacemakers

Video 16.1 Apical 4-chamber view of a TEE demonstrating circumferential pericardial effusion postimplantation of a leadless pacemaker. [00:08]

Video 16.2 LAO fluoroscopy view showing a steerable sheath positioned in the right ventricle through the leadless pacemaker delivery sheath. The orthogonal view helps in directing the Goose Neck snare over the leadless pacemaker. [00:07]

Video 16.3 Videos 16.3A and 16.3B feature RAO and LAO fluoroscopic views of the new leadless pacemaker implanted in the right ventricular apical septum. [00:06] [00:06]

Video 16.4 Video 16.4A shows 4-chamber view of a TEE demonstrating the presence of a mobile echodensity on the mechanical mitral prosthetic valve, consistent with vegetation in the clinical scenario. [00:06] Video 16.4B shows a short-axis view of a TEE demonstrating the presence of a mobile echodensity (vegetation) on the mechanical mitral prosthetic valve. [00:06]

Video 16.5 Videos 16.5A and 16.5B show RAO and LAO fluoroscopic views of the attempt to grasp the proximal retrieval knob of the leadless pacemaker using a Goose Neck snare. [00:06] [00:06]

Video 16.6 Videos 16.6A and 16.6B feature RAO and LAO fluoroscopic views showing a steerable catheter being used in an attempt to move the leadless pacemaker to make it more coaxial with the delivery sheath. [00:06] [00:06]

Video 16.7 Video 16.7A shows the LAO view showing the use of a Goose Neck snare from access obtained in the right internal jugular vein to help make the leadless pacemaker more co-axial with the sheath. [00:06] Video 16.7B shows the RAO fluoroscopic view of the leadless pacemaker being successfully withdrawn into the delivery sheath. [00:06]

Case 17: Femoral Device Extraction

Video 17.1 Selective venography from the catheter confirms complete occlusion of the SVC. Note the massively dilated azygous vein that serves as a conduit to deliver the venous drainage from the superior part of the body to the RV through azygous system that eventually drains to the right atrium through the IVC. [00:07]

Video 17.2 The SVC occlusion was crossed using a vein-finder catheter and a medium support 0.15-inch wire. [00:04]

Video 17.3 After a stiff wire was exchanged with its tip in the IVC, venoplasty was performed to open the SVC occlusion. [00:05]

Video 17.4 Mechanical extraction sheath over one of the pacemaker leads was used to break the adhesions. [00:08]

Video 17.5 As the mechanical sheath was advanced, we can notice the lead rotating in the vasculature. It points to the inadequate engagement of the scar tissue. The mechanical sheath has to be pulled back and advanced coaxially over the lead to engage the adhesion binding sites. [00:04]

Video 17.6 The presence of multiple loops, temporary pacemaker wires, and 0.35-inch wire from the SVC increases the risk of lead entanglement. The mechanical extraction sheath is currently on the ventricular leads, which is looped around the other wires. [00:14]

Video 17.7 A 14-Fr laser sheath (GlideLight, Philips Medical) was advanced over the lead to push it back to the right atrium to disentangle the loops. The lead, along with the inner sheath, was pulled back into the outer sheath. [00:02]

Case 18: Lead Extraction through the Femoral Venous Route

Video 18.1 A clinical case where a combination of ablation catheter and Goose Neck snare were used to stabilize ICD lead during the extraction of the nonfunctioning pacing lead, Model 3830 (Medtronic), attached to the ICD lead. [00:01]

Video 18.2 Intracardiac echo (open rotational) showed that the ICD and atrial leads are firmly embedded in the SVC wall. [00:06]

Video 18.3 Images are taken through a thoracoscope during the extraction of an ICD lead. The SVC is imaged while traction is applied to lead/locking stylet from the left subclavian lead entry site (Video 18.3A) [00:18] and then with the lead snared through a femoral approach (Video 18.3B) [00:20]. With subclavian traction, force is concentrated in a discreet area. With femoral traction, force is dispersed over a larger area of tissue. This difference, likely helps to preserve tissue integrity.

Video 18.4 Animation of the results of Finite element wall modeling. Vascular wall stresses subclavian (Video 18.4A) versus femoral pull (Video 18.4B). The highest stress points are denoted in white. [00:05]

Video 18.5 Technique to extract lead fragment from superior approach. Video 18.5A demonstrating 16-Fr laser sheath advanced (non powered mode) over a wire through a 18-Fr dry gore sheath. [00:01] In Video 18.5B, the lead fragment has been snared with an EnSnare. An Agilis sheath (visible within the 16-Fr laser sheath) was used to guide the EnSnare (see text). [00:29] Lead successfully removed.

Video 18.6 Video 18.6 shows the effects of traction on deployed locking stylet within a Fineline lead. Deployed stylet was unable to bind within an ETFE-coated lumen. [00:45]

Video 18.7 (A) Cine of snaring Fineline lead and locking stylet within. After snaring, the snare is first used to unscrew the lead tip from its atrial attachment. The lead and locked locking stylet are then pulled into the Cook femoral workstation inner sheath with kinking of the stylet. This snared locking stylet provides a strong rail for extraction tools to be safely advanced from above. [00:14] (B) Cine demonstrating the removal of an atrial Fineline lead. The snared locking stylet provides a safe and stable rail for the lead extraction tool's advancement to the right atrium. The lead is then released from the snare and successfully removed. Note atrial lead structure is preserved is during removal. [00:53]

Video 18.8 Snaring of ventricular lead without pulling the locking stylet into the Cook inner sheath. The lead is held but not effectively stabilized. [00:07]

Video 18.9 Without a firm grip on the lead, the locking stylet retracts with traction, coils unwind and stretch. Needle's Eye Snare is removed after failing to hold the locking stylet in place. The lead is removed despite the poor rail from the snare. [00:42]

Case 19: Coronary Sinus Lead Extraction of a Starfix Lead

Video 19.1 The deployment of a Starfix lead with lobe attachment to the vessel wall. [02:08]

Video 19.2 RAO 30 [00:03] and LAO 30 [00:04] images from a patient with device infection referred for extraction. Leads present are Medtronic 6947 dual-coil ICD lead, Medtronic 5076, and Medtronic 4195 Starfix lead.

Video 19.3 ICD lead and atrial lead have already been removed prior to attempt to remove the Starfix lead. As the powered sheath advances on the CS, traction is applied independently to the blue polyurethane tubing. This results in a partial collapse of the proximal lobes with a more favorable physical structure for removing the narrow end of a cone. [00:01]

Video 19.4 With traction applied to both the lead and blue tubing, a powered sheath is advanced in a nonpowered mode into the CS. This disrupts binding sites and allows effective traction delivery. [00:04]

Video 19.5 Coronary sinus venogram after removal of the Starfix lead demonstrating venous branch occlusion after the Starfix removal. [00:03]

Video 19.6 Video of Starfix removal. Atrial pacing and ICD lead have been removed. Temporary pacing lead in place. The laser was advanced in a non-powered mode from the innominate to the CS os and into the CS. Traction is applied to the blue tubing for lobe undeployment as the extraction sheath approaches the CS while also independently applying traction to the main lead body. [00:15]

Case 20: Extraction of Coronary Sinus Lead

Videos 20.1 and 20.2 Scout fluoroscopy showing the two retained CS leads with the pacing electrodes in separate CVs. The leads have been damaged and retained from a previous extraction attempt. The free end of one is in the left innominate vein, and the other is in the inferior vena cava. [00:09] [00:05]

Video 20.3 The first lead (with the free end in IVC) is snared using a multi-loop EnSnare. [00:18]

Video 20.4 A TightRail extraction sheath in advanced up the IVC to the right atrium. Note the calcification at the os of the CS that is visible near the end of this image. [00:13]

Video 20.5 The free end of the lead is again snared with an EnSnare that has been placed through the TightRail extraction sheath. The sheath is then advanced to the calcification at the CS os. [00:56]

Video 20.6 The TightRail is now at the os of the CS, and with traction on the lead, it begins to bore through the calcification. Not shown: The sheath eventually passes through the calcium to the takeoff of the lead into the target vessel, but due to the severe angulation, coaxial alignment could not be maintained. The decision was made to use a laser sheath to attempt to gain a better alignment. [00:18]

Video 20.7 After a laser sheath is placed into the IVC, the lead is again snared. [00:14]

Video 20.8 The laser sheath is advanced to the takeoff of the CV, and lasing with gentile traction to maintain alignment is performed. Note the tissue's hazy appearance around the distal end of the lead, consistent with calcium deposition. [00:24]

Video 20.9 The lead breaks at the takeoff point to the vein. The risk of further attempts to extract this fully embedded fragment was deemed to be higher than the risk of leaving it in place. [00:01]

Video 20.10 A Needle's Eye Snare has been placed into the right atrium. This was used to capture the body of the second lead. [00:01]

Video 20.11 The second lead was retracted into the snare, and the entire lead remnant was pulled into the sheath and out of the body. [00:18]

Video 20.12 Final fluoroscopy showing the retained end of the first lead. [00:01]

Case 21: Azygous Vein Coil and Subcutaneous Array Extraction

Video 21.1 Laser extraction sheath (GlideLight, Philips Medical) is advanced over the subcutaneous coil. The coil is eventually taken out of the tissue plane with traction. [00:02]

Case 22: Lead Extraction in a Patient with Prosthetic Valvular Endocarditis

Video 22.1 CT angiography cine showing the brachiocephalic vein obstruction due to lead adhesion. [00:01]

Video 22.2 Left femoral venogram showing occlusion at the IVC with contrast filling of the hemiazygos system (arrow). The amputated epicardial lead was seen in this view. Left femoral venogram shows complete obstruction at the IVC. [00:09]

Video 22.3 Videos 22.3A and 22.3B show the CS lead removal allowed the passing of a stiff wire and the occlusion balloon through the brachiocephalic vein. The occlusion balloon was deployed in the SVC–RA junction through the brachiocephalic vein. [00:12] [00:01]

Video 22.4 Countertraction was applied on the RV lead at the lead tip-myocardium interface and freed the lead from the myocardium. [00:11]

Case 23: A Patient with Congenital Atrioventricular Block and Severe Tricuspid Valve Regurgitation

Video 23.1 Color Doppler echocardiography of the tricuspid valve showing severe regurgitation. [00:05]

Video 23.2 2D echocardiography showing encapsulated calcification of the right ventricular pacing lead abutting the tricuspid valve causing leaflet entrapment. [00:05]

Video 23.3 Cine of chest CT (coronal view) showing the course of each lead and calcification around the leads. [00:06]

Video 23.4 Preoperative TEE showing impingement of the RV lead on the tricuspid valve and calcification (left) and severe tricuspid regurgitation (right). [00:02]

Video 23.5 Cine-fluoroscopy showing inability to pass the mechanical sheath beyond the junction of left clavicle and the first rib. [00:06]

Video 23.6 Cine-fluoroscopy showing freeing of the first RV lead down to the RA with the laser sheath. [00:14]

Video 23.7 Cine-fluoroscopy showing freeing of the second RV lead down to the RA with the laser sheath. [00:05]

Video 23.8 Intraoperative view of the calcified encapsulation of the RV lead at the tricuspid valve. Please note the calcification is being crushed. [02:15]

Video 23.9 Intraoperative view showing the RV lead embedded with the tricuspid valve leaflet and papillary muscles. [02:15]

Video 23.10 Postrepair TEE showing tricuspid valve ring (left) and trace-to-mild residual tricuspid regurgitation. [00:02]

Case 26: Lead Extraction Using Single Sheath Mechanical Dilatation

Video 26.1 Angiography performed from a left antecubital peripheral access. Patency of the central venous system is demonstrated, with the presence of adherence in the subclavian and innominate vein tract. [00:06]

Video 26.2 A fluoroscopy zoom on the coil shows no insulator defects. There is an excess lead loop before the tricuspid valve, suggesting it as the possible location of the damage. [00:10]

Video 26.3 The sheath is inserted, taking care to be coaxial with vein entrance. [00:19]

Video 26.4 The adherence in the subclavian and innominate tract, predicted by the venography, was overcome using a larger dilator (10.0-Fr Byrd Dilator Sheath Set (B) Polypropylene, Cook Vandergrift Inc.). [00:48]

Video 26.5 Another adherence, just before the atrial dipole, was overcome with larger size dilator (11.5-Fr Byrd Dilator Sheath Set (C) Polypropylene, Cook Vandergrift Inc.). The transition zone, with small caliper differences, is usually at risk for the development of adherences. [00:56]

Video 26.6 The subsequent adherences present in the atrium were easily overcome with the same dilator. [00:31]

Video 26.7 A larger dilator was repositioned to engage the strong adherence before the tricuspid valve (13.0-Fr Byrd Dilator Sheath Set (D) Polypropylene, Cook Vandergrift Inc.). [00:17]

Video 26.8 It was challenging to engage this adherence. Moreover, the lack of advancement of the stylet over the tricuspid valve added difficulties in this passage. [00:56]

Video 26.9 The externalization of a wire from the lead is visible, with a loop conformation. The wire was engaged with the oversize sheath. [00:53]

Video 26.10 The possibility of grasping the lead proximal to the site of adherence and making it free-floating was checked, in order to evaluate a cross-over to jugular approach in case subclavian access was unsuccessful. [00:17]

Video 26.11 The strong and large adherence localized just before the tricuspid valve, was overcome with the largest dilator available (13.0-Fr Byrd Dilator Sheath Set (D) Polypropylene, Cook Vandergrift Inc.). The dilator was advanced up to the tip, so the lead was totally removed only after all the lead was covered by the sheath. [00:56]

Video 26.12 Videos 26.12A and 26.12B show that after the cannulation of coronary sinus, an angiography with a Swan Ganz catheter was performed, revealing a posterior-lateral branch with a good caliper. [00:17]

Video 26.13 Videos 26.13A–C feature the final fluoroscopy showing the ipsilateral CRT-D reimplantation. [00:04]

Video 26.14 A case of despiralized dual-coil ICD removed with the internal jugular approach. [00:47]

1 Structural Basis for Lead Extraction Complications

Justin Z. Lee, MBBS; Samuel A. Shabtaie, MD; Samuel J. Asirvatham, MD

INTRODUCTION

Lead extraction has the highest complication and mortality rate among device-related procedures.[1] It is essential for the electrophysiologist who performs lead extraction to be familiar with the tools involved with lead extractions, the engineering aspects of the lead, and the anatomic basis of lead extraction. In that context, this chapter reviews the critical cardiac and venous anatomy that is essential for the electrophysiologist to keep in mind when performing the procedure. This chapter reviews the anatomic basis for complications that can happen during lead extraction, techniques to avoid the injury, and early recognition of complications when they occur.

VENOUS COMPLICATIONS

Superior Vena Cava

The anatomy of the superior vena cava (SVC) is of paramount importance as the most common cause of death related to lead extraction is SVC laceration.[2] The SVC is formed by the confluence of the right and left brachiocephalic veins, and it returns deoxygenated blood to the right atrium. Typical venous turns occur at the innominate–SVC junction and the SVC–right atrial junction. **Figure 1.1** shows the relationship of the SVC to the heart. It is unsupported in its more proximal portion, and therefore has no cushion when tension is applied to its wall. The parietal pericardial reflection can be visualized as well in Figure 1.1. It is closer to the atrium posteriorly and farther from the atrium anteriorly. When a laceration occurs above the pericardial reflection, this can lead to hemothorax and brisk bleeding into the mediastinum, requiring prompt recognition and emergent surgical repair to prevent the patient's rapid demise. Sole reliance on the presence of the development of pericardial effusion and hemopericardium for recognition of an SVC injury above the level of the pericardial reflection may be misleading. Of all vascular injuries during lead extraction, two-thirds were in the SVC, half of which were above the pericardial reflection and the other half below.[3] This also highlights the importance of ensuring that the SVC balloon is deployed with its tip beyond the brachiocephalic–SVC junction level.

Below the pericardial reflection, the SVC is contained within the pericardial space (see Figure 1.1). Therefore, if a perforation occurs below the pericardial reflection, this results in hemopericardium. The SVC is also closely related to the right superior pulmonary vein (RSPV), forming a posterior buttress (see Figure 1.1). Perforation at this level will lead to an RSPV-to-SVC fistula.

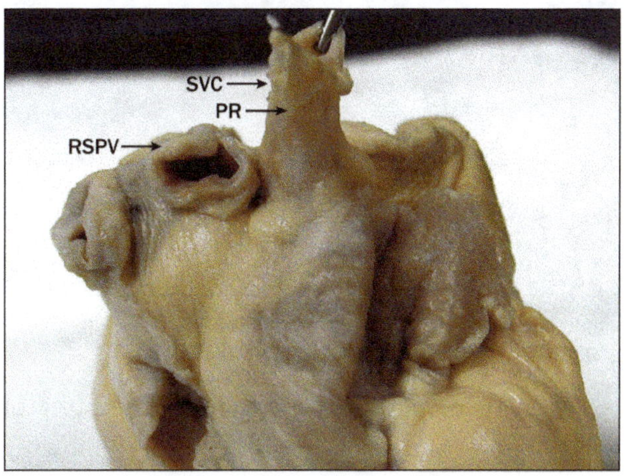

Figure 1.1 Lateral view from an autopsied heart showing the relative anatomy of the superior vena cava (SVC), pericardial reflection (PR), and the right superior pulmonary vein (RSPV).

 Cardiotext Publishing. ISBN: 978-1-942909-54-5

The challenges during extraction and the frequent need for specialized laser or mechanical sheaths are adhesions and fibrosis forming around the lead. The free wall of the SVC is one of the most frequent sites for the development of adhesions and fibrosis (**Figure 1.2**).[4] When a lead is placed via the left subclavian vein, the point where lead slack is taken up is at the free wall of the SVC. With cardiac contractility, the free wall of the SVC undergoes repeated contact and abrasions from the lead, which leads to adhesions. As opposed to left-sided leads, right-sided leads will have slack taken up by the medial portion of the SVC.

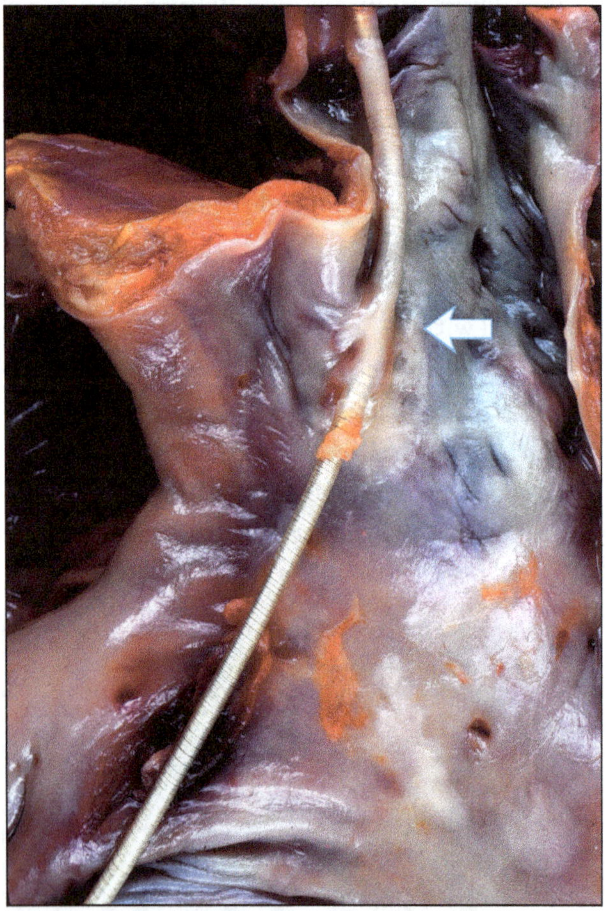

Figure 1.2 Lead adhesions (**arrow**) at the free wall of the SVC. (Anatomic image courtesy of William Edwards, MD.)

It is also worth noting that the amount of microscopic injury to venous structures following extraction may be much higher than clinically apparent. One study has shown 9.3% of extracted leads contained segments of the vein, most of which were transmural (including the adventitial layer), though only 1.1% required surgical intervention.[5] A transmural venous injury detected microscopically will not always correspond to a perforation of the SVC because of the myocardium and adipose tissue support outside the vein proper as the SVC enters the right atrium.[6]

Key Anatomic Points for the Extractionist

Superior Vena Cava

- Perforation above the pericardial reflection is catastrophic mediastinal bleeding but without pericardial effusion.
- Medial adhesions are less common likely because of aortic pulsatility in this region.
- Posterior inferior perforations may lead to fistulae with the right upper pulmonary vein.
- SVC balloons need to be sized appropriately for the larger volume extrapericardial portion.

CALCIFICATION AND LEAD-TO-LEAD INTERACTIONS

The challenges faced during lead extraction are primarily due to fibrosis and calcification, binding the leads to the surrounding tissue. Initially following lead implantation, thrombus development may occur, with subsequent fibrosis and encapsulation of a lead with a fibrin sheath within 5 days postimplantation.[7,8] As the body attempts to isolate the foreign material from the surrounding environment, acute inflammatory cells, followed by a macrophage predominate chronic inflammatory phase, ultimately results in fibroblast recruitment and proliferation, yielding a fibrotic capsule.[9,10] Binding sites have been found to contain high collagen content in addition to ongoing chronic inflammation present in leads with a long dwell time.[11]

Figure 1.3 shows that lead adhesions can also occur to a neighboring lead, resulting in lead-to-lead adherence. These make extraction challenging, especially if the adhesions and fibrosis calcify. Figure 1.3 also shows calcification between both leads. Laser energy does not penetrate calcified adhesions well, whereas mechanical sheaths and rotating metal sheaths may be more effective in traversing calcification.[12]

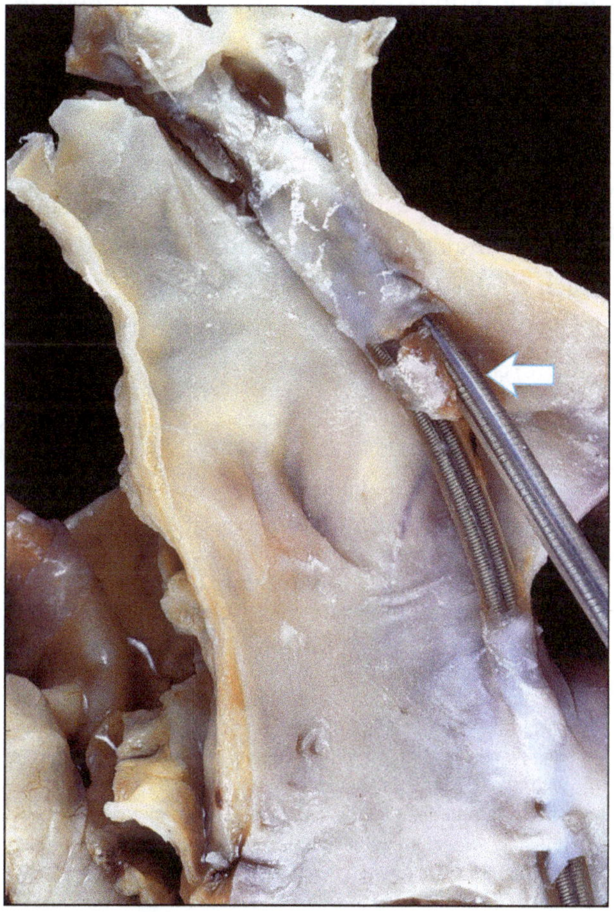

Figure 1.3 Lead-to-lead adhesions with calcification (**arrow**). (Anatomic image courtesy of William Edwards, MD.)

In cases of lead-to-lead adherence, especially if the leads are attached at multiple points, it is not possible to just extract one lead. The goal will be to separate the leads as much as possible. This will require the operator to be prepared to work back and forth between 2 or more adhered leads and be comfortable alternating between mechanical and laser extraction tools. **Figure 1.4** shows lead-to-lead adherence, which resulted in both leads coming out together during the extraction process, with the first lead pulling the second lead out at the attachment point.

RIGHT ATRIUM

The interior of the right atrium is composed of a thin posterior component in which the SVC, inferior vena cava (IVC), and coronary sinus (CS) return blood to the heart. The right atrial wall is very thin, averaging 2 mm in thickness. In contrast, the right ventricle is nearly twice as thick, which is why atrial lead perforation is more common than ventricular position.[13] **Figure 1.5** illustrates a case where a peripherally inserted central catheter line perforated the right atrial wall, resulting in saline infusion into the pericardial space and tamponade. This highlights the relative ease of right atrial perforation, even with a peripherally inserted central catheter with line

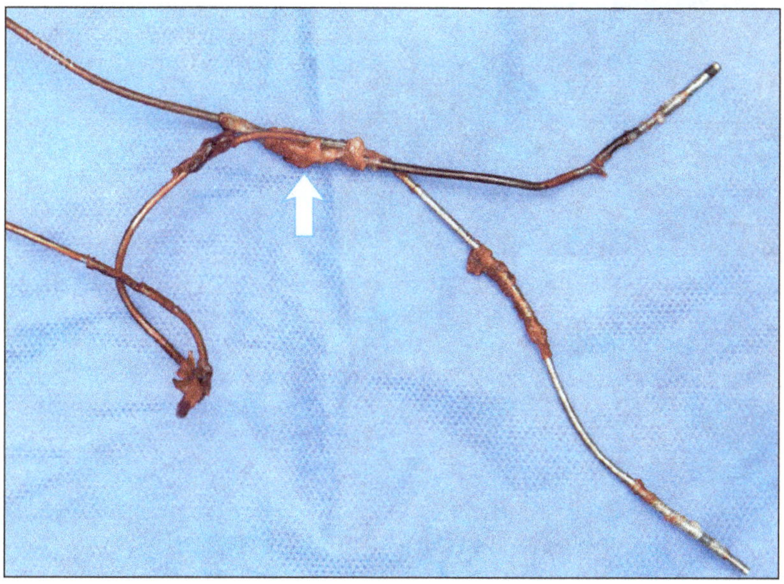

Figure 1.4 Adhesions binding leads together causing lead-to-lead adherence.

with no extendable helix. A partial perforation may heal spontaneously but can lead to cardiac tamponade following the extraction of the lead.

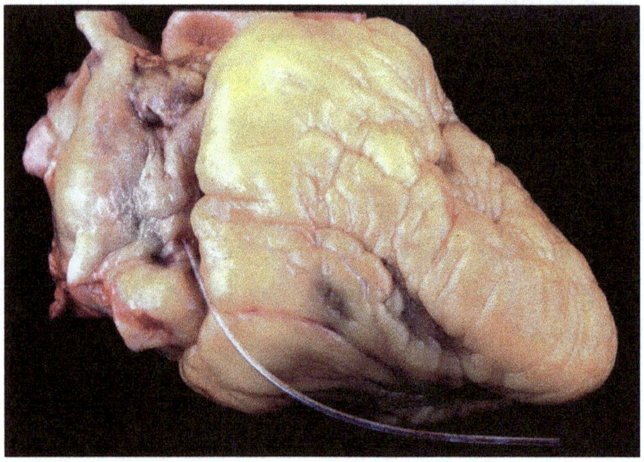

Figure 1.5 Perforation of a peripherally inserted central catheter in the right atrium. (Anatomic image courtesy of William Edwards, MD.)

Figure 1.6 demonstrates that as opposed to the thin and smooth posterior component, the anterior component of the right atrium is lined with pectinate muscles. However, in between the pectinate muscles, there is very thin atrial tissue. If a lead is placed into the thin tissue, there may be a higher risk of perforation acutely. Perforation may be small and may not be detected clinically. The patient may only have minor symptoms or pericarditis that resolves, and the lead may be left in that location. During implant, sensing and pacing thresholds may still be satisfactory because the ring electrode is still in contact with the pectinate musculature.

However, the extraction of these leads can cause a larger perforation and acute tamponade. This highlights the importance of freeing up as much tissue as possible before applying traction. It is also essential to avoid traction without some countertraction.

Key Anatomic Points for the Extractionist

Right Atrium

- The free wall of the right atrium is complex, with a paucity of myocardium between pectinates.
- The electrogram may be large with good thresholds at implant because of contact with the proximal electrode despite partial perforation of the very thin right atrial wall between pectinates.
- Right atrial lead positioning on the superior limbus and Bachmann's bundle may be less likely to lead to free wall perforation from the tip but may still occur when excessive slack leads to fibrosis on the free wall commonly employed with this type of lead positioning.
- Antero-inferior lead positioning in the atrium may cause difficulty with extraction because of the proximity of the conduction system when using thermal energy.

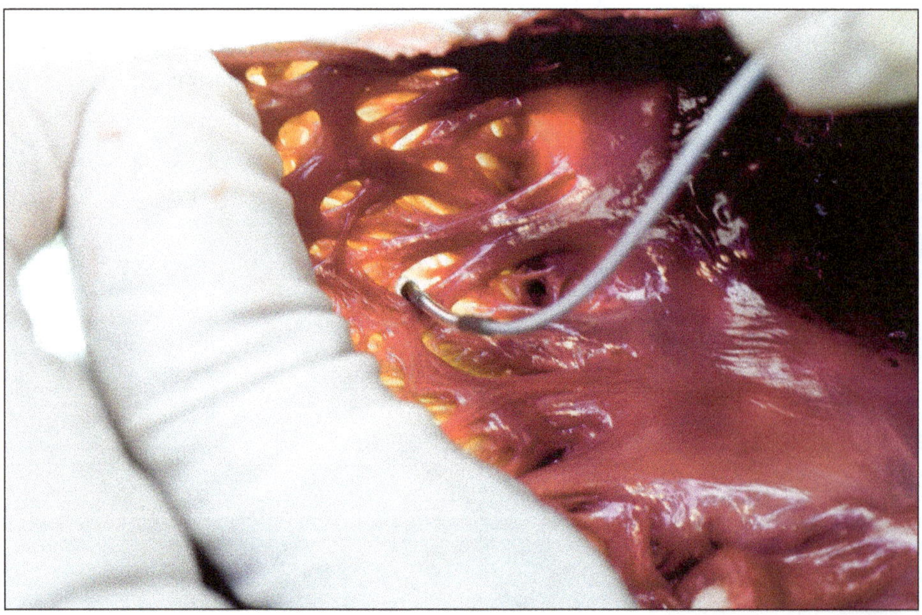

Figure 1.6 The anterior right atrial wall has interwoven pectinates, but the wall in between the pectinates is very thin.

RIGHT VENTRICLE

The right ventricle (RV) composes a significant portion of the anterior surface of the heart. It superiorly tapers into the conus arteriosus, a conal structure that leads to the pulmonary trunk. The interior of the RV is lined with irregular muscular elevations, trabeculae carnae, predominately in the inferior aspect. The RV apex and RV free wall in between trabeculae carnae are thin and are at high risk for perforation.[14] **Figure 1.7** demonstrates the thinness of the RV wall. In the image, the lead with an unextended helix is tenting the thin RV wall. With the extension of the helix, there will be a perforation.

When traction is applied during the extraction of leads, the lead comes out at the point of least resistance. Although the goal is for the lead to be released at the point of the lead–myocardial interface, it may not always happen. **Figure 1.8** illustrates that it is possible that the path of least resistance may be the interface of the myocardium to myocardium, resulting in a large perforation during extraction. This is especially likely if no countertraction is applied.

Figure 1.9 demonstrates the vector when traction is applied from the superior approach and inferior approaches. In cases where the superior approach to extraction is unsuccessful, one

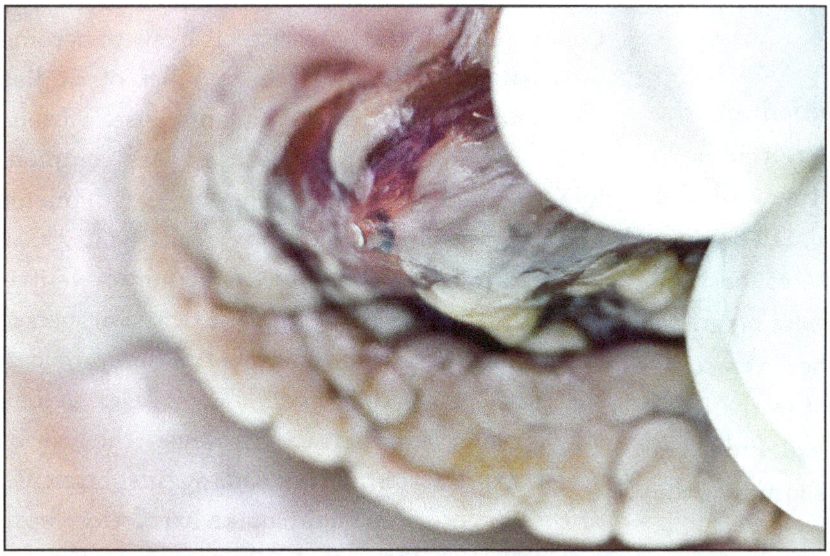

Figure 1.7 Thin right ventricular wall tented by a lead with an unextended helix.

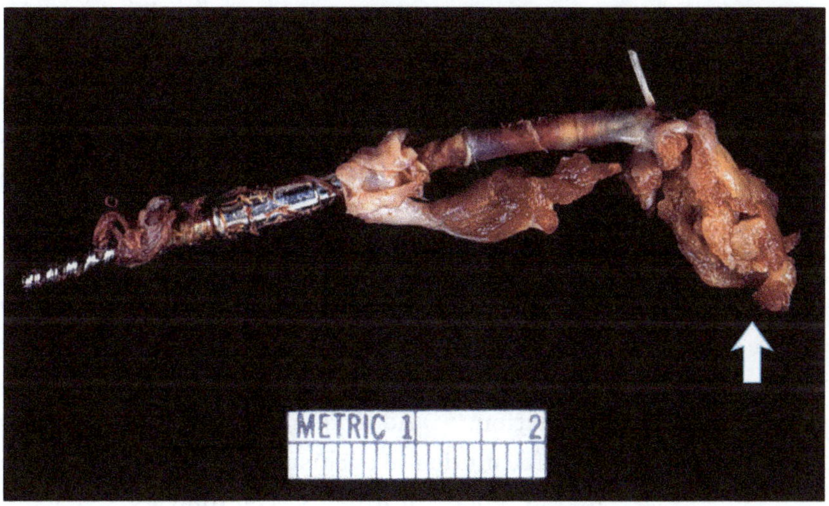

Figure 1.8 Extracted lead that was removed with a myocardial tissue (**arrow**). (Anatomic image courtesy of William Edwards, MD.)

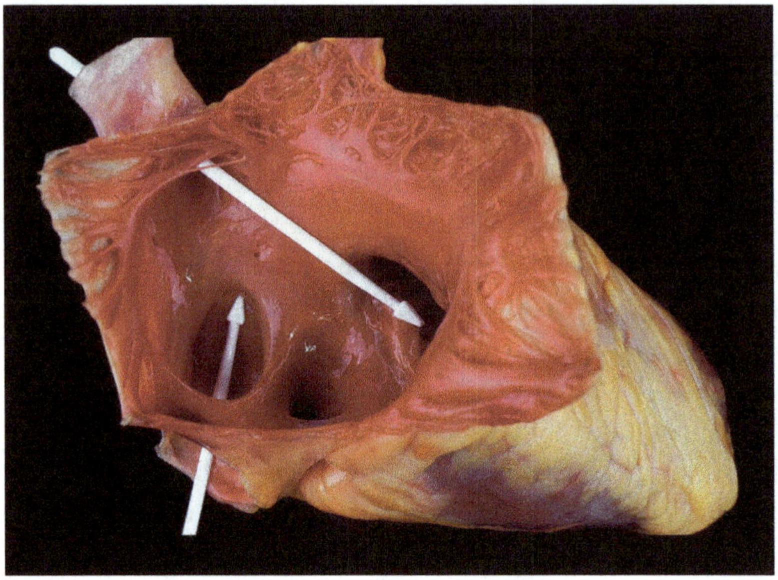

Figure 1.9 Right anterior oblique view of the heart, demonstrating the vector of traction from the superior approach compared to the inferior approach. (Anatomic image courtesy of William Edwards, MD.)

can consider using an alternative vector of traction via the inferior approach.

For leads implanted in the right ventricular outflow tract (RVOT), the direction of the implanted leads in the right anterior oblique (RAO) view can help distinguish a free wall lead versus a septal lead position. **Figure 1.10** demonstrates that in the RAO view, anterosuperiorly directed lead indicates that the lead was implanted to the RVOT's free wall and is a higher extraction risk. **Figure 1.11** demonstrates that in the RAO view, posteroinferiorly directed lead indicates that the lead was implanted to the septum of the RVOT and is a lower extraction risk.

Key Anatomic Points for the Extractionist

Right Ventricle

- Free wall of the right ventricular lead placement is far more likely to result in cardiac perforation when extracting chronic leads.
- Septal lead position should be ascertained fluoroscopically where the lead points leftward in the LAO projection but is neither close to the anterior of inferior silhouette (true mid-septal positioning).
- Chronic His bundle lead extraction has not yet been evaluated but may involve a risk of perforation of the membranous portion of the intraventricular septum.
- Free wall versus septal lead location in the RVOT is best ascertained with the RAO with anterosuperiorly directed leads involving the free wall and posteroinferiorly directed leads in the RAO, indicating septal and low extraction risk positioning.

CORONARY SINUS

Coronary sinus lead extraction is likely to become increasingly common as the number of cardiac resynchronization devices implanted rise.[2] Fibrous adhesions in the CS tend to be less common, hypothesized to be due to smaller lead diameter and lack of direct fixation mechanisms.[15] As opposed to leads placed in the atrium or ventricles, CS leads have much higher extraction success with manual traction.[16] Simple traction provided successful extraction in 91.4% of cases in one single-center experience.[17] However, the use of active fixation to stabilize leads against branches of the CS vessel wall may make extraction more difficult.[18–20] **Figure 1.12** demonstrates an active fixation CS lead (Attain Starfix, Medtronic), which provides additional support in the CS with deployable lobes. It may be more challenging to extract due to significant tissue ingrowth around fixation lobes.[21] **Figure 1.13** shows an extracted StarFix lead with tissue fibrosis preventing retraction of the active fixation lobes, with a partially torn vein adhered to the fibrosed tissue. Major complications have been reported in 15%–17% of cases of CS lead extraction.[22,23] Additionally, reimplantation may be difficult due to occlusion or thrombosis of the main CS body or direct vessel injury.[21]

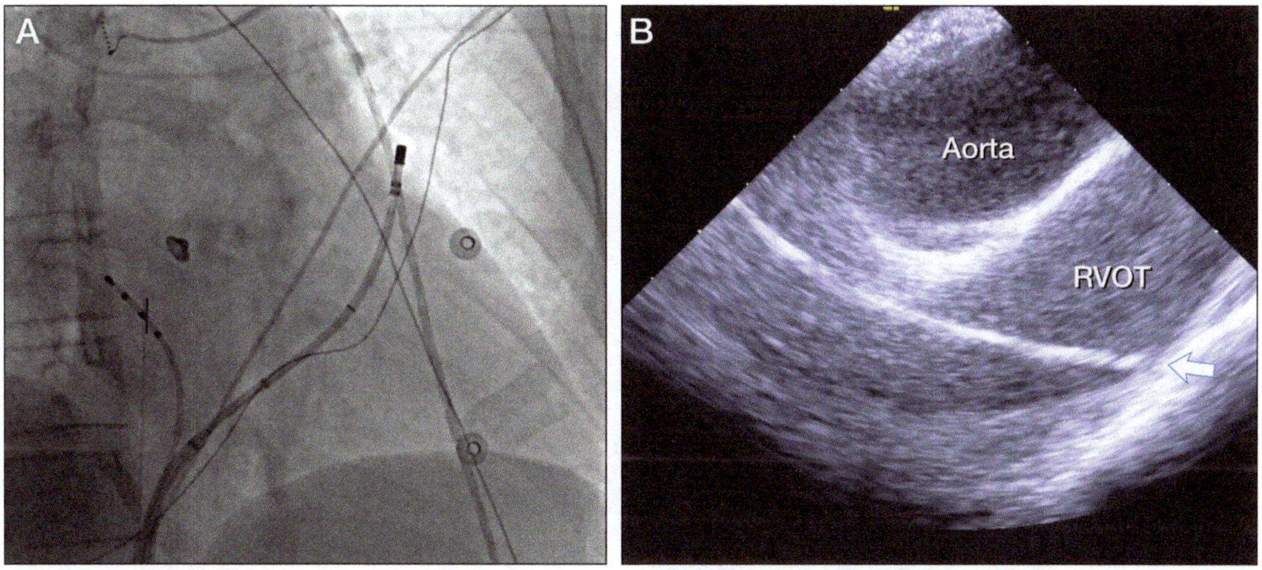

Figure 1.10 **Panel A** demonstrates that in the RAO view, anterosuperiorly directed leads or catheters point towards the free wall. **Panel B** shows intracardiac echo demonstrating the catheter (**arrow**) pointing towards the free wall of the RVOT.

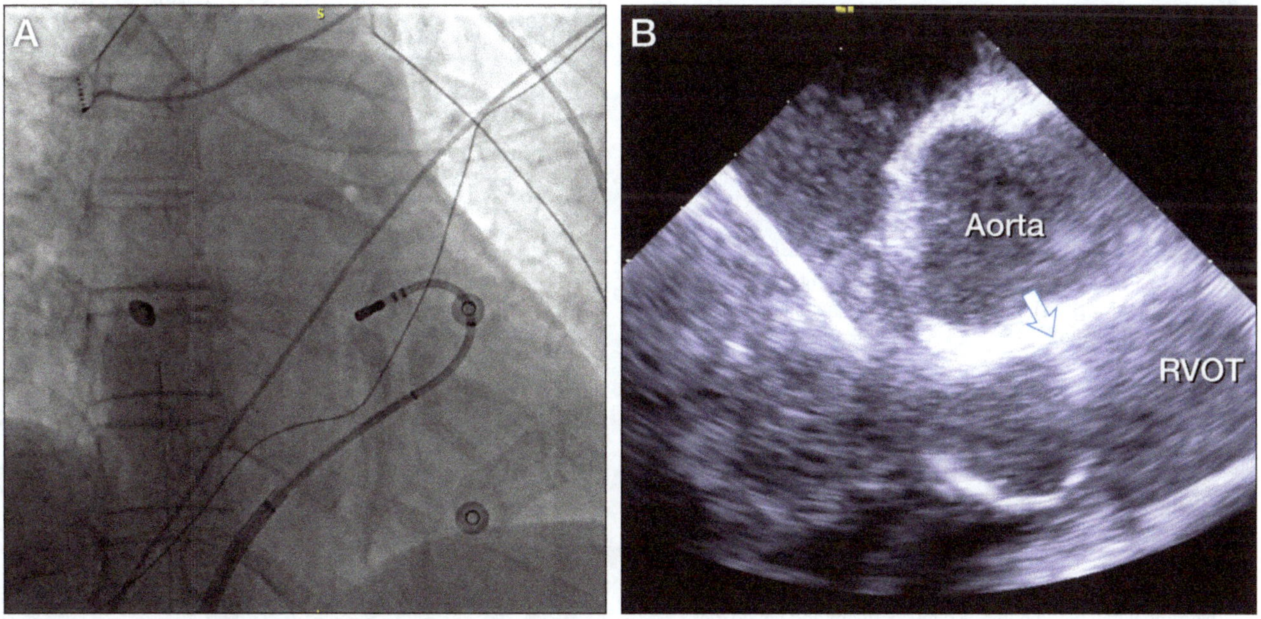

Figure 1.11 **Panel A** demonstrates that in the RAO view, posteroinferiorly directed leads or catheters point towards the septum. **Panel B** shows intracardiac echo demonstrating the catheter (**arrow**) pointing toward the septum between the RVOT and the aorta.

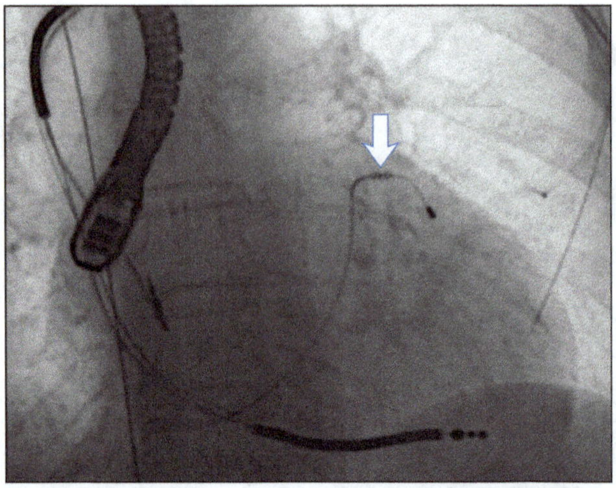

Figure 1.12 StarFix lead with active fixation lobes deployed.

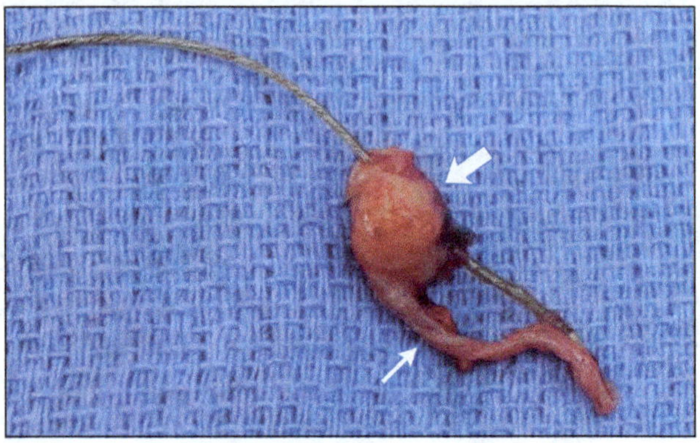

Figure 1.13 Extracted StarFix lead with tissue fibrosis around the lobes (**block arrow**). A partially torn vein is adhered to the fibrosis (**small arrow**).

Key Anatomic Points for the Extractionist

Coronary Sinus

- The CS itself has a muscular coat extending up to the first posterolateral vein and approximately 2 to 3 cm from the ostium.
- Beyond the posterolateral vein, the great cardiac vein (CV) is extremely thin with no intrinsic myocardium and a high-risk area from this site and beyond for perforation, including thermal energy or sheath deployment.
- Detailed knowledge of the type of lead and, when necessary, imaging or angiography to see if adhesions exist in the distal branches or the main CS assist with risk stratification. CS balloon preparation with CS angiography and wire placement for possible balloon deployment should a perforation occur, can be considered based on the specific anatomy akin to SVC complication prophylaxis.
- Inadvertent middle CV lead placement of ventricular leads, including implantable cardioverter-defibrillator (ICD) leads, should be considered when the distal portion of the lead appears straight and without slack. Failure to recognize this may result in venous tears, mainly when extracting coils.

TRICUSPID VALVE

The tricuspid valve lies between the right atrium and ventricle and contains 3 cusps whose bases are attached to a fibrous ring around the valve orifice. Chordae tendineae connect valve cusps to ventricular surfaces via papillary muscles, which form conical projections with their base to the ventricular wall. Typically, there are 3 papillary muscles (septal, anterior, and posterior) that correspond to tricuspid valve cusps. Given this intricate network, leads can be trapped in between the chordae during implantation (**Figure 1.14**) and complicate the extraction process. Furthermore, fibrosis forms at points of contact and abrasion of the lead and tissue.[24,25] There can be a significant amount of fibrosis that forms around the lead (**Figure 1.15**). The addition of fibrosis around the points of lead to chordae contact will add to the complexity of the extraction. Patients with leads that have gone in between the chordae can develop tricuspid regurgitation (TR) immediately after lead implantation. Tricuspid valve tear can also develop following lead extraction (**Figure 1.16**), especially if the adherence of the lead to the valve or valvular apparatus is not freed and traction is applied without adequate countertraction.

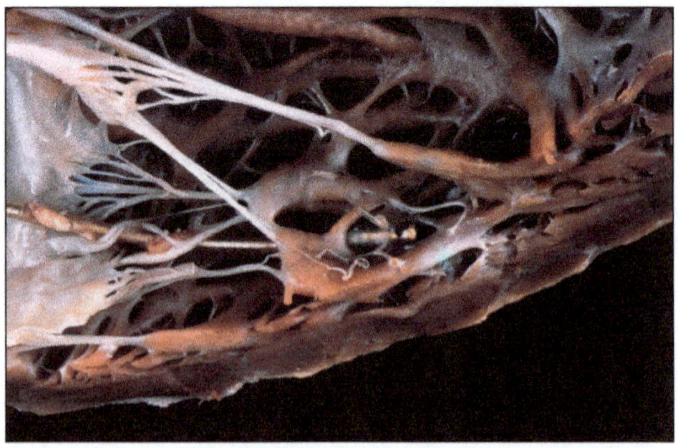

Figure 1.14 Tined lead that went in between the chordae to reach the right ventricular wall. (Anatomic image courtesy of William Edwards, MD.)

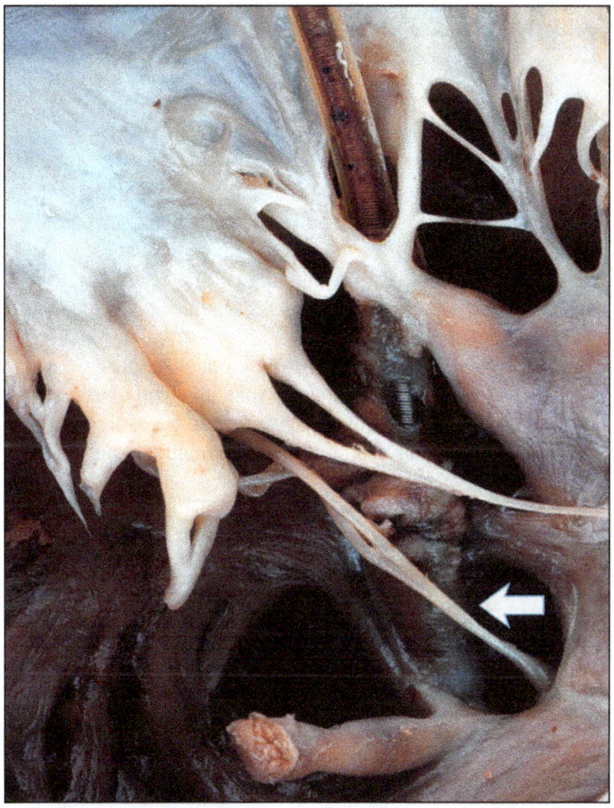

Figure 1.15 Ensheathment of a lead that has gone in between the chordae with fibrosis and calcification (**arrow**). (Anatomic image courtesy of William Edwards, MD.)

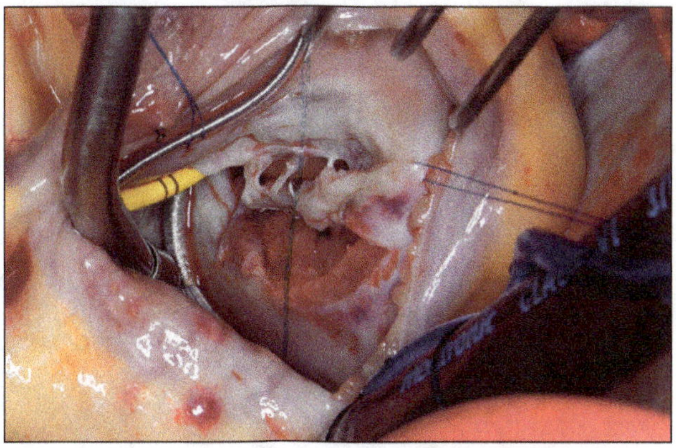

Figure 1.16 Tricuspid valve tear following lead extraction resulting in severe tricuspid regurgitation requiring surgical repair.

However, even in a central lead position, fibrosis can still occur at points where there is contact between the lead and tissue. **Figure 1.17** shows that beyond the lead tip to the myocardial interface, a centrally positioned lead can also be in contact with the chordae, the papillary muscle, and the tricuspid leaflet. Fibrosis along these points of contact can still involve the chordae, leading to delayed TR. In these scenarios, patients often have no TR immediately after the extraction, but with increasing fibrosis between the points of lead contact, they can have increasing TR. If the reason for extraction is TR, extraction itself would make the TR worse in these patients.

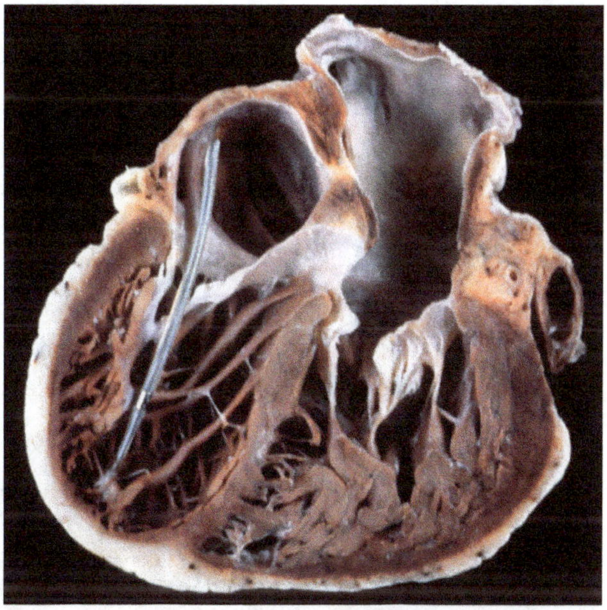

Figure 1.17 Lead with points of contact along with the tricuspid apparatus. (Anatomic image courtesy of William Edwards MD.)

Worsening tricuspid valve function following RV lead removal has been reported between 0.32%–10.0% of cases.[26–28] The incidence of flail tricuspid valve requiring invention following extraction is unknown, though it is thought to be low at 0.03%.[29] Risk factors for traumatic TR include extraction of multiple leads and the use of more than one extraction tool.[27,30] Other risk factors for traumatic TR include longer implantation time, increased age, and the presence of pacemaker leads (over ICD leads).[27,28] The presence of lead extraction-related TR has also been associated with a longer hospital stay, development of right-sided heart failure, and worse long-term prognosis.[31]

Occasionally, one will encounter exteriorized leads that require extraction. **Figure 1.18** shows the tricuspid valve during surgery with an exteriorized lead traversing outside of the annulus. Occasionally, surgeons will leave leads exteriorized after tricuspid valve repair, annuloplasty, or replacement. Exteriorized leads have the potential to reduce the interactions of a centrally positioned lead with the tricuspid valve apparatus. However, the downside is that the extraction will be challenging. In an exteriorized lead, if a laser or mechanical sheath is used all the way across the tricuspid valve and into the right ventricle, there will be a large disruption in the tricuspid valve after extraction. One technique that can be employed is to get the sheath as close to the level of the valve as possible under transesophageal or intracardiac echocardiography guidance and then try to slide the lead out. This way, there is less disruption in the tricuspid valve.

Key Anatomic Points for the Extractionist

Tricuspid Valve

- The absence of TR before extraction does not exclude significant fibrosis between the lead and the subvalvular apparatus.
- Caution when employing thermal energy on the inferior free wall and annulus is required to avoid perforation and possible arterial trauma.
- Appropriate fluoroscopic appearance of slack with a partial heel with no abrupt curves or kinks in the lead when applying slack at implant or preextraction makes adherence to free wall or papillary muscle chordae unlikely. Ventricular inversion, when applying extreme traction, should be avoided since severe tricuspid valve trauma may result even if the lead is freed without perforation from its tip.

SPECIAL SITUATIONS

Congenital Heart Disease

Patients with congenital heart disease are less likely to have successful laser lead extractions, which is thought to be due in part to increased calcification.[32] A thorough understanding of

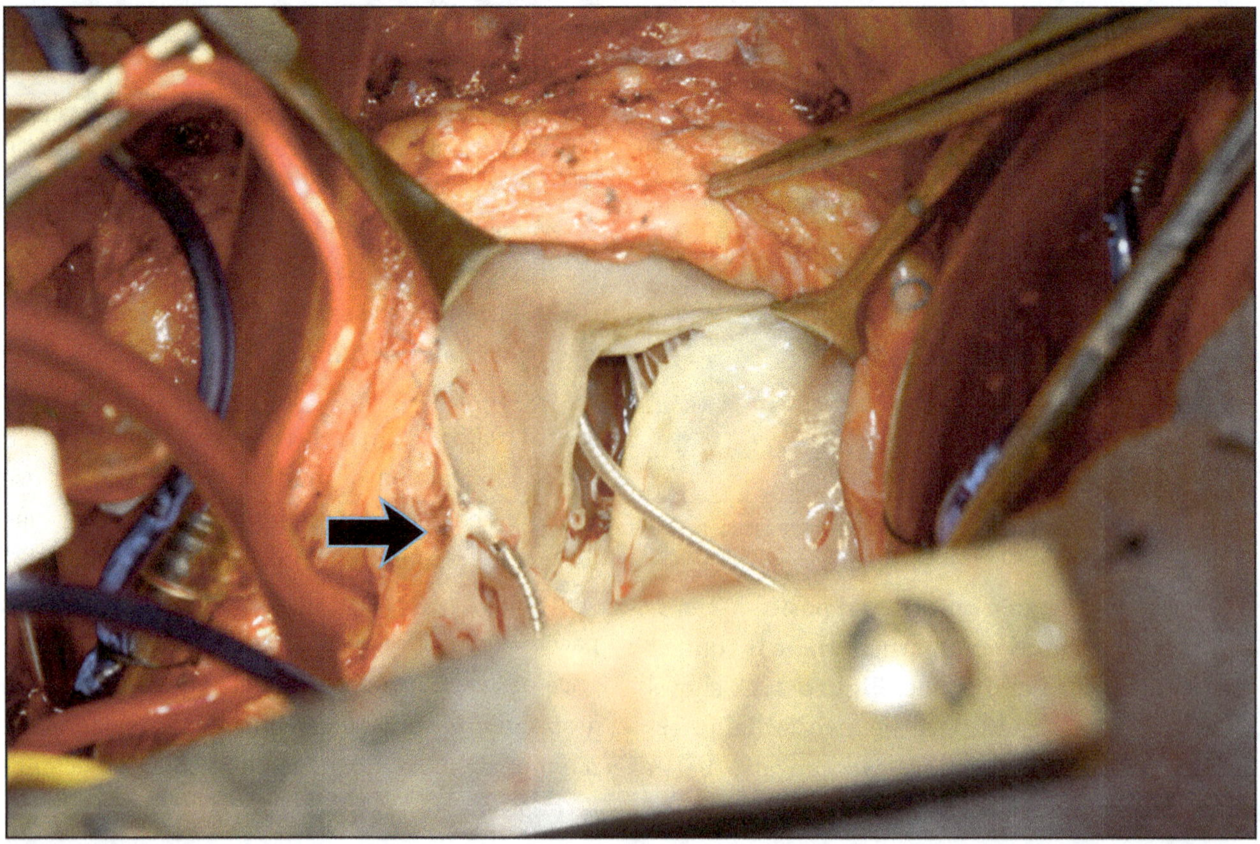

Figure 1.18 View of the tricuspid valve from the right atrium. A lead is seen exteriorized (**arrow**), and another lead is seen going through the annulus.

patient anatomy, device history, and the lead course is paramount to a successful procedure.

Figure 1.19 shows a fluoroscopy image of a patient with dextrocardia and L-transposition. The course of the CS is towards the right side. The principles of having the extraction sheath being coaxial with the lead applies as well. However, in patients with congenital heart disease, the angles of the lead will be different. Therefore, a thorough understanding of the angels and anatomy of the vascular structures and baffles when extracting leads in congenital heart disease patients is important.

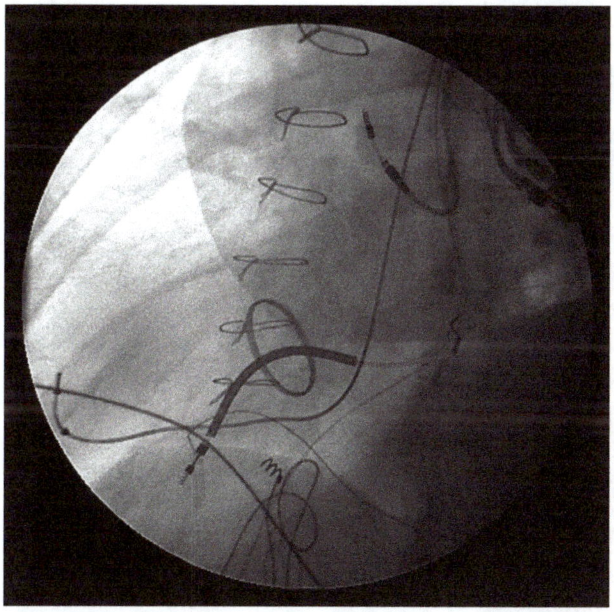

Figure 1.19 Fluoroscopy image of a patient with dextrocardia and L-transposition.

Persistent Left Superior Vena Cava

The presence of a persistent left SVC (PLSVC) presents a unique challenge during lead extraction. The PLSVC is the most common thoracic venous congenital malformation present in 0.3%–0.5% of individuals in the general population.[33] Typically with PLSVC, the SVC will drain into the right atrium through a dilated CS in 80%–90% of cases; in 10%–20% of cases, the SVC drains into the left atrium resulting in a right-to-left shunt.[34,35] A lead positioned via the left superior vena cava goes directly downwards towards the CS before making a sharp turn at the level of the CS towards the right atrium or the great cardiac vein (CV) (**Figure 1.20**). If a sheath was advanced through the left SVC and to the level of the left SVC to CS and continued forward pressure is applied, it will lead to perforation of the CS.

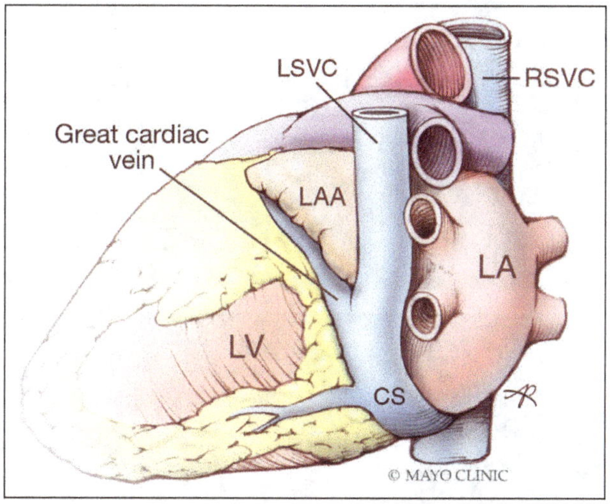

Figure 1.20 Anatomy of a persistent left superior vena cava (PLSVC). *Abbreviations:* CS, coronary sinus; LA, left atrium; LAA, left atrial appendage; LV, left ventricle; RSVC, right superior vena cava.

Leads in the Middle Cardiac Vein

The middle CV is located on the posterior interventricular groove draining directly into the CS and typically accompanies the posterior interventricular artery (posterior descending artery). **Figure 1.21** shows a patient with the placement of an ICD lead into a middle CV. We can compare this lead position to the right ventricular lead placed in the right ventricle. It is essential to recognize the close proximity of the vein to the artery as the use of laser sheaths can cause arterial thermal damage to the posterior descending artery and the posterolateral branch (**Figure 1.22**). The operator should cease the use of laser catheters near the ostium of the vein to avoid the potential for thermal injury.

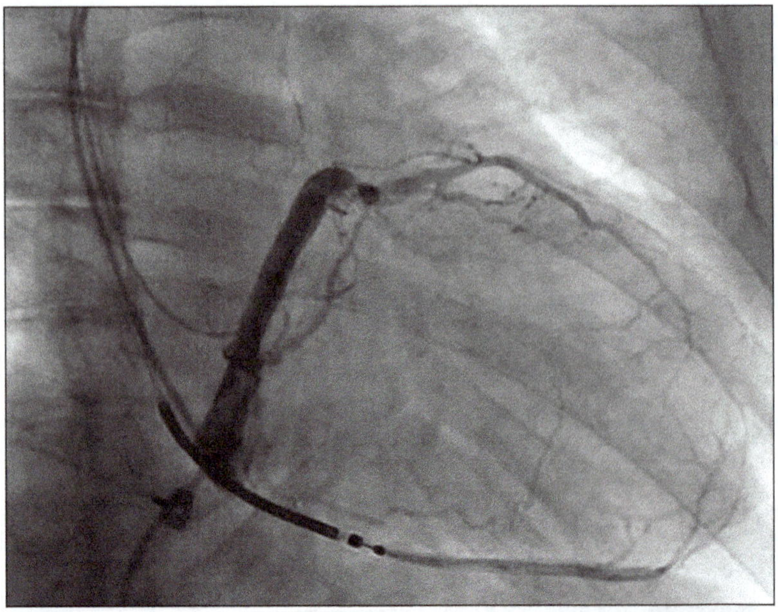

Figure 1.21 RAO view showing ICD lead in the middle CV.

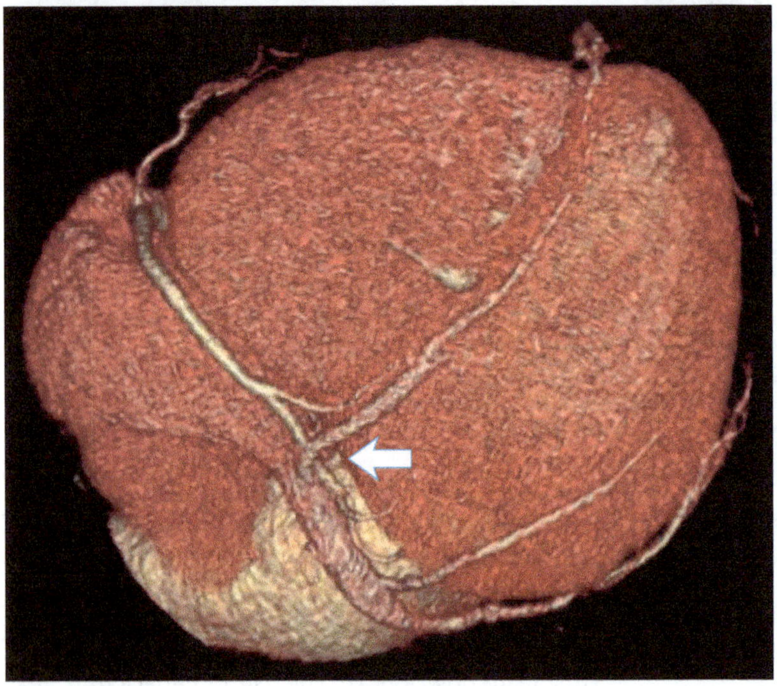

Figure 1.22 Posterior view of the heart, demonstrating the close relationship between the middle CV and the posterior descending artery and the posterolateral branch (**arrow**).

Leads in the Systemic Circulation

Rarely, leads may be placed transarterially either intentionally or inadvertently. Inadvertent lead implantation in an arterial vessel is a rare and likely underrecognized complication.[36–38] In many of these cases, anatomic variation accounts for misplacement into the left ventricle during implantation.[39] **Figure 1.23** shows a patient with the inadvertent placement of pacing lead into the left ventricle through a retro-aortic approach. If unrecognized, the extraction of a lead placed in the arterial system will lead to thromboembolism and systemic embolization.

CONCLUSIONS

An understanding of the anatomy involved during the extraction process is essential to reduce complications. It is vital to appreciate the

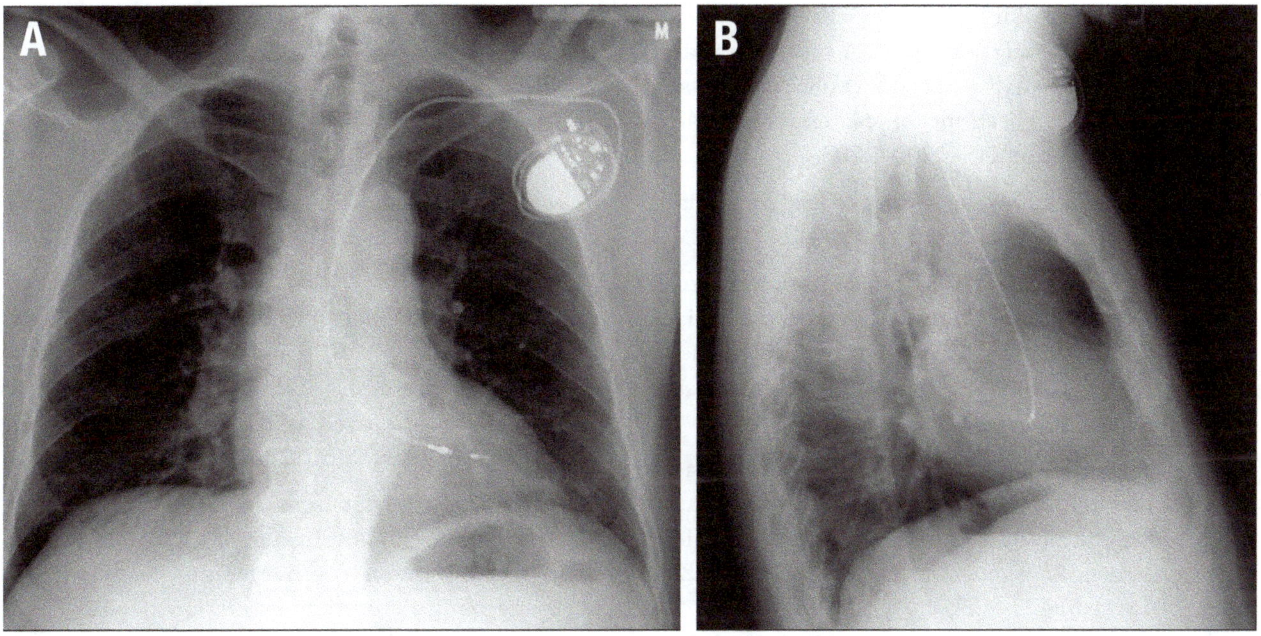

Figure 1.23 Pacing lead is seen taking a retroaortic course into the left ventricle.

relationship of the lead with the surrounding structures. This involves a thorough preprocedural preparation and comprehensive review of the clinical history and imaging data before each extraction procedure.

REFERENCES

1. Lee JZ, Agasthi P, Pasha AK, Tarin C, Tseng AS, Diehl NN, et al. Stroke in patients with cardiovascular implantable electronic device infection undergoing transvenous lead removal. *Heart Rhythm.* 2018;15(11):1593–600.
2. Wazni O, Wilkoff BL. Considerations for cardiac device lead extraction. *Nat Rev Cardiol.* 2016; 13(4):221–229.
3. Brunner MP, Cronin EM, Wazni O, Baranowski B, Saliba WI, Sabik JF, et al. Outcomes of patients requiring emergent surgical or endovascular intervention for catastrophic complications during transvenous lead extraction. *Heart Rhythm.* 2014;11(3):419–425.
4. Smith HJ, Fearnot NE, Byrd CL, Wilkoff BL, Love CJ, Sellers TD. Five-year experience with intravascular lead extraction. U.S. Lead Extraction Database. *Pacing Clin Electrophysiol.* 1994;17(11 Pt 2):2016–2020.
5. Tarakji KG, Saliba W, Markabawi D, Rodriguez ER, Krauthammer Y, Brunner MP, et al. Unrecognized venous injuries after cardiac implantable electronic device transvenous lead extraction. *Heart Rhythm.* 2018;15(3):318–325.
6. DeSimone CV, Noheria A, Lachman N, Edwards WD, Gami AS, Maleszewski JJ, et al. Myocardium of the superior vena cava, coronary sinus, vein of Marshall, and the pulmonary vein ostia: Gross anatomic studies in 620 hearts. *J Cardiovasc Electrophysiol.* 2012;23(12):1304–1309.
7. Robboy SJ, Harthorne JW, Leinbach RC, Sanders CA, Austen WG. Autopsy findings with permanent pervenous pacemakers. *Circulation.* 1969;39(4):495–501.
8. Huang TY, Baba N. Cardiac pathology of transvenous pacemakers. *Am Heart J.* 1972;83(4): 469–474.
9. Anderson JM, Rodriguez A, Chang DT. Foreign body reaction to biomaterials. *Semin Immunol.* 2008;20(2):86–100.
10. Wong VW, Rustad KC, Akaishi S, Sorkin M, Glotzbach JP, Januszyk M, et al. Focal adhesion kinase links mechanical force to skin fibrosis via inflammatory signaling. *Nat Med.* 2011; 18(1):148–152.

11. Rennert RC, Rustad K, Levi K, Harwood M, Sorkin M, Wong VW, et al. A histological and mechanical analysis of the cardiac lead-tissue interface: Implications for lead extraction. *Acta Biomater.* 2014;10(5):2200–2208.
12. Love CJ. Lead Management and lead extraction. *Card Electrophysiol Clin.* 2018;10(1):127–136.
13. Hirschl DA, Jain VR, Spindola-Franco H, Gross JN, Haramati LB. Prevalence and characterization of asymptomatic pacemaker and ICD lead perforation on CT. *Pacing Clin Electrophysiol.* 2007;30(1):28–32.
14. Li Y, Dykoski R, Li J. [Chronic transvenous pacemaker/implantable cardioverter defibrillator leads implantation induced pathological changes]. *Zhonghua Xin Xue Guan Bing Za Zhi.* 2015;43(5):423–427.
15. Bongiorni MG, Zucchelli G, Soldati E, Arena G, Giannola G, Di Cori A, et al. Usefulness of mechanical transvenous dilation and location of areas of adherence in patients undergoing coronary sinus lead extraction. *Europace.* 2007;9(1):69–73.
16. Hamid S, Arujuna A, Khan S, Ladwiniec A, McPhail M, Bostock J, et al. Extraction of chronic pacemaker and defibrillator leads from the coronary sinus: Laser infrequently used but required. *Europace.* 2009;11(2):213–215.
17. Sheldon S, Friedman PA, Hayes DL, Osborn MJ, Cha YM, Rea RF, et al. Outcomes and predictors of difficulty with coronary sinus lead removal. *J Interv Card Electrophysiol.* 2012;35(1):93–100.
18. Kowalski O, Lenarczyk R, Prokopczuk J, Pruszkowska-Skrzep P, Zielinska T, Sredniawa B, et al. Effect of percutaneous interventions within the coronary sinus on the success rate of the implantations of resynchronization pacemakers. *Pacing Clin Electrophysiol.* 2006;29(10): 1075–1080.
19. Bontempi L, Vassanelli F, Ashofair N, Inama L, Mariggio D, Cerini M, et al. The novel active fixation coronary sinus lead: Efficacy and safety of transvenous extraction procedure. *Europace.* 2016;18(2):301–303.
20. Nagele H, Azizi M, Hashagen S, Castel MA, Behrens S. First experience with a new active fixation coronary sinus lead. *Europace.* 2007;9(6): 437–441.
21. Cronin EM, Ingelmo CP, Rickard J, Wazni OM, Martin DO, Wilkoff BL, et al. Active fixation mechanism complicates coronary sinus lead extraction and limits subsequent reimplantation targets. *J Interv Card Electrophysiol.* 2013;36(1):81–86; discussion 6.
22. Crossley GH, Sorrentino RA, Exner DV, Merliss AD, Tobias SM, Martin DO, et al. Extraction of chronically implanted coronary sinus leads active fixation vs passive fixation leads. *Heart Rhythm.* 2016;13(6):1253–1259.
23. Kypta A, Blessberger H, Saleh K, Honig S, Kammler J, Steinwender C. Removal of active-fixation coronary sinus leads using a mechanical rotation extraction device. *Pacing Clin Electrophysiol.* 2015;38(3):302–305.
24. Novak M, Dvorak P, Kamaryt P, Slana B, Lipoldova J. Autopsy and clinical context in deceased patients with implanted pacemakers and defibrillators: Intracardiac findings near their leads and electrodes. *Europace.* 2009;11(11):1510–1516.
25. Lin G, Nishimura RA, Connolly HM, Dearani JA, Sundt TM, 3rd, Hayes DL. Severe symptomatic tricuspid valve regurgitation due to permanent pacemaker or implantable cardioverter-defibrillator leads. *J Am Coll Cardiol.* 2005;45(10): 1672–1675.
26. Shepherd E, Stuart G, Martin R, Walsh MA. Extraction of SelectSecure leads compared to conventional pacing leads in patients with congenital heart disease and congenital atrioventricular block. *Heart Rhythm.* 2015; 12(6):1227–1232.
27. Franceschi F, Thuny F, Giorgi R, Sanaa I, Peyrouse E, Assouan X, et al. Incidence, risk factors, and outcome of traumatic tricuspid regurgitation after percutaneous ventricular lead removal. *J Am Coll Cardiol.* 2009;53(23): 2168–2174.
28. Park SJ, Gentry JL, 3rd, Varma N, Wazni O, Tarakji KG, Mehta A, et al. Transvenous extraction of pacemaker and defibrillator leads and the risk of tricuspid valve regurgitation. *JACC Clin Electrophysiol.* 2018;4(11):1421–428.

29. Brunner MP, Cronin EM, Jacob J, Duarte VE, Tarakji KG, Martin DO, et al. Transvenous extraction of implantable cardioverter-defibrillator leads under advisory—a comparison of Riata, Sprint Fidelis, and non-recalled implantable cardioverter-defibrillator leads. *Heart Rhythm.* 2013;10(10):1444–1450.

30. Coffey JO, Sager SJ, Gangireddy S, Levine A, Viles-Gonzalez JF, Fischer A. The impact of transvenous lead extraction on tricuspid valve function. *Pacing Clin Electrophysiol.* 2014;37(1):19–124.

31. Messika-Zeitoun D, Thomson H, Bellamy M, Scott C, Tribouilloy C, Dearani J, et al. Medical and surgical outcome of tricuspid regurgitation caused by flail leaflets. *J Thorac Cardiovasc Surg.* 2004;128(2):296–302.

32. McCanta AC, Kong MH, Carboni MP, Greenfield RA, Hranitzky PM, Kanter RJ. Laser lead extraction in congenital heart disease: A case-controlled study. *Pacing Clin Electrophysiol.* 2013;36(3):372–380.

33. Tyrak KW, Holda J, Holda MK, Koziej M, Piatek K, Klimek-Piotrowska W. Persistent left superior vena cava. *Cardiovasc J Afr.* 2017;28(3):e1–e4.

34. Goyal SK, Punnam SR, Verma G, Ruberg FL. Persistent left superior vena cava: A case report and review of literature. *Cardiovasc Ultrasound.* 2008;6:50.

35. Granata A, Andrulli S, Fiorini F, Logias F, Figuera M, Mignani R, et al. Persistent left superior vena cava: What the interventional nephrologist needs to know. *J Vasc Access.* 2009;10(3):207–211.

36. Issa ZF, Rumman SS, Mullin JC. Inadvertent transarterial insertion of atrial and ventricular defibrillator leads. *J Interv Card Electrophysiol.* 2009;24(1):63–66.

37. Van Gelder BM, Bracke FA, Oto A, Yildirir A, Haas PC, Seger JJ, et al. Diagnosis and management of inadvertently placed pacing and ICD leads in the left ventricle: A multicenter experience and review of the literature. *Pacing Clin Electrophysiol.* 2000;23(5):877–883.

38. Lepore V, Pizzarelli G, Dernevik L. Inadvertent transarterial pacemaker insertion: An unusual complication. *Pacing Clin Electrophysiol.* 1987;10(4 Pt 1):951–954.

39. Rovera C, Golzio PG, Corgnati G, Conti V, Franco E, Frea S, et al. A pacemaker lead in the left ventricle: An "unexpected" finding? *J Cardiol Cases.* 2019;20(6):228–231.

2 | Clinical Assessment

Kunal Shah, MD; Ulrika Birgersdotter-Green, MD

INTRODUCTION

Over 1 million new cardiovascular implantable electronic devices (CIEDs) are inserted yearly across the globe.[1–4] Consequently, lead management is becoming an increasingly vital component of patient care.[1] A critical component of lead management is understanding when lead extraction is necessary and indicated. In addition to understanding the guidelines, it is also imperative to incorporate the patient's profile in the overall clinical assessment. This section will address guidelines for lead extraction, clinical assessment, and shared decision making.

INDICATIONS FOR LEAD EXTRACTION

The indications for extraction can be broadly separated into infectious and noninfectious categories.

Infection-Related Indications

Infection remains the most common reason for extraction. Over 60,000 patients with CIEDs develop new infections every year worldwide, and there has been a 320% increase in hospitalizations for CIED infections from 1996 to 2006.[5–9]

The infection-related indications for extraction and subsequent device management are reviewed in the 2010 American Heart Association (AHA) Update to the CIED Infection Scientific Statement.[10] A practical algorithm from this statement is presented in **Figure 2.1**.

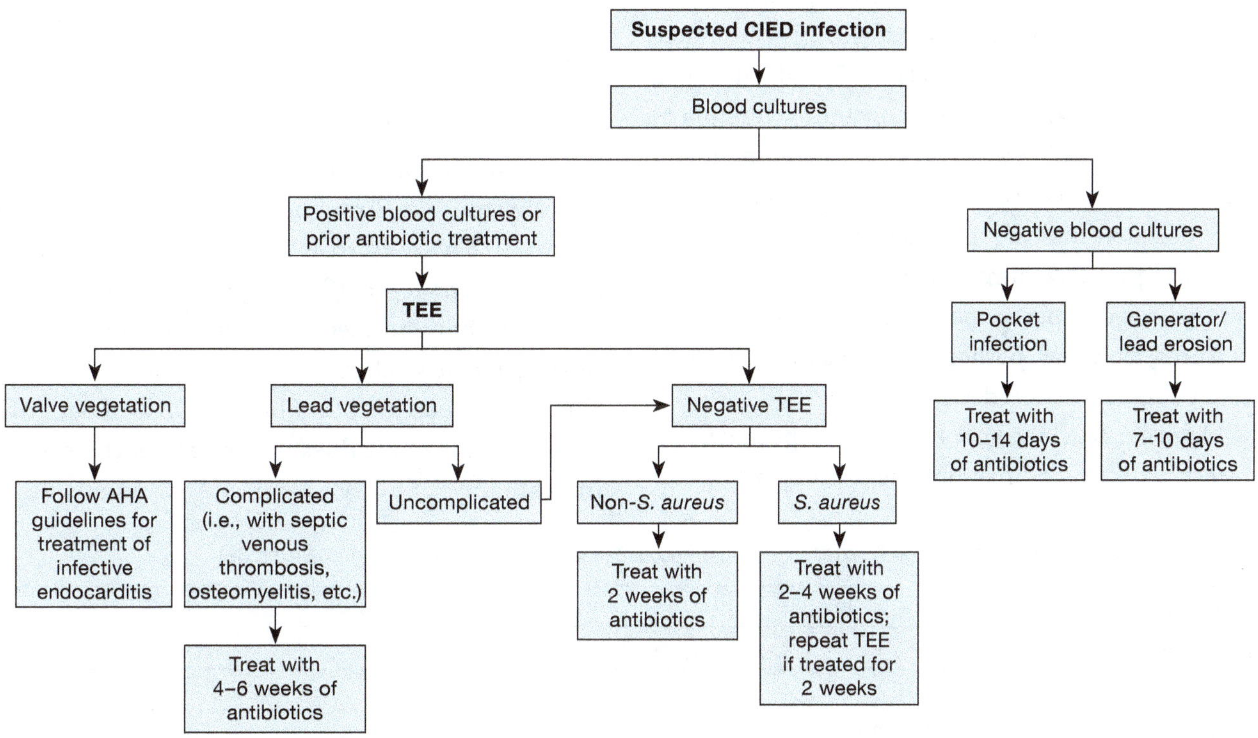

Figure 2.1 Workflow summary of how to manage suspected CIED infection.[10]

Cardiac Lead Extraction: A Case-Based Contemporary Approach.
 ISBN: 978-1-942909-54-5

Table 2.1 summarizes the infectious indications for lead extraction based on current Heart Rhythm Society (HRS) guidelines and is further detailed in the subsequent text.[1]

Pocket infections are the most clinically apparent CIED issue during follow-up. They necessitate complete CIED extraction but can have highly variable clinical presentations. Less than half of patients present with classic inflammatory changes such as erythema, swelling, pain, warmth, or drainage.[1,10,11] Device erosion through the skin is less common, and it mandates CIED extraction as any external exposure allows local pathogens to enter the pocket and vasculature.[1,10,11]

Clinicians should also have a high suspicion for CIED infection in any patient who presents with systemic symptoms such as fever, chills, anorexia, or malaise. However, the absence of these symptoms does not exclude CIED infection. When any CIED infection is suspected, it is imperative to obtain two sets of blood cultures, which will help guide extraction decisions, antibiotic choice, and treatment duration.[1,10]

If bacteremia is discovered in any patient with a CIED, clinicians may evaluate if CIED is the source of or involved in the infection. Specifically, if a patient has unexplained or recurrent bacteremia or fungemia, CIED extraction is recommended.[1] Infectious disease consultation ultimately guides the decision-making process of the extraction team. **Figure 2.2** summarizes workflow with various pathogen species potentially found in blood cultures; however, pathogen alone should not dictate CIED extraction decision.[1,10,12]

Another crucial component of a suspected CIED infection is the transesophageal echocardiogram (TEE). The TEE can help visualize vegetations, valvular dysfunction, and perivalvular abscesses with a high specificity.[1,14] CIED extraction is recommended if endocarditis or lead vegetations are present, regardless of pathogen species. If the diagnosis of CIED infection is in doubt, additional imaging modalities such as FDG-PET/CT or tagged white blood cell (WBC) scan may be useful.[1,15]

In summary, CIED extraction is recommended for definite system infection, endocarditis (even without device involvement), and unexplained bacteremia/fungemia[1] (see Table 2.1).

Noninfectious Related Indications

The growing need for CIED extraction in patients without infection (**Table 2.2**) largely stems from patients living longer and increased implantation of defibrillator systems.[1,7,13,16] High-voltage leads tend to fail at higher rates, and cardiac resynchronization therapy (CRT) systems involve an additional left ventricular (LV) lead, which occupies more intravenous space.[1,17]

The reasons for extraction fall into three major categories: vascular issues, intrinsic lead issues, and miscellaneous issues summarized in **Table 2.3** and detailed in the subsequent text.

Vascular Issues

Transvenous leads can cause fibrosis, stenosis, and thrombosis throughout their implanted life span.[1,17,18] Severe fibrosis and stenosis can lead to superior vena cava (SVC) syndrome. This syndrome is characterized by persistent shortness of breath, facial swelling, and migraines. Although this is only seen in approximately 0.1% of patients with CIED, when it does occur, lead extraction is indicated.[1,19,20] SVC syndrome may be amenable to

Table 2.1 Infectious indications for CIED extraction, class of recommendation (COR), and level of evidence (LOE)

Indication	COR	LOE
Infectious		
Definite CIED infection	I	B
Endocarditis (+/– device or lead involvement)	I	B
Unexplained persistent/recurrent bacteremia/fungemia	I	B

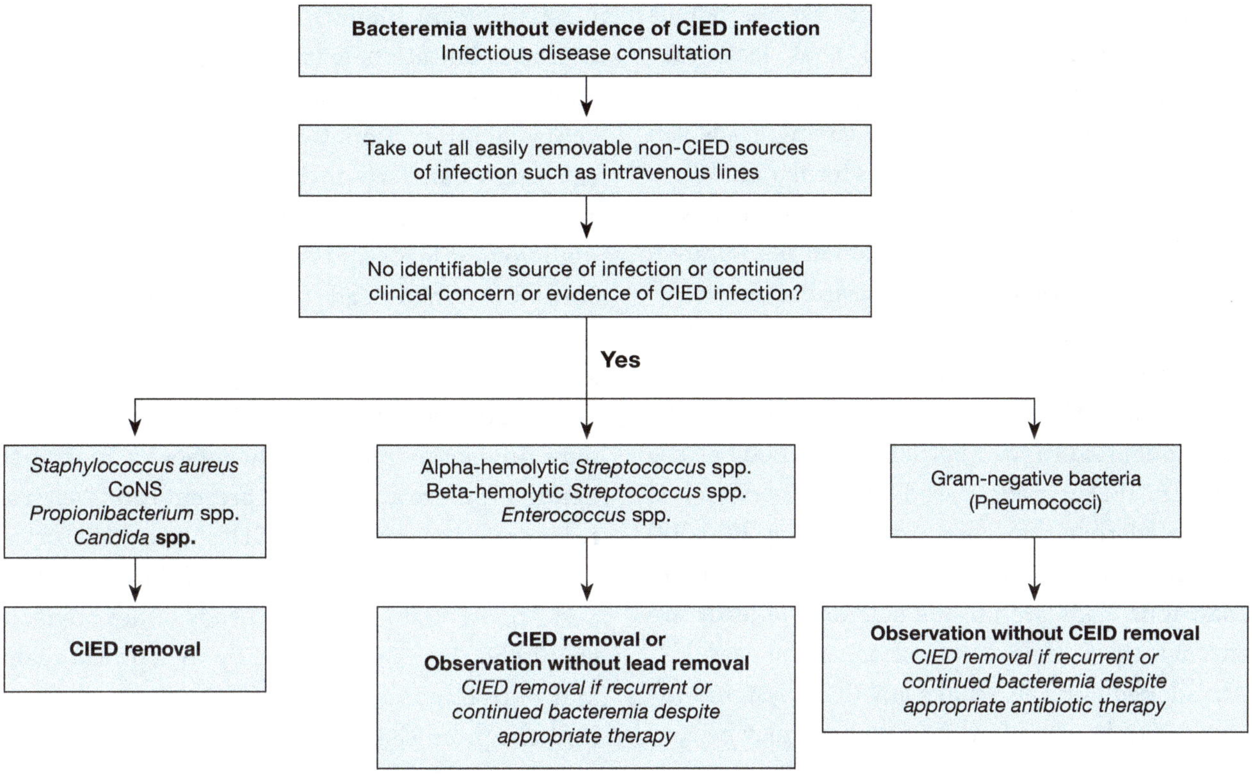

Figure 2.2 Workflow summary from the 2017 HRS expert consensus on lead extraction detailing management of bacteremia and common pathogens.[1]

Table 2.2 Noninfectious indications for CIED extraction, class of recommendation (COR), and level of evidence (LOE)

Indication	COR	LOE
Noninfectious		
Vascular Issue		
Lead thrombus + related embolization	I	C
SVC syndrome	I	C
Planned venous stent deployment around lead	I	C
SVC occlusion and need for a new lead	I	C
Ipsilateral venous occlusion and need for a new lead	IIA	C
> 4 leads on one side or > 5 leads through SVC	IIA	C
Lead Issue		
Lead failure of pace-sense circuit or shock ability	IIA	B
Lead under advisory + evidence of lead compromise	IIB	B
Other		
RV lead causing life-threatening arrhythmias	I	C
Chronic pain due to CIED	IIA	C
Radiation therapy planned in the path of the lead	IIA	C
Severe tricuspid regurgitation due to lead	IIB	C
To facilitate access to MRI	IIB	C

percutaneous stent implantation. Before venous stenting, it is recommended that leads are extracted to avoid entrapment.[1,20,21]

In addition to stenosis and scarring, leads can also serve as a nidus for thrombus formation. When a clinically significant thrombotic event occurs secondary to lead thrombus, extraction is indicated, especially in patients with intracardiac shunts.[1,22] Often, these shunts may need to be closed before extraction to avoid thrombotic debris.[1,22]

Abandoned leads are leads that are deemed nonfunctional and capped but left in the body at the time of CIED upgrade. Based on registry data, it is estimated that there are approximately 600,000 abandoned leads in the United States.[1,23,24] If more than four leads are on one side or five leads are through the SVC, lead extraction can be useful.[1,25] Abandoned leads also make any CIED system MRI incompatible. Therefore, lead removal may be considered to facilitate access to an MRI.[1,26]

Lead-Related Issues

After implantation, leads are exposed to the constant flow of blood, muscular contraction, and vein wall interaction. Occasionally, this mechanical stress can lead to insulation breakdown or conductor fracture. This is more common in high-voltage leads and can result in inappropriate shocks.[27] When lead failure compromises the pace-sense circuit or ability to appropriately shock, extraction can be useful.[1] In addition, the Food and Drug Administration (FDA) will produce advisories on leads that show a high incidence of failure and clinical presentations such as recurrent, inappropriate ICD shocks. Historical examples include the Medtronic Sprint Fidelis and Abbott Riata leads.[28,29] Leads under advisory should be closely monitored by the clinical team, and extraction can be useful in those showing lead compromise in the appropriate patient.[1]

Table 2.3 Summary of major indications for CIED extraction, class of recommendation (COR), and level of evidence (LOE)

Indication	COR	LOE
Infectious		
Definite CIED infection	I	B
Endocarditis (+/– device or lead involvement)	I	B
Unexplained persistent/recurrent bacteremia/fungemia	I	B
Noninfectious		
Vascular Issue		
Lead thrombus + related embolization	I	C
SVC syndrome	I	C
Planned venous stent deployment around lead	I	C
SVC occlusion and need for a new lead	I	C
Ipsilateral venous occlusion and need for a new lead	IIA	C
> 4 leads on one side or > 5 leads through SVC	IIA	C
Lead Issue		
Lead failure of pace-sense circuit or shock ability	IIA	B
Lead under advisory + evidence of lead compromise	IIB	B
Other		
RV lead causing life-threatening arrhythmias	I	C
Chronic pain due to CIED	IIA	C
Radiation therapy planned in the path of the lead	IIA	C
Severe tricuspid regurgitation due to lead	IIB	C
To facilitate access to MRI	IIB	C

Other

Rarely, the generator or leads can cause significant pain and discomfort due to musculoskeletal issues or possibly occult infections.[30] Chronic pain attributed to the CIED and not amenable to other medical treatment can be an indication for lead extraction.[1] Patients undergoing external beam radiation for cancer therapy have dramatically risen in the last two decades.[33] If the CIED is in the radiation beam's path and could attenuate the therapeutic dose, device and lead extraction can be considered.[1,33]

CLINICAL ASSESSMENT

A thorough assessment of the patient and their device is at the center of lead management and extraction. **Table 2.4** summarizes the general workflow when working up patients for extraction.

Table 2.4 Clinical assessment workflow for CIED extraction

Step	Assessment
History	• Age, gender • Comborbidities: specifically assess for LV function, diabetes, prior sternotomy, and prior stroke • Allergies • Medication list, including anticoagulants • Device and lead history, current settings, pacemaker dependency
Physical Exam	• BMI • Baseline vitals to assess for systemic inflammatory response • Asssesment of hemodynamic status • Wound inspection
Blood Work	• Blood cultures 2 sets for microbial speciation • CBC to assess for anemia and thrombocytopenia • BMP to assess for kidney function, fluid/electrolyte status • Type and screen in preparation for possible blood loss during extraction • ESR
Imaging	• CXR: assess for total number of of leads • TEE: identify vegetations, thrombi, valvular dysfunction • CT: assess binding sites, possible perforation • Other: if difficulty identifying source of infection • PET • WBC Scan

RISK ASSESSMENT

After putting together the clinical assessment, it is vital to understand the various risk factors and their unique impact on each patient. The risks can be globally divided into patient factors and device factors. **Table 2.5** summarizes the various risks and the relative weight of their severity based on retrospective data and expert consensus. It is essential to understand that this is an inexact science, and care must be tailored for each patient.

Patient Factors

The main clinical contributors to increased risk at the time of extraction include: age, female sex, renal dysfunction, left ventricular dysfunction, diabetes mellitus, anemia, thrombocytopenia, prior stroke, prior sternotomy, current CIED infection, and low body mass index.[34–39] While some risk factors may not have been conclusively shown to worsen mortality or complication rates, it is essential to pull all this information together to make a complete plan for the patient. One example of this is patients who have had a prior sternotomy for cardiovascular surgery. While one study showed the lack of complications with prior sternotomy, it is vital to know this information and prepare for arterial and venous access if an emergent cardiopulmonary bypass is needed.[40]

Lead Factors

Lead factors that increase risk include: lead implant duration, type of lead, presence of dual-coil ICD lead, and the number of leads being extracted.[35–37] It logically follows that longer lead dwell time within the blood pool will lead to more time for adhesions, fibrous formation, and potential damage.[1,37,40] A combined age of all the leads greater than ten years can predict procedural complications, and extra precautions should be taken during these cases.[37] The type of lead can also impact extraction, as ICD leads are typically larger and more complex than pacemaker leads. ICD dual coil leads, especially the superior vena cava (SVC) coil, can lead to increased adhesions at the SVC-right atrial junction and lead-to-lead binding.

Extraction risk models weighing the above factors have been created to quantify the risk factors previously described above.[41] While risk modeling is not entirely predictive of outcomes, it can be a useful tool to weigh the patient data alongside the indication and urgency of lead extraction.

Table 2.5 Summary of risk factors for CIED extraction

Risk Factor	Mortality Risk	Complication Risk
Patient profile		
Advanced age > 65	+	+
Low BMI	+	++
Prior sternotomy	+	++
Female gender	++	+++
Renal dysfunction/ESRD	++	+++
Heart failure (> NYHA II or recent admission)	+++	+++
CIED infection	++++	++++
Lead factors		
Dual-coil ICD lead	++	++
Combined lead age > 10 years	++	+++
3 or more leads present	++	++++

The number of '+' signs indicates an estimate of relative risk[34–40]

SHARED-DECISION MAKING AND REFERRALS

Ultimately, the patient is at the core of lead management and decision for extraction. They must be educated on risks, benefits, and alternatives of the extraction procedure and intimately involved in the shared decision-making process. It is also recommended to discuss operator volume, success rates, and complication rates with patients during this process.[1] A referral to an experienced, high-volume extraction center will help facilitate the best patient outcomes.

REFERENCES

1. Kusumoto FM, Schoenfeld MH, Wilkoff BL, et al. 2017 HRS expert consensus statement on cardiovascular implantable electronic device lead management and extraction. *Heart Rhythm.* 2017;14(12):e503–e551.
2. Greenspon AJ, Patel JD, Lau E, et al. Trends in permanent pacemaker implantation in the United States from 1993 to 2009: Increasing complexity of patients and procedures. *J Am Coll Cardiol.* 2012;60(16):1540–1545.
3. Mond HG, Proclemer A. The 11th world survey of cardiac pacing and implantable cardioverter-defibrillators: Calendar year 2009—a World Society of Arrhythmia's project. *Pacing Clin Electrophysiol.* 2011;34(8):1013–1027.
4. Camm J, Nisam S. Implantable cardioverter-defibrillator utilization. *Europace.* 2011;13(3): 448.
5. Joy PS, Kumar G, Poole JE, London B, Olshansky B. Cardiac implantable electronic device infections: Who is at greatest risk? *Heart Rhythm.* 2017;14(6):839–845.
6. Sohail MR, Eby EL, Ryan MP, Gunnarsson C, Wright LA, Greenspon AJ. Incidence, treatment intensity, and incremental annual expenditures for patients experiencing a cardiac implantable electronic device infection: Evidence from a large US payer database 1-year post implantation. *Circ Arrhythm Electrophysiol.* 2016;9(8).
7. Voigt A, Shalaby A, Saba S. Rising rates of cardiac rhythm management device infections in the United States: 1996 through 2003. *J Am Coll Cardiol.* 2006;48(3):590–591.
8. Voigt A, Shalaby A, Saba S. Continued rise in rates of cardiovascular implantable electronic device infections in the United States: Temporal trends and causative insights. *Pacing Clin Electrophysiol.* 2010;33(4):414–419.
9. Cantillon DJ, Exner DV, Badie N, et al. Complications and health care costs associated with transvenous cardiac pacemakers in a nationwide assessment. *JACC Clin Electrophysiol.* 2017;3(11):1296–1305.
10. Baddour LM, Epstein AE, Taubert KA, et al. Update on cardiovascular implantable electronic device infections and their management: A scientific statement from the American Heart Association. *Circulation.* 2010;121:458–477.
11. Sohail MR, Uslan DZ, Khan AH, et al. Management and outcome of permanent pacemaker and implantable cardioverter-defibrillator infections. *J Am Coll Cardiol.* 2007;49(18): 1851–1859.
12. Rodriguez Y, Garisto J, Carrillo RG. Management of cardiac device-related infections: a review of protocol-driven care. *Int J Cardiol.* 2013;166(1): 55–60.
13. Wilkoff BL. How to treat and identify device infections. *Heart Rhythm.* 2007;4(11):1467–1470.
14. Dumont E, Camus C, Victor F, et al. Suspected pacemaker or defibrillator transvenous lead infection. Prospective assessment of a TEE-guided therapeutic strategy. *Eur Heart J.* 2003; 24(19):1779–1787.
15. Juneau D, Golfam M, Hazra S, et al. Positron emission tomography and single-photon emission computed tomography imaging in the diagnosis of cardiac implantable electronic device infection: A systematic review and meta-analysis. *Circ Cardiovasc Imaging.* 2017;10(4).
16. Field ME, Jones SO, Epstein LM. How to select patients for lead extraction. *Heart Rhythm.* 2007;4(7):978–985.
17. Kramer DB, Hatfield LA, McGriff D, et al. Transvenous implantable cardioverter-defibrillator lead reliability: Implications for postmarket surveillance. *J Am Heart Assoc.* 2015;4(6):e001672.

18. Swerdlow CD, Ellenbogen KA. Implantable cardioverter-defibrillator leads: Design, diagnostics, and management. *Circulation.* 2013;128(18):2062–2071.

19. Abu-El-Haija B, Bhave PD, Campbell DN, et al. Venous stenosis after transvenous Lead Placement: A study of outcomes and risk factors in 212 consecutive patients. *J Am Heart Assoc.* 2015;4(8):e001878.

20. Fu HX, Huang XM, Zhong L, et al. Outcome and management of pacemaker-induced superior vena cava syndrome. *Pacing Clin Electrophysiol.* 2014;37(11):1470–1476.

21. Riley RF, Petersen SE, Ferguson JD, Bashir Y. Managing superior vena cava syndrome as a complication of pacemaker implantation: A pooled analysis of clinical practice. *Pacing Clin Electrophysiol.* 2010;33(4):420–425.

22. Khairy P, Landzberg MJ, Gatzoulis MA, et al. Transvenous pacing leads and systemic thromboemboli in patients with intracardiac shunts: A multicenter study. *Circulation.* 2006;113(20):2391–2397.

23. Amelot M, Foucault A, Scanu P, et al. Comparison of outcomes in patients with abandoned versus extracted implantable cardioverter defibrillator leads. *Arch Cardiovasc Dis.* 2011;104(11):572–577.

24. Suga C, Hayes DL, Hyberger LK, Lloyd MA. Is there an adverse outcome from abandoned pacing leads? *J Interv Card Electrophysiol.* 2000;4(3):493–499.

25. Gula LJ, Ames A, Woodburn A, et al. Central venous occlusion is not an obstacle to device upgrade with the assistance of laser extraction. *Pacing Clin Electrophysiol.* 2005;28(7):661–666.

26. Russo RJ, Costa HS, Silva PD, et al. Assessing the risks associated with MRI in patients with a pacemaker or defibrillator. *N Engl J Med.* 2017;376(8):755–764.

27. Kleemann T, Becker T, Doenges K, et al. Annual rate of transvenous defibrillation lead defects in implantable cardioverter-defibrillators over a period of >10 years. *Circulation.* 2007;115(19):2474–2480.

28. Hauser RG, Maisel WH, Friedman PA, et al. Longevity of Sprint Fidelis implantable cardioverter-defibrillator leads and risk factors for failure: Implications for patient management. *Circulation.* 2011;123(4):358–363.

29. Sung RK, Massie BM, Varosy PD, et al. Long-term electrical survival analysis of Riata and Riata ST silicone leads: National Veterans Affairs experience. *Heart Rhythm.* 2012;9(12):1954–1961.

30. Celikyurt U, Agacdiken A, Bozyel S, et al. Assessment of shoulder pain and shoulder disability in patients with implantable cardioverter-defibrillator. *J Interv Card Electrophysiol.* 2013;36(1):91–94.

31. Al-Mohaissen MA, Chan KL. Prevalence and mechanism of tricuspid regurgitation following implantation of endocardial leads for pacemaker or cardioverter-defibrillator. *J Am Soc Echocardiogr.* 2012;25(3):245–252.

32. Lee JC, Epstein LM, Huffer LL, Stevenson WG, Koplan BA, Tedrow UB. ICD lead proarrhythmia cured by lead extraction. *Heart Rhythm.* 2009;6(5):613–618.

33. Grant JD, Jensen GL, Tang C, et al. Radiotherapy-induced malfunction in contemporary cardiovascular implantable electronic devices: Clinical incidence and predictors. *JAMA Oncol.* 2015;1(5):624–632.

34. Tarakji KG, Wazni OM, Harb S, Hsu A, Saliba W, Wilkoff BL. Risk factors for 1-year mortality among patients with cardiac implantable electronic device infection undergoing transvenous lead extraction: The impact of the infection type and the presence of vegetation on survival. *Europace.* 2014;16(10):1490–1495.

35. Agarwal SK, Kamireddy S, Nemec J, Voigt A, Saba S. Predictors of complications of endovascular chronic lead extractions from pacemakers and defibrillators: A single-operator experience. *J Cardiovasc Electrophysiol.* 2009;20(2):171–175.

36. Merchant FM, Levy MR, Kelli HM, et al. Predictors of long-term survival following transvenous extraction of defibrillator leads. *Pacing Clin Electrophysiol.* 2015;38(11):1297–1303.

37. Brunner MP, Cronin EM, Duarte VE, et al. Clinical predictors of adverse patient outcomes in an experience of more than 5000 chronic

endovascular pacemaker and defibrillator lead extractions. *Heart Rhythm*. 2014;11(5):799–805.

38. Polewczyk A, Rinaldi CA, Sohal M, et al. Transvenous lead extraction procedures in women based on ESC-EHRA EORP European Lead Extraction ConTRolled ELECTRa registry: Is female sex a predictor of complications? *Europace*. 2019;21(12):1890–1899.

39. Sood N, Martin DT, Lampert R, Curtis JP, Parzynski C, Clancy J. Incidence and predictors of perioperative complications with transvenous lead extractions: Real-world experience with National Cardiovascular Data Registry. *Circ Arrhythm Electrophysiol*. 2018;11(2): e004768.

40. Tsang DC, Perez AA, Boyle TA, Carrillo RG. Effect of prior sternotomy on outcomes in transvenous lead extraction. *Circ Arrhythm Electrophysiol*. 2019;12(9):e007278.

41. Bontempi L, Vassanelli F, Cerini M, et al. Predicting the difficulty of a transvenous lead extraction procedure: Validation of the LED index. *J Cardiovasc Electrophysiol*. 2017;28(7): 811–818.

3 | Lead Extraction Imaging

Pierce J. Vatterott, MD; Imran S. Syed, MD; Akbar H. Khan, MD

INTRODUCTION

Soon after cardiac implantable electronic devices (CIED) lead implantation, a fibrous growth process is initiated to bind sites along the intravascular lead path and at the distal electrode myocardial interface. Scar formation progresses from a soft to solidified scar and is often calcified.[1,2] Clinical factors can help predict fibrous adherences, but considerable individual patient-to-patient variance exists.[2–4] Removal of CIED leads is more challenging and carries increased risk when significant scar adhesions and/or perforation of vascular and cardiac tissue are present.[3] Removal can result in significant complications such as superior vena cava (SVC) tear, cardiac avulsion, and death.[3,4]

Imaging's role is to define lead extraction tasks and challenges. To assist the lead extraction, imaging helps physicians in planning the procedure and during the procedure. The critical role of imaging is in defining the number of leads, lead path, vascular adhesions, lead-to-lead adherence, cardiac perforations, and specific CIED lead issues.[3,4] Information is gathered from multiple modalities, with each modality either adding its unique findings or confirming other modalities' findings. Both preoperative and procedural imaging are used. **Table 3.1** lists imaging studies that can be utilized preprocedure.

PREPROCEDURAL IMAGING

Preprocedural Chest X-Ray

Posterior-anterior (PA) and lateral chest X-rays (CXRs) are simple and widely available tools that contain a wealth of information.[5,6] An early review of the CXR is essential and can aid in directing other preprocedural imaging. The extractor may also recognize inaccuracies in reported lead information, lead damage, and unusual lead course, among other findings (**Table 3.2**). Information obtained can impact procedural strategies. An example is finding sternal wires, and evidence of prior coronary artery bypass graft (CABG) should direct the CT image reader to define graft locations in case of urgent sternotomy.

Table 3.1 Preprocedural and procedural imaging tests

Preprocedural imaging tests	• CXR • Echocardiogram • CT scan • Subclavian venogram
Procedural imaging tests	• Subclavian venogram • Cine imaging fluoroscopy • SVC angiography • RV angiography • Transthoracic echocardiography • Intracardiac echocardiography

Table 3.2 Checklist for reviewing CXR prior to lead extraction

- Passive, fixed-screw, or extendable/retractable leads
- Unusual lead requiring special extraction technique (i.e., Medtronic LV Starfix lead)
- Any unaccounted-for leads
- Abandoned leads
- Damaged leads
- Prior approach for implantation
    - Bilateral subclavian
    - Tunneled leads
    - Medial access with possible clavicular crush injury
    - Epicardial leads. Is the exit site from the thorax remote from the pocket?
- Unusual lead loop or course
- Pacing or ICD leads
- Single- or dual-ICD coil
- SVC coil location
- Evidence of extruded cables
- Twiddler's syndrome
- Inadequate connector pin seating
- Cardiac perforation

 Cardiotext Publishing. ISBN: 978-1-942909-54-5

The following cases are clinical vignettes that feature examples of information available in the CXR.

Clinical Vignettes

Figure 3.1 shows a CXR of a 60-year-old male referred for extraction and upgrade to a biventricular implantable cardioverter-defibrillator (ICD). He has a history of a dilated cardiomyopathy (ejection fraction [EF] 25%), complete heart block, and permanent atrial fibrillation. In reviewing the CXR, 2 abandoned unipolar, right-sided leads implanted 16 years before are visualized, with the right ventricular (RV) lead severed. The distal end is in the SVC. The atrial lead is an extendable retractable lead, and the RV unipolar lead is passive. A left-sided single pacemaker generator is connected to a bipolar extendable retractable lead (implanted 5 years before) with the tip in the RV apex. The distal portion of the severed lead was successfully removed via a snare placed within a powered sheath. All other leads were removed using standard techniques. Identification of the severed right-sided implanted RV lead allowed preprocedure development of an appropriate extraction strategy.

Figure 3.2 shows another patient with multiple bilateral subclavian-placed leads. A left-sided pacing lead is severed, likely due to a clavicular crush. The distal portion lies within the vasculature, and likely a femoral approach is required to remove this lead (after others have been extracted). In comparison, the preoperative CXR in **Figure 3.3** views a subcutaneous ICD placed with prior abandoned leads for a dual-chamber ICD. Upon closer analysis, the atrial pacing lead is compromised at the clavicle, but the ICD lead fracture is related to the suture sleeve (these were confirmed at the procedure). Once again, a review of the CXR led to appropriate preprocedural planning with our cardiovascular surgeon's involvement to access the lead compromised at the clavicle. We were able to maintain the superior approach, prep leads in a standard fashion, and successfully remove both leads.

The CXRs in **Figure 3.4** are from a frail, pacemaker-dependent, 86-year-old male who presented with a failing ventricular pacing lead and

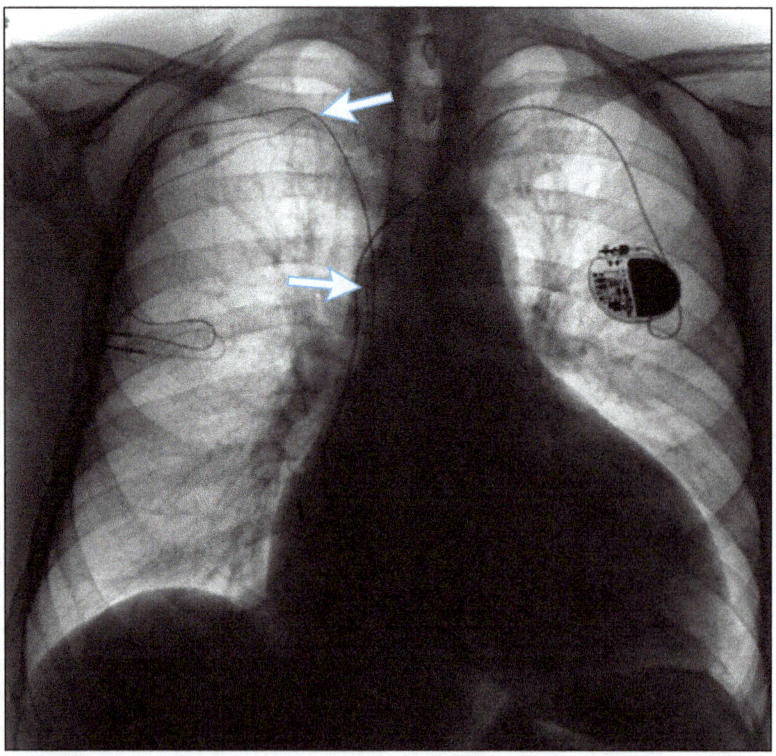

Figure 3.1 PA CXR in a 60-year-old male referred for a device upgrade. Note the right chest abandoned unipolar pacing leads. **Arrows** point out the 2 ends of a severed RV lead.

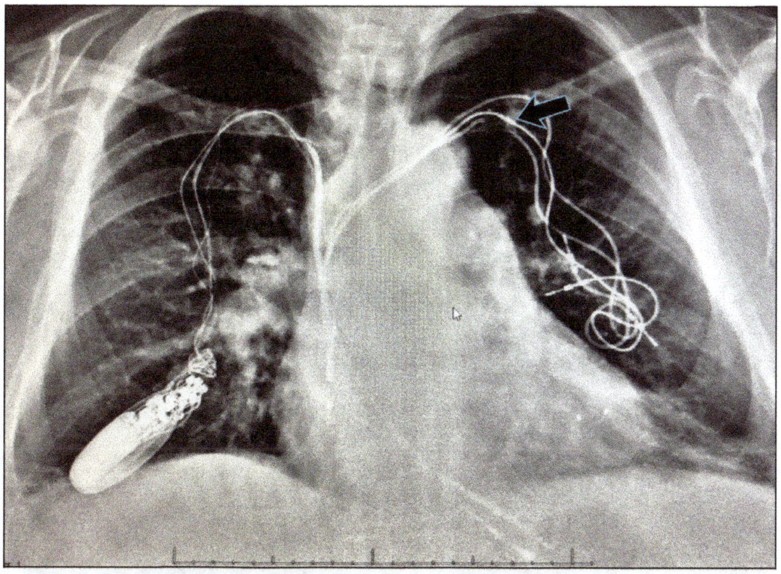

Figure 3.2 PA CXR showing a severed lead (**arrow**), likely due to clavicular crush injury.

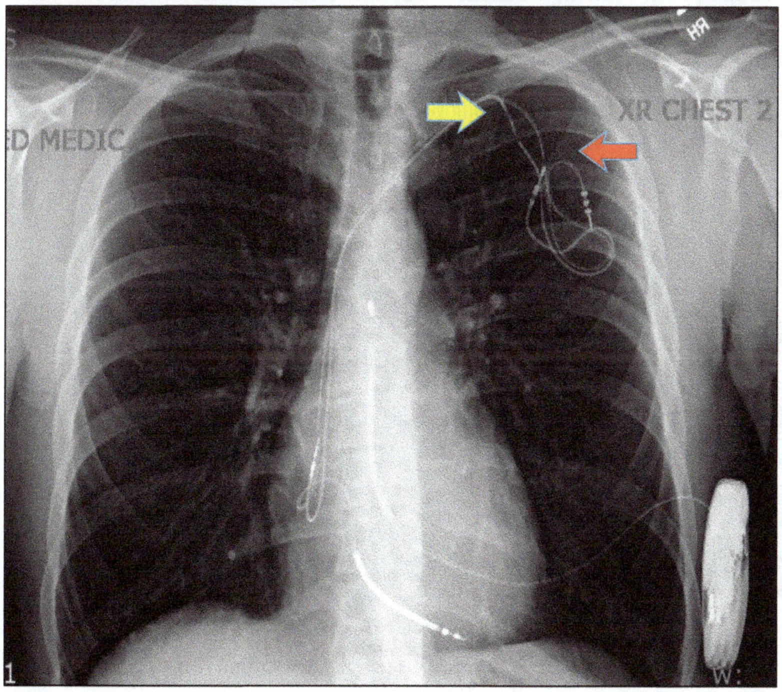

Figure 3.3 PA CXR showing fractures in both a transvenous pacing lead and an ICD lead. The **yellow arrow** points to a clavicular crush injury of the pacing lead and the **red arrow** points to an ICD lead fracture associated with a suture sleeve.

near syncopal spells. He has a history of prior CABG, EF 40%, chronic atrial fibrillation, and Class 3 congestive heart failure symptoms. Device interrogation during left arm movement demonstrated ventricular electrogram noise with pacing inhibition. A previously placed dual-chamber pacemaker system is seen on a PA CXR (Figure 3.4, Panel A). Digital magnification (Figure 3.4, Panel B) highlights a clavicular lead crush as the probable cause of the failing lead. Not only does this define the issue, but it also defines a challenge to lead removal. A tight space between the first rib and clavicle and lead ossification may make it difficult to advance an extraction sheath. The extraction approach would require a powered sheath-cutting tool such as a Philips TightRail Sub C, Cook Shortie, or the use of a Bone Rongeur.

In addition, it is critical to review the lateral CXR prior to extraction. In the same patient, the lateral CXR (Figure 3.4, Panel C) shows that the ventricular lead courses to an atypical posterior location. 2D echocardiography demonstrated the

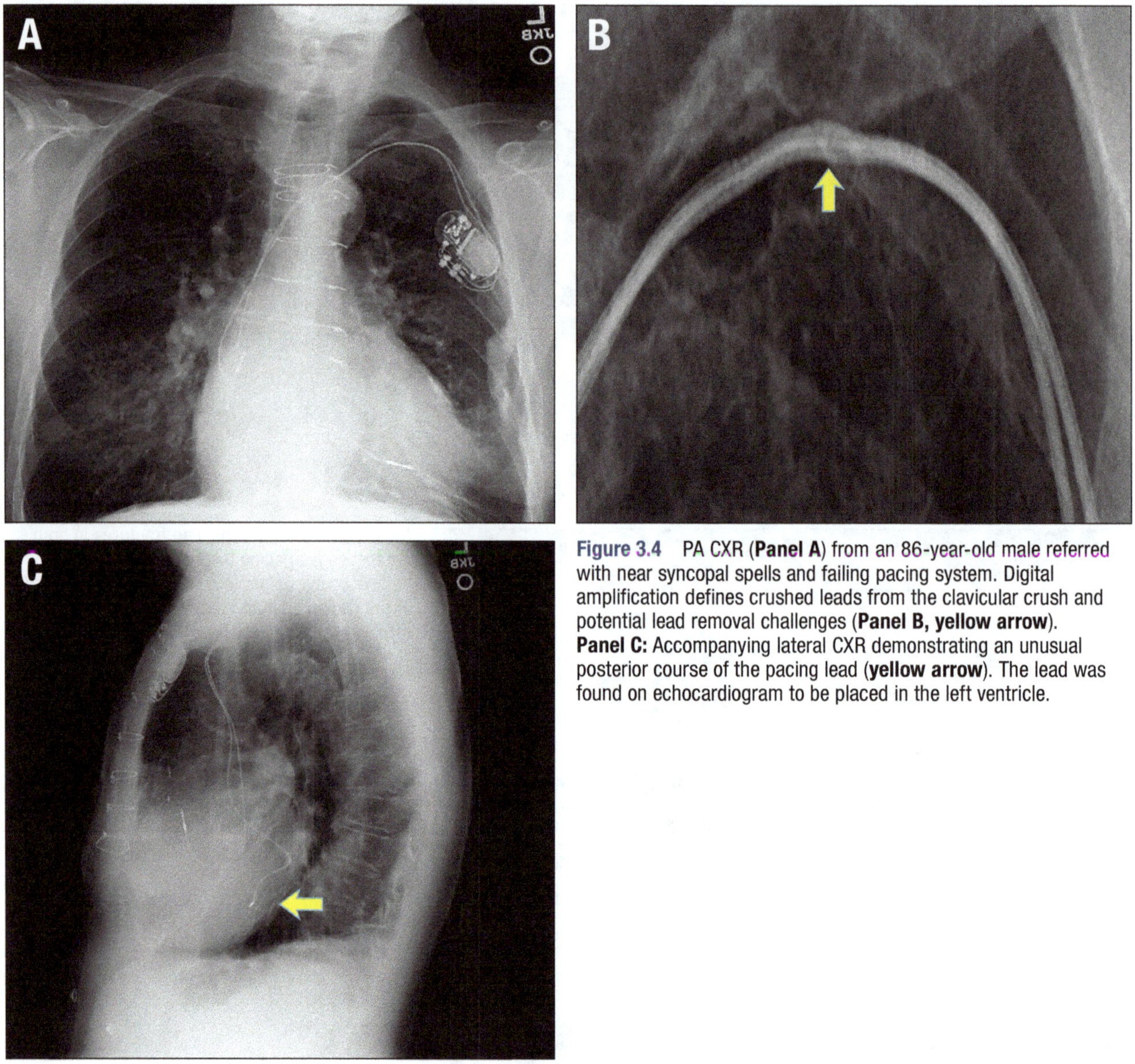

Figure 3.4 PA CXR (**Panel A**) from an 86-year-old male referred with near syncopal spells and failing pacing system. Digital amplification defines crushed leads from the clavicular crush and potential lead removal challenges (**Panel B, yellow arrow**). **Panel C:** Accompanying lateral CXR demonstrating an unusual posterior course of the pacing lead (**yellow arrow**). The lead was found on echocardiogram to be placed in the left ventricle.

lead course through a patent foramen ovale into the left ventricle (LV). No extraction was performed considering his age and overall health. For reference, the postpacing system revision CXR (**Figure 3.5**) delineates appropriately placed new RV and LV leads in comparison. It is noteworthy that extraction of leads inadvertently placed in the LV is possible with cerebral protection devices placed in the bilateral carotids or as an open-heart procedure.

Unusual intravascular CIED lead courses may be seen as in these 2 patients (**Figure 3.6**) with device infection for extraction. In Figure 3.6, Panel A, an LV lead placed 6 years prior dislodged with the lead tip at the right pulmonary artery. Or it may show excessive lead slack (Figure 3.6, Panel B) with redundant lead in the RV outflow tract (RVOT). Once again, preprocedural imaging allowed time to problem solve, use other imaging modalities to study further, and accomplish safe and successful extractions.

An ICD SVC coil increases vascular binding sites. Extraction of these ICD leads is associated with a higher incidence of vascular tears.[7,8] Preprocedure, the physician should note lead course, coil location, and potential vascular binding sites. A

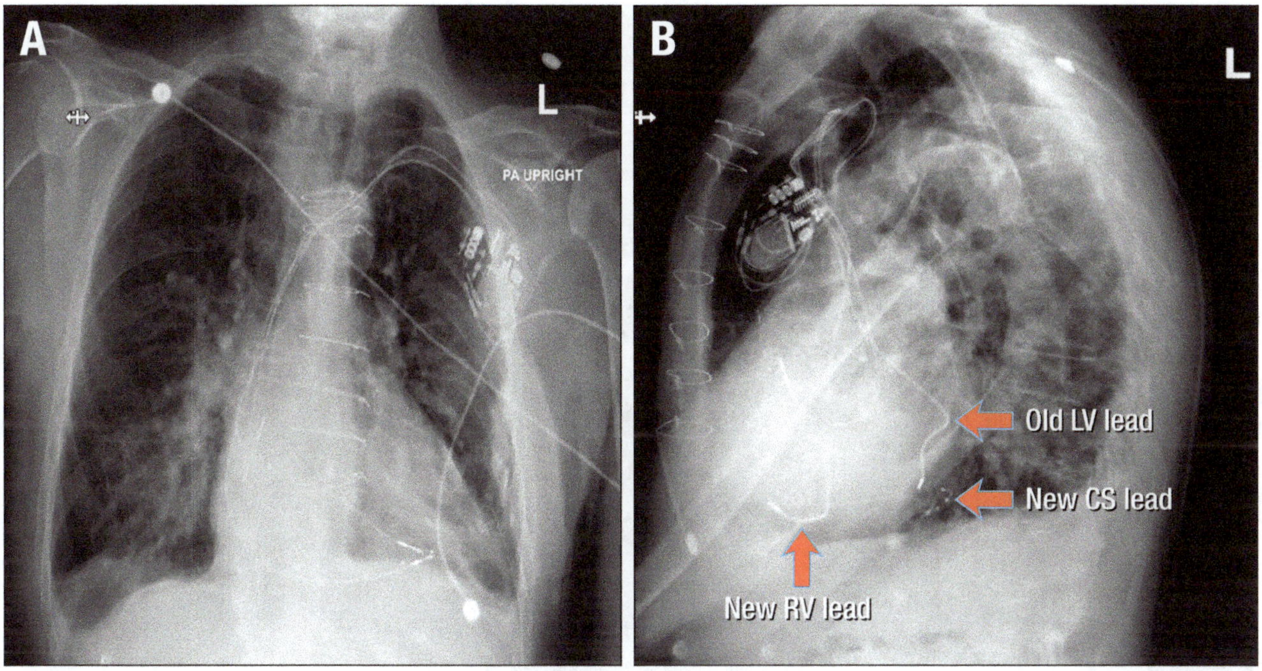

Figure 3.5 PA and lateral CXR after placement of a biventricular pacemaker in the same patient as seen in Figure 3.4. Compare the correctly placed RV and CS leads with the prior placed lead in the LV.

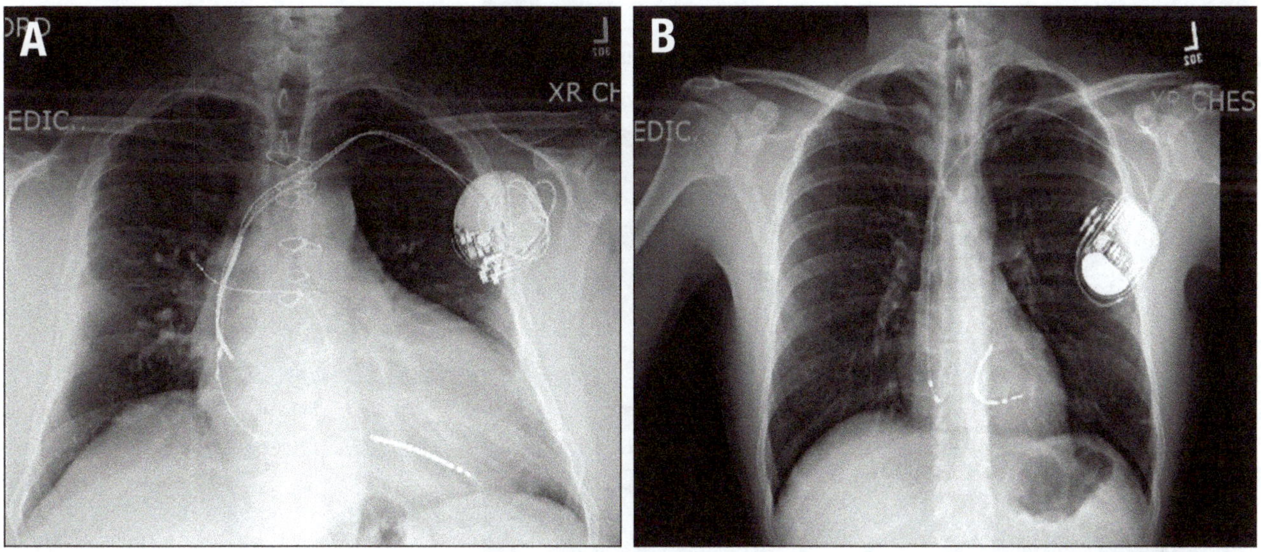

Figure 3.6 Two patients referred for extraction of infected systems. **Panel A** demonstrates an LV lead likely dislodged shortly after implant 6 years prior. The possibility of vascular attachment in the right pulmonary artery should be recognized. In **Panel B**, this ICD lead has been buckled into the RVOT to accommodate an atrial sensing electrode. Pulmonic valve functional regurgitation was corrected with extraction.

review of the lateral CXR (**Figure 3.7**) may demonstrate a course and angulation not noted on the PA film that should be taken into account during the extraction. Lead-to-lead interaction with an SVC coil increases the complexity of extraction with a potential need to stabilize a lead with a femoral snare. **Figure 3.8** is taken from a patient with 2 potentially entangled, nonfunctioning ICD leads. It is easy to imagine multiple potential lead-to-lead binding sites with potential additional vasculature binding sites. During extraction, traction on one lead may affect the other lead and its vascular binding sites. Chest computed tomography (CT) and intracardiac echocardiogram were used for further study and guide a successful extraction of both fractured leads.

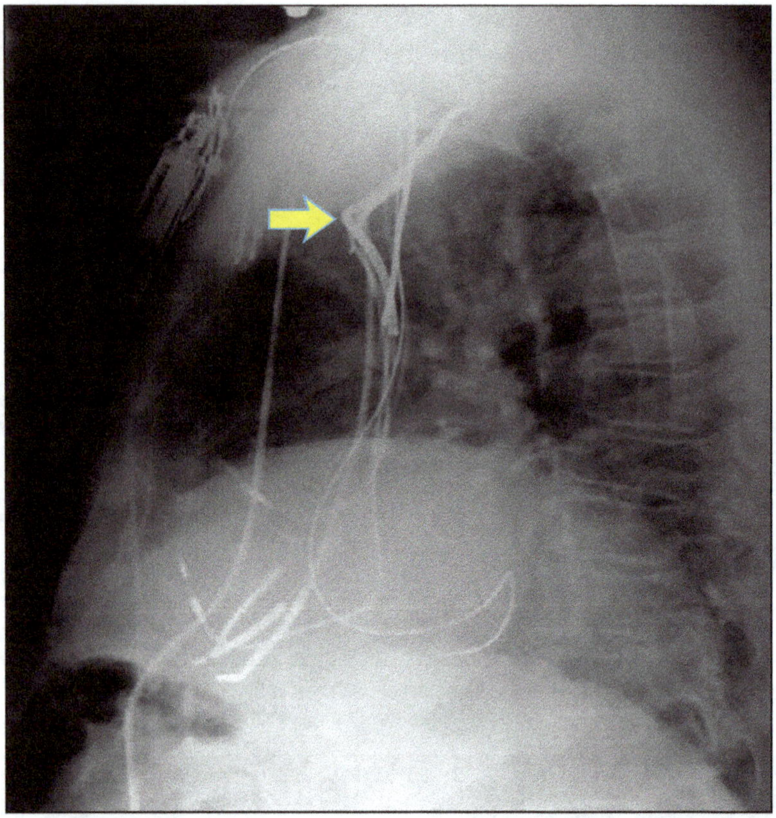

Figure 3.7 Lateral CXR film from a patient with multiple prior ICD lead placements. Note several ICD leads have a steep angulated posterior to the anterior course with possible SVC wall adherence at the point of angulation (**yellow arrow**).

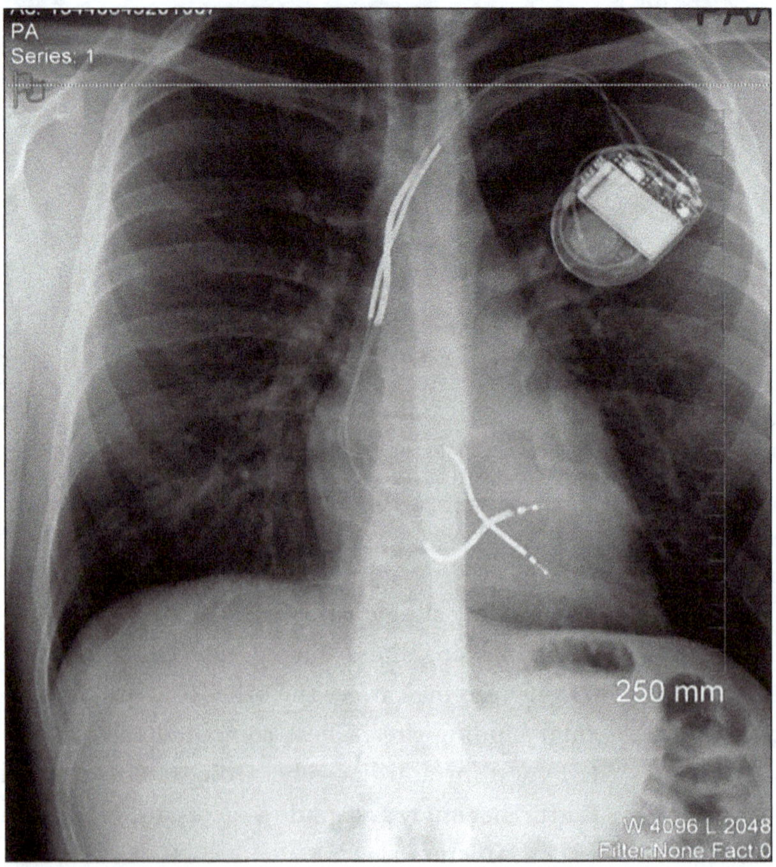

Figure 3.8 PA CXR from a 26-year-old male referred with 2 fractured ICD leads. Note both ICD lead SVC coils and distal leads are intertwined with each other. SVC coils may be adhered to each other and also to the SVC wall.

Cardiac Computed Tomography

Cardiac CT has an emerging role in preprocedural risk assessment before lead extraction. CT allows for noninvasive preprocedural assessment of venous stenosis and occlusion, fibrotic and calcific adhesions of leads to vascular walls, lead position in the cardiac chambers, and cardiac lead perforation. The benefits of obtaining this information need to be weighed against the potential risks of contrast media and radiation exposure associated with CT on an individual basis. However, the potential severity of the complications related to lead extraction means that preprocedural CT scanning's potential benefit often outweigh the risks in many patients.

Certain patient populations (long lead dwell times, female gender, low body mass index, prior stroke, diabetes mellitus, hemodialysis-dependent end-stage renal failure, oral anticoagulation, infection-related indication for lead extraction) are recognized to have increased risk during lead extraction. However, clinical risk factors have varied across studies, and their practical utility in risk assessment is limited. It is not clear whether these clinical factors in themselves cause complications or are, in fact, a surrogate for other variables (e.g., fibrosis) that more directly cause complications. Several anatomic factors have been recognized to contribute to risk during lead extraction. One of the most important is fibrotic lead encapsulation that binds the lead to the vessel wall or myocardium, leading to a risk of vascular tears as an extraction sheath is advanced over these sites. Another important risk factor is chronic lead perforation through the myocardium, which may result in myocardial avulsion. While real-time imaging (fluoroscopy, venography, RV angiography, intravascular and intracardiac ultrasound) can visualize these anatomic factors, the primary advantage of cardiac CT lies to noninvasively provide information about these anatomic factors in advance of a procedure.

Assessment of Venous Stenosis and Occlusion

Contrast-enhanced CT allows for accurate assessment of venous patency (SVC, brachiocephalic, and subclavian veins) and detection of stenosis sites and occlusions (**Figure 3.9**). Studies in

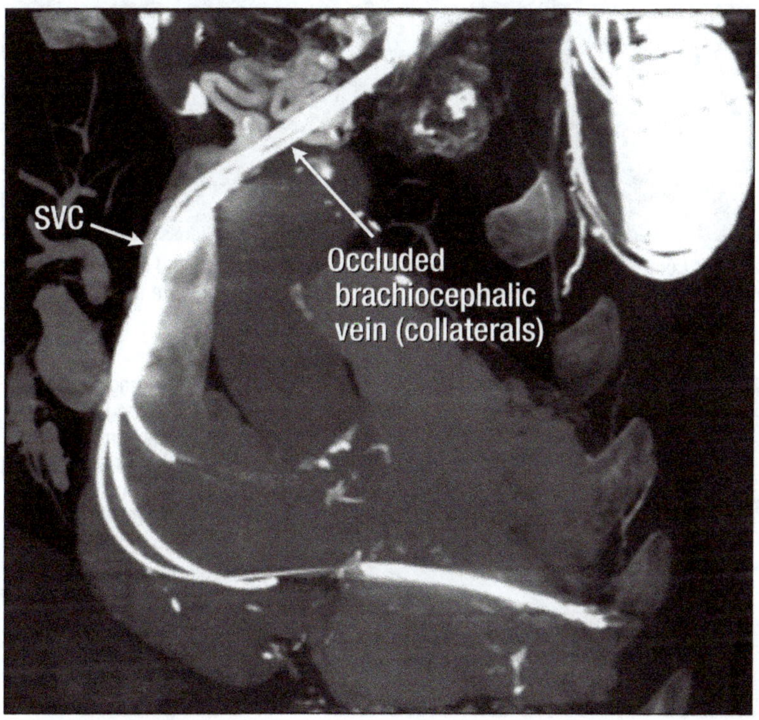

Figure 3.9 CT parasagittal maximal intensity projection demonstrating occlusion of the right brachiocephalic vein with development of collateral venous channels.

patients undergoing lead extraction have demonstrated the incidence of ipsilateral stenosis/occlusion to range between 25% and 44%.[9,10] Several points are worth mentioning regarding a structured CT protocol to detect venous stenosis/occlusion. Contrast administration is necessary—either delayed (venous) phase imaging after administration of contrast or early (arterial) phase imaging with diluted contrast may be performed. Contrast should usually be administered via the ipsilateral arm to detect ipsilateral stenosis/occlusion. In cases where ipsilateral occlusion has already been diagnosed, contrast may be administered via the contralateral arm to detect contralateral venous patency, which may be relevant if a new device is to be reimplanted on that side.

Assessment of Device Lead Position in the Right Atrium and Right Ventricle

Identification of lead tip position in the RV has a bearing on the risk of complications such as perforation. The risk is present with nonseptal insertion and highest with apical insertion where the RV wall is thinnest. Cardiac CT is considered the gold standard for assessing lead position in the geometrically complex RV and is superior to other modalities.[11] Multiple studies have demonstrated that CXR and fluoroscopy are inaccurate in reliably distinguishing septal from nonseptal insertion with only 21%–56% concordance with CT.[11,12] In particular, device leads demonstrated by CT to be on the anterior free wall are often misidentified on CXR and fluoroscopy as having septal insertion. An RV segmentation technique using multiplanar reformatting is recommended for assessment (**Figure 3.10**). A 2-chamber long-axis view of the RV is reconstructed and then further segmented into orthogonal basal, mid, and apical short-axis slices. Abnormal lead locations (e.g., pulmonary artery) or valve interactions (**Figure 3.11**) can be identified. Right atrial (RA) leads and coronary sinus leads can also be reliably identified using a multiplanar technique (**Figure 3.12**).

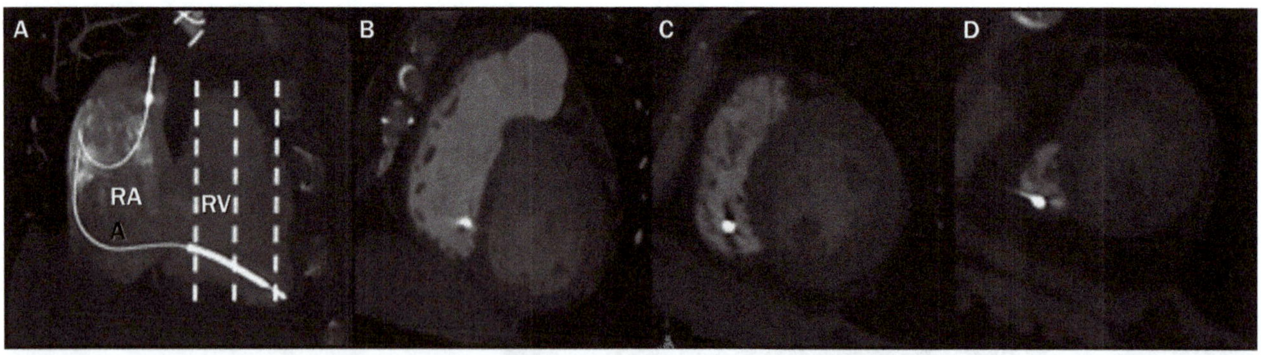

Figure 3.10 CT assessment of RV lead tip position. **Panel A:** Long axis view of the RV is reconstructed. Basal, mid, and apical slices are obtained (**blue lines**). **Panel B:** Basal RV short axis. **Panel C:** Mid RV short axis. **Panel D:** RV lead tip is seen to terminate in the RV apex in the RV apical inferior segment.

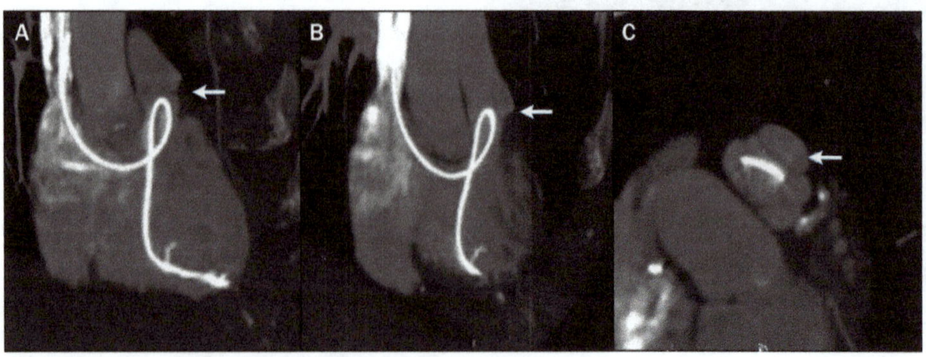

Figure 3.11 CT images of the device lead in the RV. **Panel A:** RVOT view in diastole demonstrating the RV lead looping in the RVOT at the pulmonic valve level. **Panel B:** RVOT view in systolic demonstrating the RV lead prolapsing further across the pulmonic valve. Short-axis view of the pulmonic valve demonstrating a prolapsing RV lead. **Arrows** indicate a pulmonic valve.

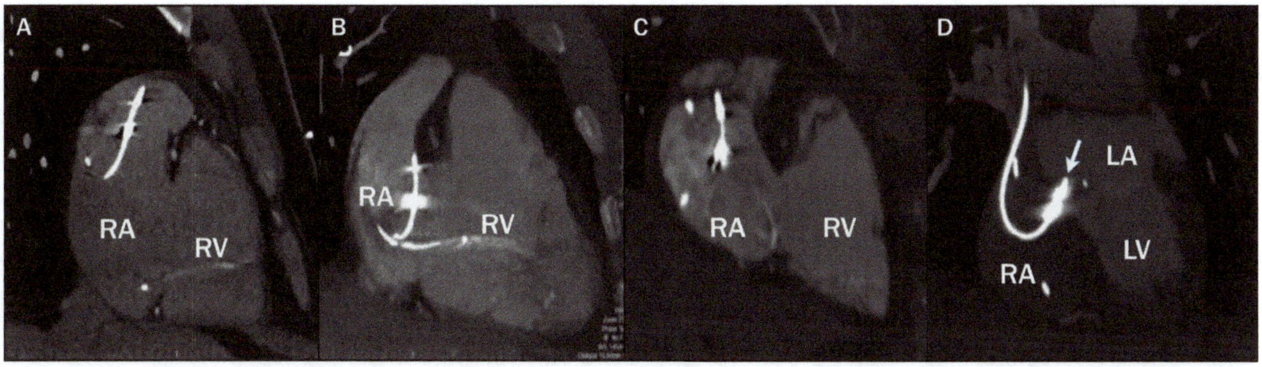

Figure 3.12 CT images from 4 patients demonstrating RA lead tip position assessment. **Panel A:** RA lead tip in a normal location in the right atrial appendage (RAA). **Panel B:** RA lead tip is at the base of the RAA. **Panel C:** RA lead tip is inserted in pectinate muscle in the RAA. **Panel D:** Modified 4-chamber view demonstrating RA lead tip (**arrow**) crossing a patent foramen ovale to reach into the left atrium.

Assessment of Device Lead Perforation in the Right Atrium and Right Ventricle

CT is currently recommended in the Heart Rhythm Society's expert consensus document to identify lead perforation in the heart. Importantly, patients with late lead perforation may be asymptomatic without significant abnormalities in electrophysiologic parameters. Early CT studies used non-ECG gated techniques and noncontrast CT to determine lead perforation and reported relatively high "occult" perforation rates. The primary challenge with identifying lead perforation relates to metal (blooming, beam hardening, and streak artifacts) and motion artifacts. A dedicated lead extraction protocol, as described below, helps to minimize artifacts and produce high-quality diagnostic images. Blended contrast protocols have uniform contrast opacification in the right-sided chambers and improve blood pool–myocardial interface identification.

Recent studies have utilized contrast-enhanced ECG-gated CT and defined significant lead perforation as a lead perforating ≥ 5 mm (due to blooming artifact). In a study by Pang et al., 4% of patients had clinically significant RV lead perforation with leads tips ≥ 5 mm beyond the epicardium, and no patient had RA lead perforation.[13] Eheili et al. used a similar threshold and detected a perforation rate of 5% in the RV and 1% in the RA, which often impacted the removal strategy.[9] Svennberg et al. detected lead perforations ≥ 5 mm in 9% of patients.[10] Some studies have distinguished "radiologic" from "clinical" perforation, with the latter described as perforation with associated pericardial effusion or changes in pacing parameters. High-risk features are evidence of definite RV lead perforation or lead tip in the true RV apex.

The incidence of RA lead perforation is rare in recent CT studies. RA leads are typically positioned in the RAA, trabeculated, and thicker than the RA's remainder. An autopsy study demonstrated active fixation RA leads typically exhibit superficial penetration into the epicardium compared to RV leads.[14] Although RA tenting is sometimes noted and considered by some extractors to be a high-risk feature, many of these leads can be safely removed without complications in clinical practice.[15] Overall, the clinical significance of isolated radiologic perforations without pericardial effusion or changes in pacing parameters remains uncertain. However, the potential risk of myocardial avulsion and cardiac tamponade may impact the decision to extract and the method and techniques chosen for extraction. **Figures 3.13** and **3.14** demonstrate the assessment of RA and RV lead perforation.

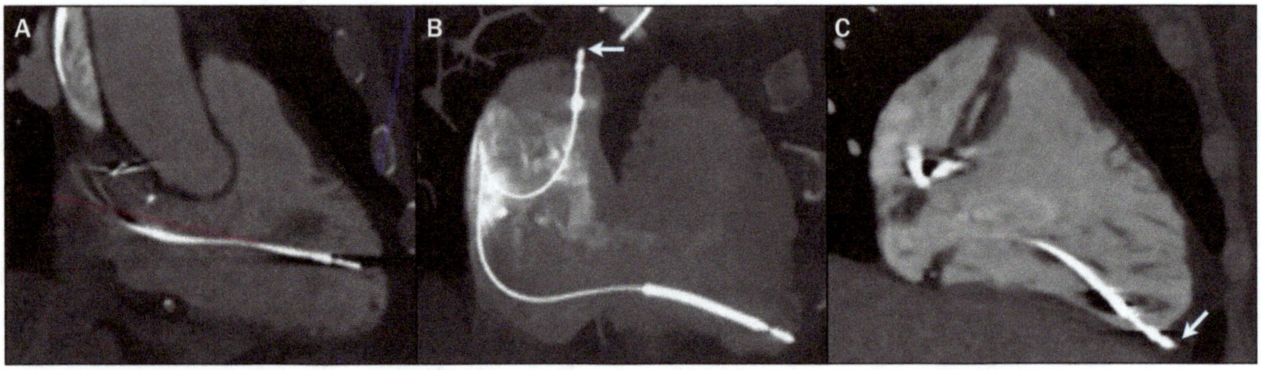

Figure 3.13 Assessment of RA and RV lead tip penetration into the RV myocardium in 3 different patients (RV long-axis view). **Panel A:** Single RV lead tip inserts into RV trabeculation. **Panel B:** Dual lead system with RA lead tip perforating the RA by ≥ 5 mm (**arrow**) and normal RV lead position in the RV apex without evidence of perforation. **Panel C:** RV lead tip (**arrow**) perforates the RV myocardium by ≥ 5 mm without evidence of pericardial effusion.

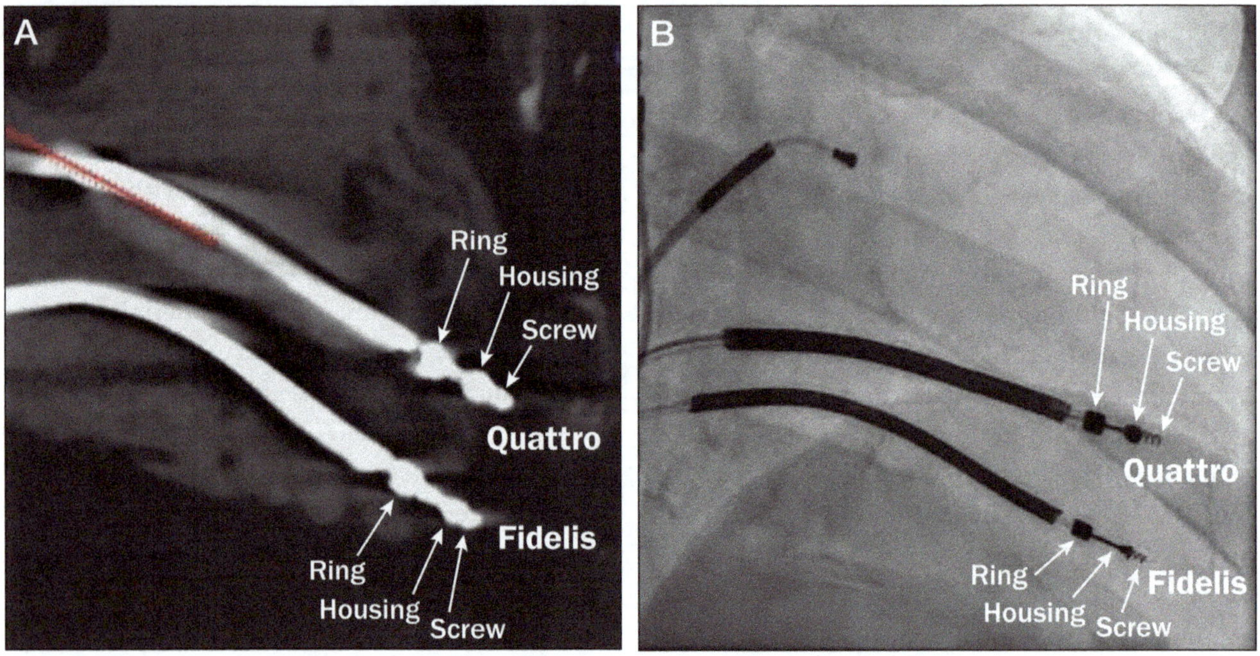

Figure 3.14 High-resolution imaging of device leads can often be obtained with a structured cardiac CT protocol. **Panel A:** Multiplanar reformatted long-axis view of the RV in a patient with Sprint Quattro and Fidelis leads. Device lead components corresponding to the ring, housing, and screw can be identified. The presence of the housing component within the RV cavity rules out significant device lead perforation. **Panel B:** Corresponding image of leads on fluoroscopy.

ASSESSMENT OF LEAD ADHERENCE TO VASCULAR STRUCTURES

After implantation, leads often undergo some degree of fibrotic encapsulation in venous structures by activating different cellular and humoral responses. Fibrotic lead encapsulation, sometimes with associated calcification, results in lead adherence to the venous wall. Sites subject to contact pressure, such as the brachiocephalic veins, the arch into the SVC, and the SVC–RA junction, are most typically involved. CT's potential to preoperatively identify lead adherence areas may enable identifying patients at risk for complex procedures and vascular complications.

In one study of 30 patients, 43% had evidence of possible lead adherence to the SVC (defined as a lead abutting the SVC wall), associated with significantly longer laser times and larger sheath sizes.[16] Two recent studies have further added to our understanding of CT's role in assessing lead adherence. In both of these studies, the presence of a centrally located lead in the lumen or a lead adjacent to the vessel wall ≤ 1 cm were categorized as low-risk findings, a lead adjacent to the vessel wall for > 1 cm was categorized as a moderate risk finding, and a lead completely embedded in the vessel wall outside the vein contour without contact with the contrast-enhanced lumen was categorized as a higher-risk finding representing severe lead adhesion. Patel et al. was limited by noncontrast CT in the majority of patients and demonstrated that a lead outside the vein contour was associated with longer fluoroscopy and procedural times.[16] The study by Svennberg et al., which utilized a structured CT protocol in the majority of patients, showed cases with severe lead adhesion had more complex procedures, as defined by an upgrade in sheath size, combination of laser and mechanical tools, a femoral snare, or prolonged fluoroscopy time > 90th percentile.[10] The absolute risk of major vascular complications was low in both single-center studies and not associated with CT findings. Please see **Figure 3.15** for representative images of none, mild, and significant lead adherence. **Figure 3.16** demonstrates CT, venography, and intracardiac ultrasound images of a patient with significant device lead adherence.

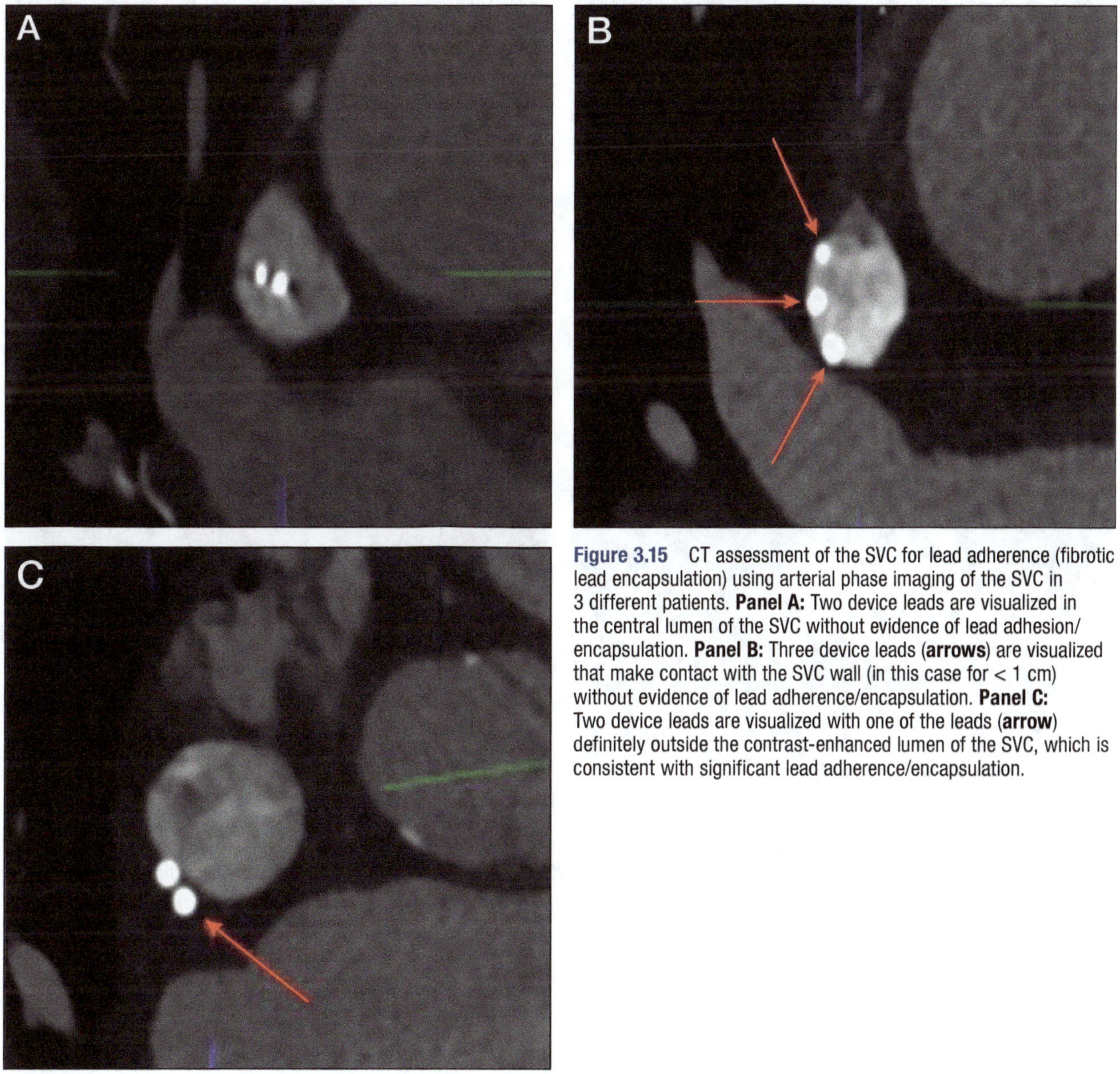

Figure 3.15 CT assessment of the SVC for lead adherence (fibrotic lead encapsulation) using arterial phase imaging of the SVC in 3 different patients. **Panel A:** Two device leads are visualized in the central lumen of the SVC without evidence of lead adhesion/encapsulation. **Panel B:** Three device leads (**arrows**) are visualized that make contact with the SVC wall (in this case for < 1 cm) without evidence of lead adherence/encapsulation. **Panel C:** Two device leads are visualized with one of the leads (**arrow**) definitely outside the contrast-enhanced lumen of the SVC, which is consistent with significant lead adherence/encapsulation.

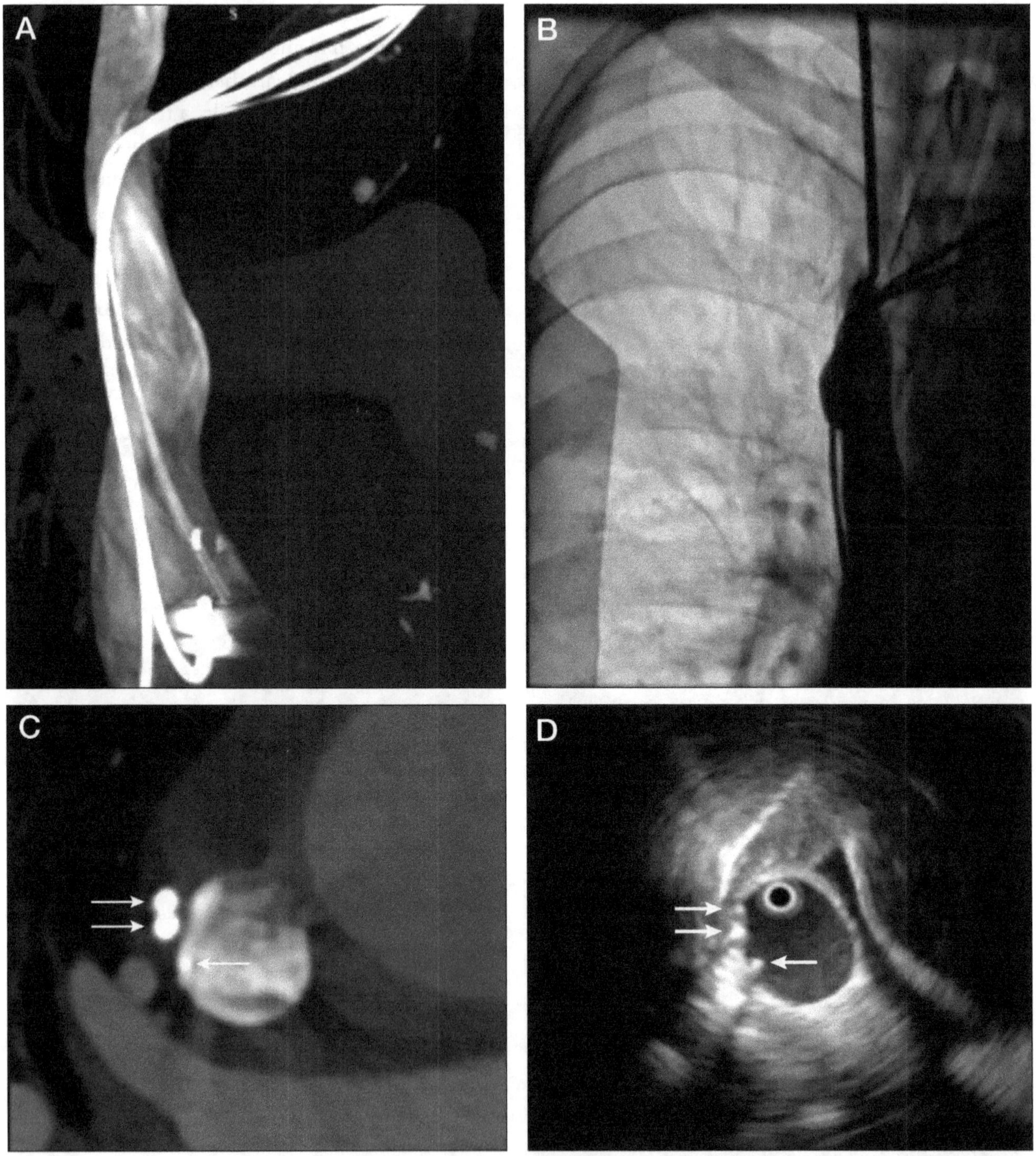

Figure 3.16 Example of vascular adherence of 2 out of 3 device leads at the level of the SVC. **Panel A:** CT venogram long-axis view of SVC with RA and RV leads outside the contrast lumen. The coronary sinus (CS) lead is within the contrast lumen of the SVC. **Panel B:** SVC venography confirms CT findings. **Panel C:** CT short-axis image of the SVC demonstrates significant vascular adherence with RA and RV leads outside the contrast-enhanced lumen of the SVC. The CS lead is within the contrast lumen of the SVC. **Arrows** indicate leads. **Panel D:** Intravascular ultrasound of the SVC confirms CT findings.

At this time, CT's primary role for assessment of lead adherence is preprocedural identification of patients who may have more (or less) complex procedures based on the presence or absence of severe adhesions. This may help estimate procedural difficulty and identify cases requiring specialized tools and/or referral to more experienced operators. Further prospective multicenter studies will be helpful to clarify further the role of CT in predicting vascular complications.

STRUCTURED CARDIAC CT PROTOCOL FOR PREPLANNING PRIOR TO LEAD EXTRACTION

Early CT studies frequently utilized non-ECG gated techniques without contrast and were hindered by significant motion- and metal-related artifacts and the inability to reliably assess vascular adherence and lead perforation due to poor blood pool discrimination from the vascular wall and myocardium. A structured CT protocol is recommended for preplanning purposes. The field of view should encompass the entire thorax from the clavicle to the bottom of the heart to determine the entire lead course. ECG gating, typically with a diastolic acquisition, should be performed to minimize motion and metal artifacts. Contrast should be administered—either a late (venous) phase acquisition with pure contrast or an early (arterial) phase acquisition with blended (diluted) contrast to minimize contrast mixing artifact. Postprocessing techniques with appropriate windowing and "sharp kernels" reduce metal blooming artifact. Metal streak artifacts are typically worst in axial projections and reduced with multiplanar image reformatting. Multiplanar reconstructions are necessary for accurate assessment of lead–vascular adherence and lead perforation.

PREPROCEDURAL ECHOCARDIOGRAPHY

Echocardiography is an established modality that provides a comprehensive structural and functional cardiac assessment. The preprocedural transthoracic echocardiogram (TTE) provides a baseline assessment of cardiac function, valvular pathology, and pericardial disease. It informs us of any tricuspid valve regurgitation (TR), its severity, and the mechanism of the regurgitation. Device leads are increasingly being recognized as a cause of significant TR.[17] The leads may result in impingement of the valve leaflets, entanglement within the chordal apparatus, cause leaflet perforation, or result in malcoaptation related to single or multiple leads.[18,19] (**Video 3.1**, **Figure 3.17**). Device lead-related TR is associated with increased morbidity and mortality.[20] 3D echocardiography is increasingly being utilized to provide information on the spatial relationship between the valvular apparatus and leads and aiding with an assessment of regurgitation severity.[20] Inadvertent damage to the tricuspid valve and resultant significant TR is a known complication of lead extraction.[21] This underscores the importance of an accurate preprocedural assessment of the structure and function of the tricuspid valve.

In cases where device infection is suspected, TTE can provide information regarding the presence or absence of vegetation involving the valves and leads, valvular dysfunction related to the vegetation, and vegetation characteristics such as size and mobility. Historically, when vegetation size has exceeded 1 cm, surgical extraction had been recommended out of concern for septic pulmonary embolization. Recent data, however, have shown that even patients with larger vegetation up to 3 or 4 cm can safely undergo percutaneous lead extraction.[22,23] At our institution and others, patients with a large burden of vegetations undergo AngioVac (AngioDynamics) removal of vegetation as part of the extraction procedure. Although the specificity of TTE for detection of lead and valvular vegetations is high (> 98%), a lower sensitivity (75%) does not allow for confidence in the exclusion of vegetations. Transesophageal echocardiography (TEE), with a greater than 90% sensitivity, is the preferred imaging modality in evaluating endocarditis, especially when TTE images are

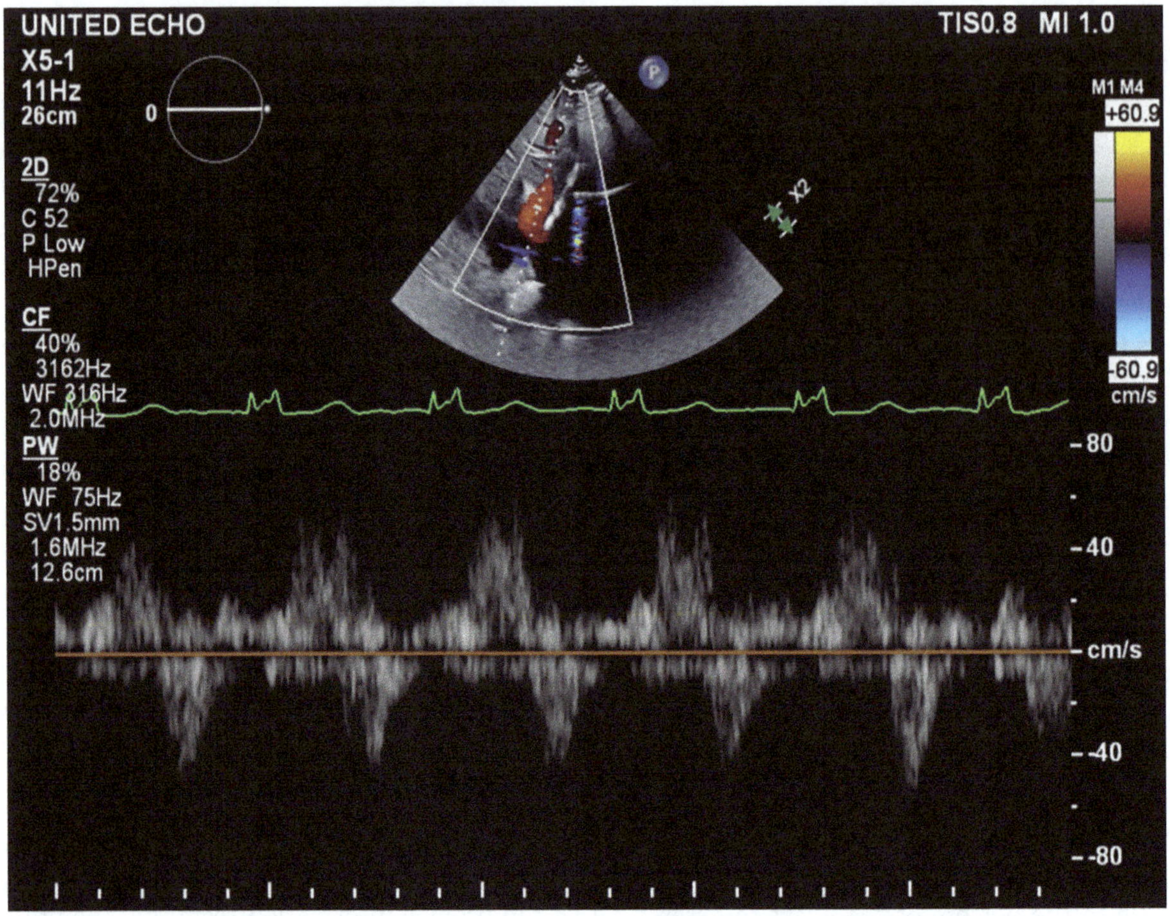

Figure 3.17 Doppler evaluation of the hepatic vein with systolic flow reversal consistent with severe TR.

suboptimal or when the suspicion for endocarditis remains high despite the absence of vegetation on the TTE.[24]

SUBCLAVIAN VENOGRAM

A subclavian venogram can be obtained preprocedure, during the procedure, or sometimes accomplished with the preprocedure CT scan. Partial occlusion with leads outside the contrast lumen illustrates subclavian and innominate vasculature binding sites.[25,26] Total vessel occlusion requires planning for any implantation of new leads after extraction. During the procedure, the extraction sheath can be used after lead removal as a conduit for a long wire to assist with subsequent new lead placement.

INTRAPROCEDURAL IMAGING

Procedural imaging has 3 purposes: (1) Further delineation of any concerns brought up by preprocedural imaging; (2) procedural guidance during extraction, such as actively examining SVC lead adherence during extraction; and (3) early detection of complications such as pericardial effusion.

Subclavian Venogram

The subclavian cine venogram in **Video 3.2** is taken from a patient referred after a failed attempt at manual extraction. Preprocedure PA and lateral CXR raised concerns over a damaged and stretched proximal ICD coil. Here the cine image demonstrates the uncoiling of the ICD SVC coil and its relationship to the subclavian scar. After careful prepping of the damaged lead, a powered sheath freed the lead from its subclavian scar entrapment, and the lead was easily removed.

Video 3.3 and **Video 3.4** are procedural cine subclavian venograms from a dependent patient with 2 failing pacing leads. Video 3.3 is at procedure initiation, and Video 3.4 shows the procedure end and placement of a new pacing system. In Video 3.3, several features are demonstrated. The vessel is patent. Lead discontinuity is seen near the clavicle. The leads are placed proximally, suggesting clavicular crush, and there appears to be bony growth associated with the leads entry into the vessel. Procedural planning incorporated separating bony growth from already damaged pacing leads with the use of a Bone Rongeur. This allowed proper lead prep to preserve lead lumens and a path for a powered extraction sheath to advance over the leads easily. For comparison, Video 3.4 is from the same patient at the procedural end. A more lateral approach first rib approach should protect lead integrity.

Cine Imaging

High-quality fluoroscopic imaging is required for lead extraction procedures.[4] Cine imaging taken at the beginning of the extraction procedure can demonstrate lead-to-lead binding, unusual lead paths, lead tip locations, and calcified scar tissue along the lead. Noting lead-to-lead binding is critical in situations of hoping to retain leads while removing others. In addition, lead integrity issues can be defined, such as fracture, insulation disruption, and ICD cable externalization in compromised Riata and Biotronik leads.[4,27] **Videos 3.5–3.10** compare cine images obtained in AP, RAO, and LAO from 2 separate patients. Videos 3.5–3.7 cine images were obtained from a 63-year-old female with pacing leads placed 16 years earlier. Cine imaging demonstrates how these leads move freely within the cardiovascular system. Little lead-to-lead or vascular adherence was found at extraction. For comparison, Videos 3.8–3.10 cine images were obtained from a 36-year-old female with leads placed 8 years earlier. Considerable, less free lead movement is seen despite normal cardiac function. In the RAO view, classic "railroad tracking" demonstrates lead-to-lead adherence from the subclavian to the distal SVC. A steep LAO cine reveals the distal portion of the ventricular lead adheres to the ventricular septum. This information at procedure initiation set expectations, assisted with tool choices for extraction, and defined challenges. Extraction of the leads placed 16 years prior was accomplished with locking stylets only, while the 8-year-old leads required a long and complex procedure for successful lead removal.

Unusual lead path or loops with possible lead adherence to the inferior vena cava (IVC) or jugular vessels have been seen. **Video 3.11** and **Video 3.12** are taken from a 73-year-old patient with a Medtronic 4193 lead implanted 9 years previously. Preprocedure CXR suggested lead dislodgement with a "funny" loop. A procedural cine taken prior to extraction outlined the lead loop presence in the IVC. Any lead adherence to the IVC puts a patient at risk of IVC tear during an extraction procedure, much as with lead adherence to the SVC.

Significant calcified lead binding sites can be picked up by cine imaging. **Video 3.13** shows a line of calcification along with the pacing leads (red arrow) and a calcified mass bridging the gap between leads at the innominate SVC junction (yellow arrow). These findings foreshadow a challenging extraction procedure to free the implanted pacing leads from a sizeable calcified scar burden. A laser-powered sheath has little effect on a calcified scar, and a cutting tool such as Philips TightRail or Cook Evolution was required.

Echocardiography

The use of TEE during extraction is a routine at many centers. It allows rapid assessment of intraprocedural complications such as pericardial effusion, tamponade, acute valve disruption, pulmonary embolism, and vascular injury.[28,29] TTE is not practical considering the limited imaging windows available during the procedure. Our center uses intracardiac echo (ICE). The most significant benefit of ICE is in delineating sites of lead vascular binding sites and lead-to-lead binding. This information is additive to other imaging modalities such a CT.[30,31] As stated earlier, vascular binding sites are associated with more complex procedures and higher procedural complications.[22,23] At other institutions, phased-array ICE is the dominant modality used during electrophysiological procedures.[30]

Our laboratory has used rotational ICE during extraction for more than 25 years, which provides a high-resolution near-field image. Through a femoral placed deflectable sheath, an ICE catheter is advanced to the innominate/SVC junction. The catheter is then gradually pulled down through the SVC to the RA evaluating potential lead vascular binding sites and lead-to-lead binding (**Figure 3.18**). After SVC scanning, the ICE

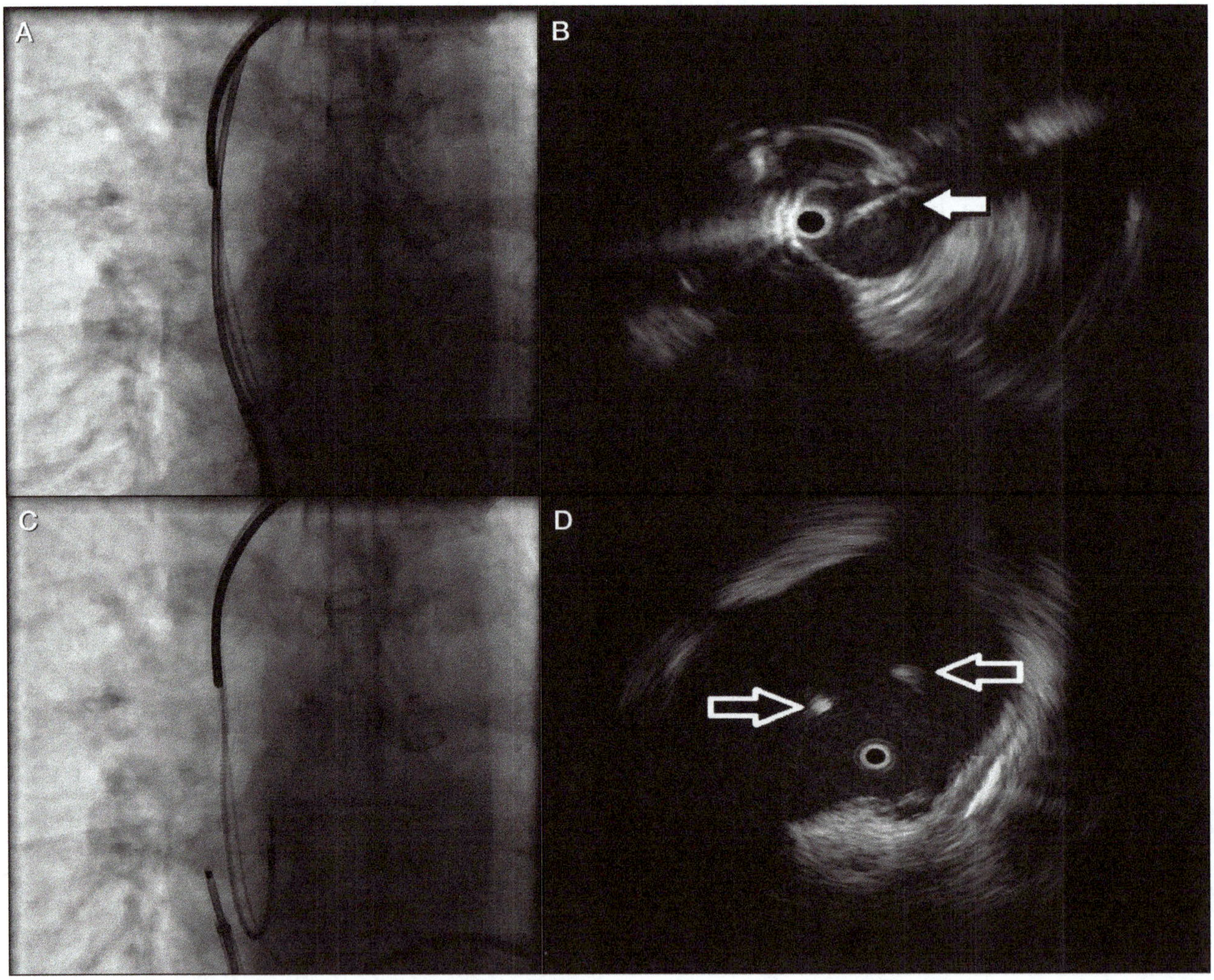

Figure 3.18 Static fluoroscopic and corresponding ICE images illustrating the SVC region surveyed for lead–SVC wall adherence and lead-to-lead binding. This encompasses the SVC innominate junction (**Panel A**) to the mid-RA (**Panel C**). **Arrows** point out leads bound together but not to the vessel wall as they exit the innominate (**Panel B**). Leads are separated and move freely within the RA (**Panel D**). *Note:* Video 3.14 is the corresponding ICE video from the same patient.

catheter is stationed within the RA. From here, the catheter can be used for pericardial space monitoring during the extraction procedure or advanced back to the SVC for observation during lead removal.

The corresponding video, **Video 3.14**, is from the same patient as Figure 3.18, illustrating pacing leads adhered to each other but no SVC binding sites. There is eventual lead separation in the RA. For comparison, **Video 3.15** is a video from a different patient that illustrates pacing leads adhered to the vasculature wall within a scarred mass. For removal, ICE can be used as a procedural guide for the removal of SVC adhered leads. **Figure 3.19** is taken from such a patient. Here an ICE scan of the SVC was used first to document and define the area of lead–SVC wall adherence (**Video 3.16** and **Video 3.17**). The decision was made to remove the lead closest to the lumen center (ICE used to choose this lead; Figure 3.19, Panel A) and monitor the progress. A Philips TightRail cutting tool was chosen. In Figure 3.19, Panel B, the lead is bound to the SVC before extraction. **Video 3.18** shows postextraction. Two pacing leads have been removed, with the remaining scar still visible within the SVC. The former path of the leads is visible.

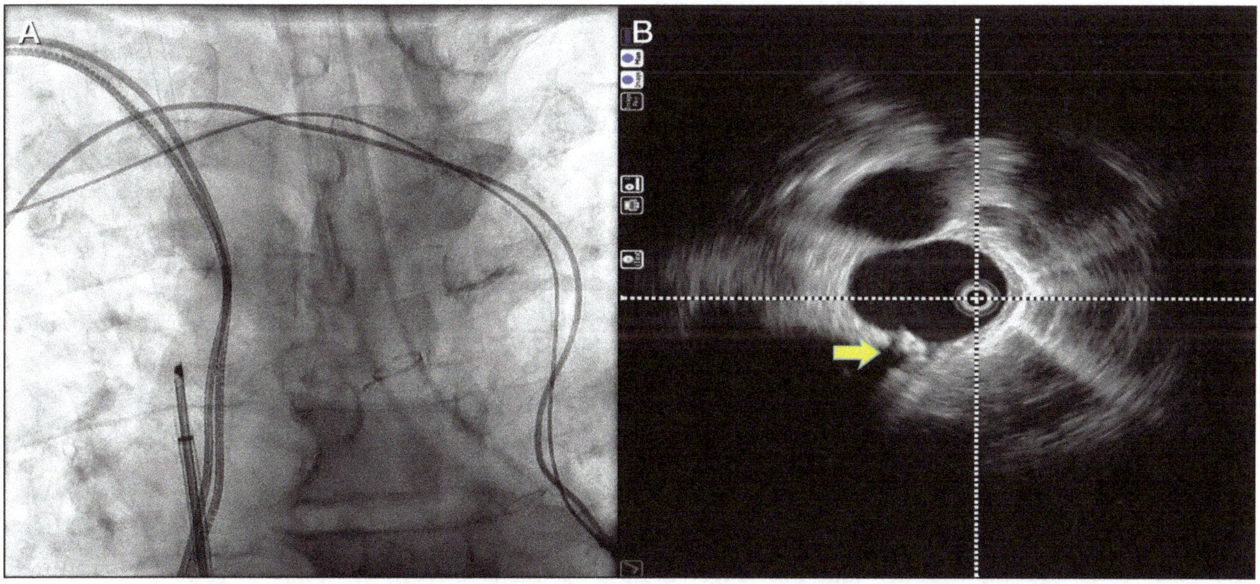

Figure 3.19 Fluoroscopic image (**Panel A**) of the position of ICE catheter for ICE image taken before lead removal and video after (see Videos 3.16–3.18). Prior to lead removal (**Panel B**), leads are incorporated by scar within the SVC wall. Using ICE and fluoroscopy, the lead body closest to the lumen center was chosen first for extraction.

CT and ICE Correlations

ICE can be used to study SVC areas of concern when the preprocedural CT scan illustrates leads outside the SVC contrast lumen. CT scans and ICE typically correlate well in demonstrating lead position within the lumen and possible vascular binding sites in the authors' experience. **Figure 3.20** contains static CT and ICE images, showing a correlation between CT and ICE. However, contrast studies appear to be limited by how contrast flows within the SVC, whereas ICE provides a high-resolution local image. **Figure 3.21** is from a 68-year-old female implanted with an ICD 2 years prior and now referred for lead endocarditis. Here is a comparison of an extraction CT scan to a corresponding ICE video (**Video 3.19**). CT suggests leads outside the contrast lumen.

ICE demonstrated significant vegetations obstructing contrast flow and no lead vascular binding sites. Contrast flow can also be affected by large amounts of scar bound to leads near the SVC wall so that flow is directed away from the wall, suggesting lead adherence to the wall (boundary layer rules). ICE video images (**Video 3.20** and **Video 3.21**) are from 2 individual patients in which the CT scan suggested leads outside the contrast lumen and potentially adhered to the SVC wall. Video 3.20 illustrating leads bound in scar and adhered to the SVC wall. For comparison, Video 3.21 reflects a complex scar binding leads near the SVC wall. On close examination, there was no lead adherence to the SVC wall. It is easy to understand how in a CT contrast study, a scarred mass directs the contrast bolus flow away from the leads and vessel wall. With little contrast near the vessel wall, the study falsely suggests adherence to the vessel wall. The near-field findings of ICE defined the true relationship. In summary, a preprocedural extraction CT scan defines areas of concern with the procedural ICE imaging, further defining those concerns. Such findings illustrate extraction challenges that allow the extraction physician to adjust their approach for a safe and successful procedure.

POSTPROCEDURAL IMAGING

Echocardiography

The postprocedural echocardiogram can be utilized for the assessment of potential procedural complications. TTE can be used to rapidly assess the presence and hemodynamic significance of any pericardial effusion. It allows for repeat evaluations to assess for any interval change in the size and significance of the effusion and aids in the management of the effusion by guiding pericardiocentesis if indicated. New or worsening tricuspid regurgitation (TR) is a known complication of lead extraction. TTE can assess this well. This inadvertent damage to the tricuspid valve is more common with the usage of laser sheaths. Motor force, photochemical destruction, and mechanical damage from the outer sheaths have been described as a possible tricuspid valve injury.[32] Lastly, suppose there is clinical concern for septic embolization of the vegetations with lead extraction. In that case, the postprocedural TTE can help assess the hemodynamic effect by evaluating the RV size and function.

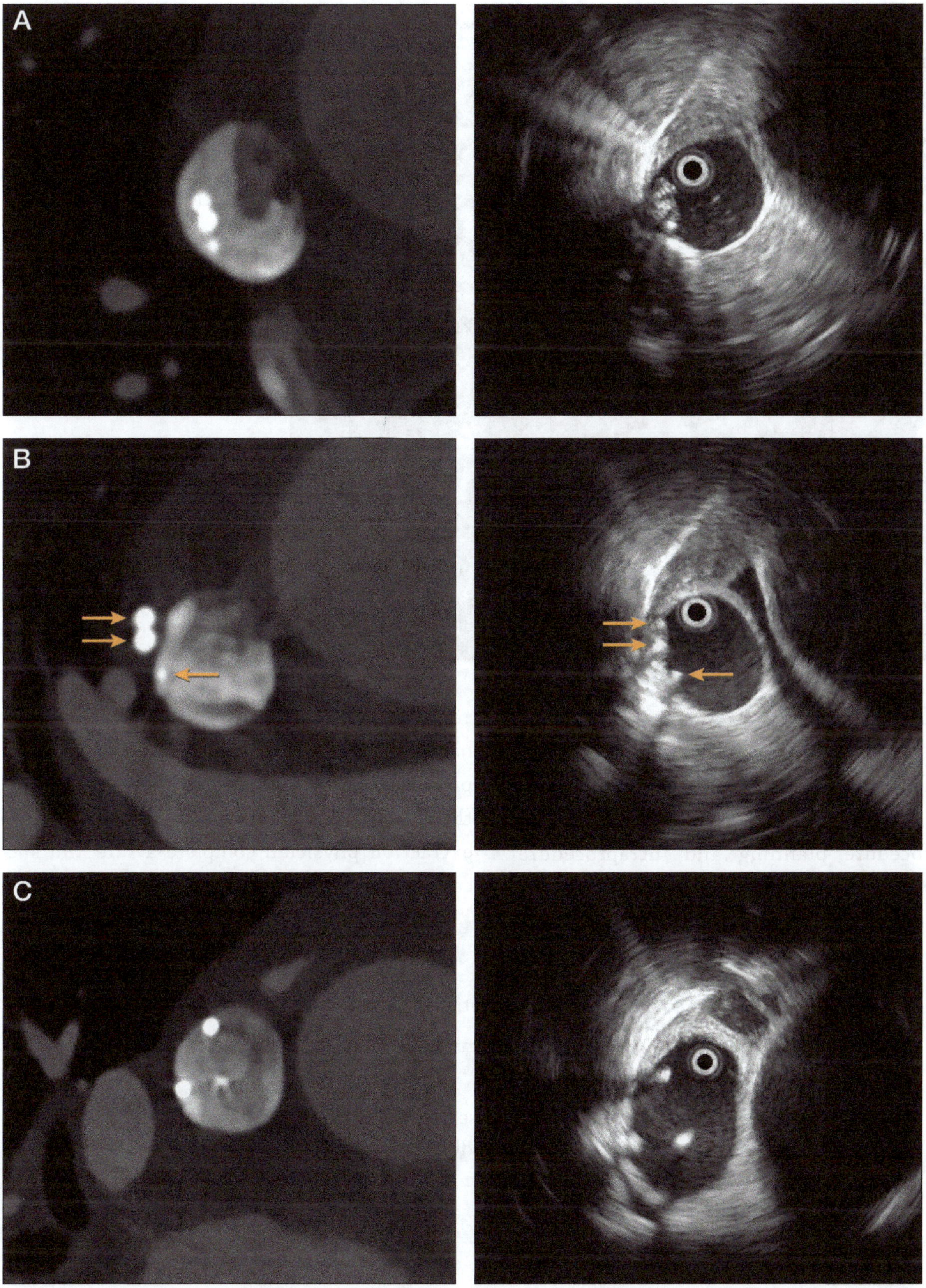

Figure 3.20 Comparison of patient findings on CT scan with ICE image taken from the superior to the inferior scan of the SVC. CT and ICE images were taken at the same level of SVC. In **Panel A**, the leads are entirely within the SVC lumen, **Panel B** two leads are incorporated within the SVC wall and the third in the lumen but associated with the SVC wall, and **Panel C** leads within the lumen, and the third associated with the SVC wall.

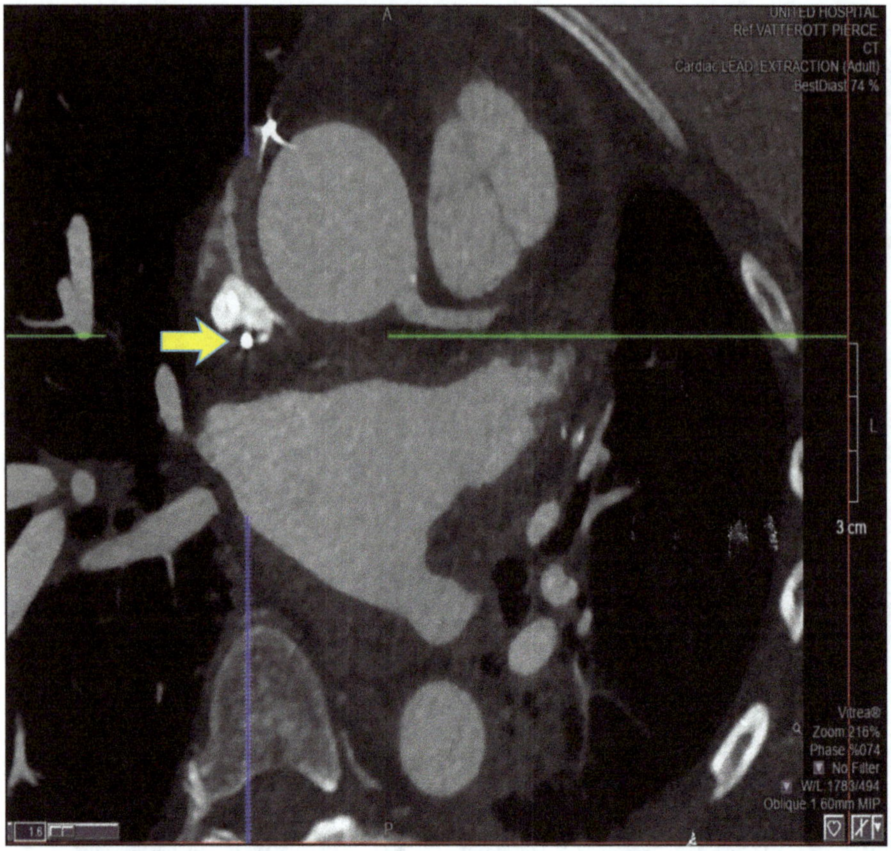

Figure 3.21 CT scan and accompanying ICE image (Video 3.19) taken from a 68-year-old patient with prior ICD system implant 2 years prior. CT scan suggests leads outside contrast lumen whereas ICE scan (Video 3.19) of SVC finds large burden of vegetations (not scar) affecting contrast flow.

CONCLUSION

Imaging is a critical part of the lead extraction process. Multiple imaging modalities can be used to create a wealth of information for both preprocedure planning and intraprocedural procedure adjustments. The extraction physician should understand how each imaging modality can assist them with an extraction procedure. Incorporating the knowledge gained through various imaging modalities helps the extraction physician complete a safe and successful extraction.

SUMMARY POINTS

- Imaging is an integral part of any lead extraction program.
- Preprocedural imaging guides procedural planning by defining challenges, patient risk, and issues needing further evaluation.
- Intraprocedural imaging further defines those potential issues bought up by preprocedural imaging. It defines lead integrity, lead–scar adhesions, lead path, and lead tip adherence. It can be used to guide the extraction procedure actively and provides monitoring for early detection of complications.

REFERENCES

1. Epstein AE, Kay GN, Plumb VJ, et al. Gross and microscopic pathological changes associated with nonthoracotomy implantable defibrillator leads. *Circulation*. 1998;98(15):1517–1524.
2. Segreti L, Di Cori A, Soldati E, et al. Major predictors of fibrous adherences in transvenous implantable cardioverter-defibrillator lead extraction. *Heart Rhythm*. 2014;11(12):2196–2201.
3. Kennergren C, Bjurman C, Wiklund R, et al. A single-center experience of over one thousand lead extractions. *Europace*. 2009;11(5):612–617.
4. Kusumoto FM, Schoenfeld MH, Wilkoff BL, et al. 2017 HRS expert consensus statement on cardiovascular implantable electronic device lead management and extraction. *Heart Rhythm*. 2017;14(12):e503–e551.
5. Burney K, Burchard F, Papouchado M, et al. Cardiac pacing systems and implantable cardiac defibrillators (ICDs): A radiological perspective of equipment, anatomy and complications. *Clin Radiol*. 2004;59(8):699–708.
6. Furman S. Chest PA and lateral. *Pacing Clin Electrophysiol*. 1993;16(5 Pt 1):953.
7. Brunner MP, Cronin EM, Wazni O, et al. Outcomes of patients requiring emergent surgical or endovascular intervention for catastrophic complications during transvenous lead extraction. *Heart Rhythm*. 2014;11(3):419–425.
8. Epstein LM, Love CJ, Wilkoff BL, et al. Superior vena cava defibrillator coils make transvenous lead extraction more challenging and riskier. *J Am Coll Cardiol*. 2013;61(9):987–989.
9. Eheili WL, Boll DT, Marin D, et al. Use of preprocedural MDCT for cardiac implantable electric device lead extraction: Frequency of findings that change management. *Am J Roentgenol*. 2017;208:770–776.
10. Svennberg E, Jacobs K, McVeigh E, et al. Computed tomography-guided risk assessment in percutaneous lead extraction. *J Am Coll Cardiol EP*. 2019;5:1439–1446.
11. Moore P, Coucher J, Ngai S, et al. Imaging and right ventricular pacing lead position: A comparison of CT, MRI, and echocardiography. *Pacing Clin Electrophysiol*. 2016;39(4):382–392.
12. Pang BJ, Joshi SB, Lui EH, et al. Validation of conventional fluoroscopic and ECG criteria for right ventricular pacemaker lead position using cardiac computed tomography. *Pacing Clin Electrophysiol*. 2014;37(4):495–504.
13. Pang BJ, Lui EH, Joshi SB, et al. Pacing and implantable cardioverter defibrillator lead perforation as assessed by multiplanar reformatted ECG-gated cardiac computed tomography and clinical correlates. *Pacing Clin Electrophysiol*. 2014;37:537–545.
14. Dvorak P, Novak M, Kamaryt P, et al. Histological findings around electrodes in pacemaker and implantable cardioverter-debrillator patients: Comparison of steroid-eluting and non-steroid-eluting electrodes. *Europace*. 2012;14: 117–123.
15. Lewis RK, Pokorney SD, Greenfield RA, et al. Preprocedural ECG-gated computed tomography for prevention of complications during lead extraction. *Pacing Clin Electrophysiol*. 2014;37: 1297–1305.
16. Patel D, Sripariwuth A, Abozeed M, et al. Lead location as assessed on cardiac computed tomography and difficulty of percutaneous transvesous extraction. *J Am Coll Cardiol EP*. 2019;5:1432–1438.
17. Lin G, Nishimura RA, Connolly HM, et al. Severe symptomatic tricuspid valve regurgitation due to a permanent pacemaker or implantable cardioverter-defibrillator leads. *J Am Coll Cardiol*. 2005;45(10):1672–1675.
18. Medriatta A, Addetia K, Yamat M, et al. 3D echocardiographic location of implantable device leads and mechanism of associated tricuspid regurgitation. *JACC Cardiovasc Imaging*. 2014;7(4):337–347.
19. Seo Y, Ishizu T, Nakajima H, et al. Clinical utility of 3-dimensional echocardiography in evaluating tricuspid regurgitation caused by pacemaker leads. *Circ J*. 2008;72(9):1465–1470.
20. Hoke U, Auger D, Thijssen J, et al. Significant lead-induced tricuspid regurgitation is associated with poor prognosis at long term follow up. *Heart*. 2014;100(12):960–968.
21. Coffey JO, Sager SJ, Gangireddy S, et al. The impact of transvenous lead extraction on

tricuspid valve function. *Pacing Clin Electophysiol.* 2014;37(1):19–24.

22. Grammes JA, Schulze CM, Al-Bataineh M, et al. Percutaneous pacemaker and implantable cardioverter-defibrillator lead extraction in 100 patients with intracardiac vegetations defined by transesophageal echocardiogram. *J Am Coll Cardiol.* 2010;55(9):886–894.

23. Meier-Ewert HK, Gray ME, John RM. Endocardial pacemaker or defibrillator leads with infected vegetations: A single center experience and consequences of transvenous extraction. *Am Heart J.* 2003;146(2):339–344.

24. De Castro S, Cartoni D, d'Amati G, et al. Diagnostic accuracy of transthoracic and multiplane transesophageal echocardiography for valvular perforation in acute infective endocarditis: Correlation with anatomic findings. *Clin Infect Dis.* 2000;30(5):825–826.

25. Abu-El-Haija B, Bhave PD, Campbell DN, et al. Venous stenosis after transvenous lead placement: A study of outcomes and risk factors in 212 consecutive patients. *J Am Heart Assoc.* 2015;4(8): e001878.

26. Li X, Ze F, Wang L, et al. Prevalence of venous occlusion in patients referred for lead extraction: Implications for tool selection. *Europace.* 2014;16(12):1795–1799.

27. Liu J, Rattan R, Adelstein E, et al. Fluoroscopic screening of asymptomatic patients implanted with the recalled Riata lead family. *Circ Arrhythm Electrophysiol.* 2012;5(4):809–814.

28. Hilberath JN, Burrage PS, Shernan SK, et al. Rescue transoesophageal echocardiography for refractory haemodynamic instability during transvenous lead extraction. *Eur Heart J Cardiovasc Imaging.* 2014;15(8):926–932.

29. Regoli F, Caputo M, Conte G, et al. Clinical utility of routine use of continuous transesophageal echocardiography monitoring during transvenous lead extraction procedure. *Heart Rhythm.* 2015;12(2): 313–320.

30. Sadek MM, Cooper JM, Frankel DS, et al. Utility of intracardiac echocardiography during transvenous lead extraction. *Heart Rhythm.* 2017; 14(12):1779–1785.

31. Yakish SJ, Narula A, Foley R, et al. Superior vena cava echocardiography as a screening tool to predict cardiovascular implantable electronic device lead fibrosis. *J Cardiovasc Ultrasound.* 2015;23(1):27–31.

32. Roeffel S, Bracke F, Meijer A, et al. Tranesophageal evaluation of tricuspid valve regurgitation during pacemaker and implantable cardioverter defibrillator lead extraction. *Pacing Clin Electrophysiol.* 2002;25(11):1583–1586.

VIDEO LEGENDS

Video 3.1 (A) 2D RV inflow with device lead causing impingement of the septal leaflet of the tricuspid valve. (B) Color Doppler interrogation of the RV inflow view showing severe TR. [00:03]

Video 3.2 Cine venogram demonstrating a patent subclavian vein with scar adherence to SVC coil. Prior traction on the ICD lead entrapped within scar resulted in uncoiling of the SVC coil. [00:12]

Video 3.3 Subclavian venograms from procedure initiation. A medial approach for placement resulted in clavicular crush and bony growth along the lead. [00:04]

Video 3.4 Subclavian venograms from procedure end. At extraction a Bone Rongeur used to allow advancement of extraction tool. For comparison, the new system is implanted with the more lateral first rib approach. [00:04]

Video 3.5 AP view Cine images obtained from a 63-year-old female with pacing leads placed 16 years earlier. Imaging demonstrates free lead movement, suggesting little lead-to-lead or vascular adherence. [00:03]

Video 3.6 RAO 30 degree Cine images obtained from a 63-year-old female with pacing leads placed 16 years earlier. Imaging demonstrates free lead movement, suggesting little lead-to-lead or vascular adherence. [00:03]

Video 3.7 LAO 30 degree Cine images obtained from a 63-year-old female with pacing leads placed 16 years earlier. Imaging demonstrates free lead movement, suggesting little lead-to-lead or vascular adherence. [00:02]

Video 3.8 AP view cine images obtained from a 36-year-old female with pacing leads placed 8 years earlier. There is little free lead movement suggestive of a heavy scar burden with lead adherence. [00:03]

Video 3.9 RAO view cine images obtained from a 36-year-old female with pacing leads placed 8 years earlier. There is little free lead movement suggestive of a heavy scar burden with lead adherence. Classic "railroad tracking" is seen in the RAO view demonstrating lead-to-lead adherence from the subclavian to the distal SVC. [00:03]

Video 3.10 LAO view cine images obtained from a 36-year-old female with pacing leads placed 8 years earlier. There is little free lead movement suggestive of a heavy scar burden with lead adherence. LAO cine reveals the distal portion of the ventricular lead adhered to the ventricular septum. [00:03]

Video 3.11 RAO view cine images taken just prior to extraction of a dislodged nonfunctioning LV lead. Note the redundant lead loop extending into the IVC with concerns over possible adherence to the IVC. [00:01]

Video 3.12 LAO view cine images taken just prior to extraction of a dislodged nonfunctioning LV lead. Note the redundant lead loop extending into the IVC with concerns over possible adherence to the IVC. [00:03]

Video 3.13 AP view vine images taken demonstrating calcified scar along pacing leads. The red arrow points out calcium along the lead while the yellow arrow points out a heavy band of calcified scar binding the 2 leads as they exit the innominate into the SVC. These images influence tool selection (please see text). [00:03]

Video 3.14 The corresponding video taken from the patient illustrated in Figure 3.18. This ICE video demonstrates the lack of any lead SVC wall adherence. [00:59]

Video 3.15 In comparison to Video 3.14, this ICE video shows a different patient's pacing leads adhered to the SVC wall within a scar. [02:17]

Video 3.16 Fluoroscopic position of the ICE catheter in the SVC region. [00:02]

Video 3.17 ICE video of pacing leads bound within a scar adhered to SVC wall. Wire for possible use of an SVC balloon seen on ICE video but not included on X-ray image. [00:31]

Video 3.18 After both leads were removed, residual scar is seen within the SVC lumen illustrating prior SVC attachment points and lead path. [00:20]

Video 3.19 ICE scan of SVC finds large burden of vegetations (not scar) affecting contrast flow. [00:15]

Video 3.20 ICE images from a patient that preprocedure contrast CT scan suggested SVC lead adherence. In this patient the SVC ICE images illustrate leads encased in a scar adhered to the SVC wall. [00:06]

Video 3.21 ICE images from a patient that preprocedure contrast CT scan suggested SVC lead adherence. In this patient, leads are encased in scar and adhered to each other but not to the SVC wall. Note the leads move independent of the SVC wall. The scar mass directs the bolus of contrast away from the vessel wall imitating adherence. [00:19]

4 | Extraction Planning and Preparation

Yong-Mei Cha, MD; Siva K. Mulpuru, MD, MPH

RISK STRATIFICATION FOR EXTRACTION

The need to remove cardiac implantable electronic devices (CIEDs) has steadily increased over the years. This outcome is due to an increase in device infections,[1] structural defects in leads, and the need for device upgrades in parallel to a larger aging population in the United States with more significant comorbidities. Despite improvements in extraction techniques and tools, lead extraction continues to be a challenging procedure with the potential for death.[2–4] The 2017 updated HRS consensus statement further addresses the importance of the availability of a cardiac surgeon and team, with access to equipment to perform emergent sternotomy or thoracotomy within 5 to 10 minutes, with a focus on maximizing procedure safety and efficacy, irrespective of the location of the procedure.[5] The logistical approach to lead extraction differs across institutions. Some institutions that provide surgical backup use an operating room or hybrid facility exclusively; others conduct extractions in the device or electrophysiology laboratory. Extraction in the device laboratory affords superior fluoroscopy, immediate access to percutaneous tools and staff experienced in their use, and schedule flexibility. However, cardiac surgical support is generally available less promptly. After a retrospective review[6] of patients who underwent CIED lead removal from January 2001 to October 2012 at Mayo Clinic (Rochester, MN), and based on previous reports on risk factors, we propose a risk stratification scheme (**Table 4.1**) to identify patients at intermediate and high risk for lead extraction as a guide to performing the extraction in the device laboratory versus the operating room. We defined patients as being at intermediate risk for lead extraction if their oldest implanted pacing leads were 1 to 10 years since implant or their oldest intracardiac converter-defibrillator (ICD) leads were 1 to 5 years since implant. Patients classified as high risk were those whose oldest pacing lead was more than 10 years or oldest ICD lead was more than 5 years. The risk of major complications potentially requiring surgical

Table 4.1 Risk stratification scheme for lead extraction

Procedural Risk	Management Plan
Low risk	Pacemaker or ICD lead < 1 year postimplant
Intermediate risk	Pacemaker lead 1–10 years postimplant ICD lead 1–5 years postimplant
High risk	Pacemaker lead > 10 years (≥ 1 lead) ICD lead > 5 years (≥ 1 lead) postimplant *or* Pacemaker lead 1–10 years postimplant or ICD lead 1–5 years postimplant, with: • Congenital heart disease • Initial implant when the patient was age < 15 years (growth into vessel wall) • Hemodialysis • Chest radiograph/CT scan showing calcified superior vena cava (SVC) or myocardium adjacent to lead • Active sepsis • Heart failure, NYHA functional class IV

intervention is estimated as 1.2% for intermediate-risk procedures and 5.3% for high-risk procedures based on the initial retrospective study from our institution. Since 2013, patients are prospectively stratified using this risk scheme, and procedures are performed in the device laboratory with stabilization and rescue strategy for low- and intermediate-risk patients and the operating room for high-risk patients.

EXTRACTION PLAN BASED ON RISK STRATIFICATION SCHEME

Before the procedure, all patients are thoroughly evaluated in the device clinic or by the inpatient service. The evaluation includes a comprehensive clinical and device history, procedural risk stratification, determination of cardiovascular surgical candidacy, and assessment of reimplantation need. For the intermediate-risk group, the procedure is performed in the device laboratory with surgical backup. Detailed planning is listed in **Table 4.2**. This approach involves alerting a cardiovascular surgical team who are physically available at any moment for immediate surgical rescue but not required to be available in the procedure room at the time of the procedure. The designated surgeon is dedicated to responding immediately to performing an emergency surgical procedure for superior vena cava (SVC) tear or myocardial tear. For SVC tear, a balloon occlusion is planned to stabilize the patient before transfer to the operating room. For myocardial tear, pericardiocentesis is planned to stabilize the patient before transfer to the operating room. Suppose the procedure is perceived to be higher risk based on the intraprocedural assessment and difficulty in extracting. In that case, the procedure is abandoned in the device laboratory and performed in the operating room. For the high-risk group, the procedure is undertaken in a hybrid operating room with a surgical team and perfusion services, with a pump primed and immediately available.

Table 4.2 Extraction plan based on risk stratification scheme

Procedural Risk	Management Plan
Low risk Perform extraction in device lab	• Type and screen • Conscious sedation • Intracardiac echocardiography (ICE) or transthoracic echocardiography (TTE) availability
Intermediate risk Perform extraction in device lab	*Before the procedure day* • Charge nurse or lab manager inform the operating room • General surgery consult for wound debridement • Cardiovascular surgery consult if there is specific concern in case of needing surgery • A clinical note needs to be documented if patient is not considered (service, patient, and family) for surgical resuscitation • Notify interventional echo lab if operator prefers intraoperative TEE • Type and crossmatch blood *The procedure day* • Device operator meets patient and address any issues • General anesthesia • Cardiovascular surgeon standby • Blood ready in the procedure room (2 units) • Arterial line • Bilateral femoral vein accesses • Rapid transfusion equipment (Level 1) in room • Cell saver on call • Bridge Occlusion Balloon for SVC occlusion in room, a long wire is ready on the table • Sternotomy/thoracotomy equipment (sternal saw, retractors, etc.) in room • Intraoperative ICE or TEE upon the operator's preference • Place temporary pacemaker (PM-dependent patient)

(continued)

(continued)

Procedure Risk	Management Plan
Intermediate risk *(continued)*	*Myocardial rupture* • Anesthesiology manage hemodynamics and vital support • Cardiovascular surgeon perform emergency sternotomy or thoracotomy to control bleeding • Transfer patient to OR for bypass and surgery *SVC tear* • Anesthesiology manage hemodynamics and vital support • Deploy Bridge Occlusion Balloon for SVC occlusion • SVC stent or transfer patient to OR for bypass and surgery
High risk Perform extraction in the OR	*Before the procedure day* • Charge RN or lab manager inform OR • General surgery consult for wound debridement • Cardiovascular surgery consult if there is specific concern in case of needing surgery or surgical lead removal is highly possible • Procedure will not be performed in the OR if patient is not considered (service, patient, and family) for surgical resuscitation • Type and crossmatch blood *The procedure day* • Device operator meets patient and addresses any issues • General anesthesia • Cardiovascular surgeon standby • Blood ready in the procedure room (2 units) • Arterial line • 1 large left femoral access for transfusion • Rapid transfusion equipment (Level 1) • Bridge Occlusion Balloon for SVC occlusion on the table, a long wire is placed from femoral vein to jugular vein • Bypass perfusion • Intraoperative TEE • Place temporary pacemaker (PM-dependent patient) *Myocardial rupture or SVC tear* • Cardiovascular surgeon perform sternotomy • Cardiovascular surgeon perform repair
Anesthesia preparation	Refer to Chapter 5, *Anesthetic Considerations and Preparation for Lead Extraction*, p. 65.
Sterilization and dripping	Refer to Chapter 6, *Room and Equipment Preparation*, p. 69.
Vascular access setup	Refer to Chapter 6, *Room and Equipment Preparation*, p. 69.

POCKET DISSECTION AND PREPARATION

Although the patient is under general anesthesia, 1% lidocaine 10–20 mL is usually injected at the incisional scar area. The scar (or opened incision in the setting of device infection or erosion) is incised. A cautery pen is used for tissue dissection and to achieve hemostasis in the pulse generator pocket. Often, the leads are looped with significant adhesion below the generator capsule. Careful blunt dissection is required to free the leads without damaging the lead insulation. The cautery pen in cutting mode is recommended for the dissection. The coagulation for hemostasis delivers higher voltages than the cutting. Since the goal is to minimize voltages near the lead, the cut waveform should be used when using electrosurgery near any lead. The lead damage is more significant with the active edge than using the flat orientation. PhotonBlade (Invuity Inc.) is associated with less damage to leads than PlasmaBlade (Medtronic).[7] For an infected CIED pocket, a swab and tissue samples should be sent for culture and antibiotic sensitivity. All sutures on the sleeve should be removed. A standard stylet is placed to the lead tip to retract the lead helix completely under the fluoroscopy. It may require more than 20 counterclockwise turns to achieve a complete retraction. At this point, a gentle pulling of the lead can be applied to remove the lead manually for those leads in a shorter indwelling duration. More often, the first encountered lead adhesion is at the subclavian vein. When the lead adhesion to the vasculature entrance is apparent, the next step is to prepare the lead for extraction. The lead will be cut to remove the connector pin and to inset the locking stylet.

LOCKING STYLET

A locking stylet is critical to transmitting the traction force along the long axis of the lead. Once the locking stylet is in place, the locking mechanism should be activated. Expanding the wire coil binds the locking stylet to the inner conductor coil and transmits the traction force to the lead distal end. The Liberator locking stylet (Cook Medical) and LLD EZ and LLD E (Philips) locking stylets accommodate a wide range of leads with inner lumen diameters from 0.38 mm (inactivated) to 0.58 mm (activated); they are shown in **Figure 4.1**, Panels A and B. The stylet has a highly visible radiopaque marker at the tip under the fluoroscopy. **Table 4.3** lists the available locking stylet features that can be selected for various commercially available leads. For example, LLD EZ locking stylet is for atrial and ventricular pacing or defibrillation leads. LLD E stylet has a length of 85 cm, made for a left ventricular lead. LLD #1 (Philips) stylet has a smaller inner lumen diameter of 0.33 mm, suitable for 5-Fr Fineline lead (Boston Scientific). Liberator Locking Stylet

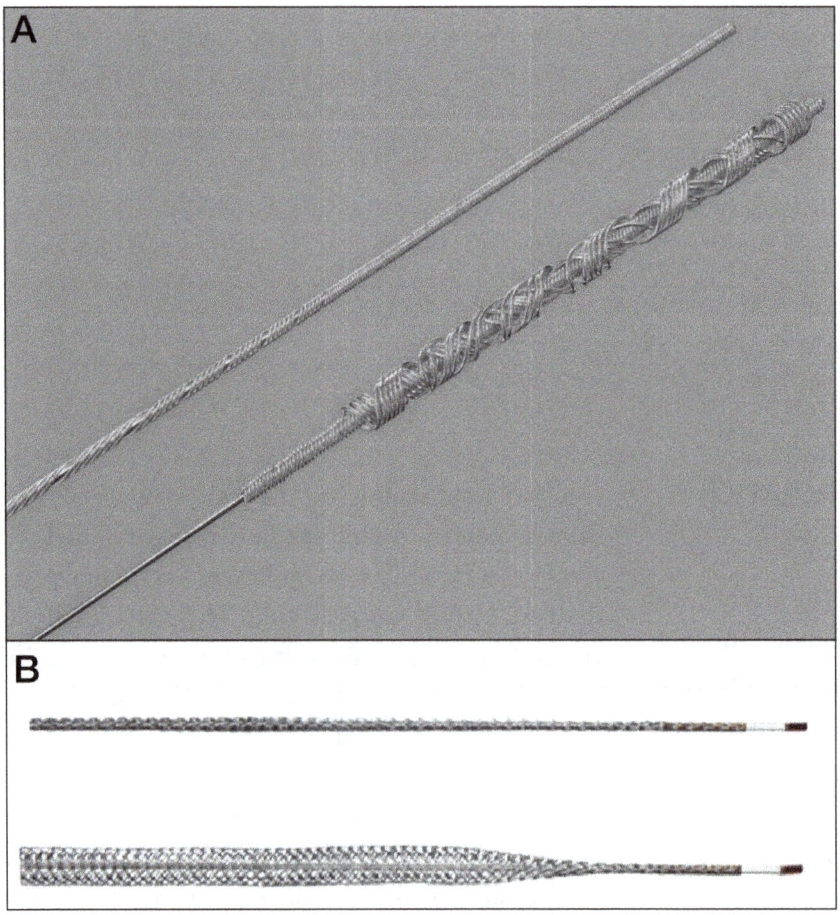

Figure 4.1 Various types of locking stylets. **Panel A:** The Liberator locking stylet (Cook Medical). **Panel B:** The Lead Locking Device (LLD) EZ. (Courtesy of Royal Philips.) In contrast to the Liberator locking stylet, the LLD locking stylet has a braided mesh over the entire length of a solid lead that expands when deployed.

Table 4.3 Locking stylet features and selection

	Philips Medical					Cook Medical
Feature	**LLD EZ**	**LLD**	**LLD #1**	**LLD #2**	**LLD #3**	**Liberator**
Model Number	518-062	518-039	518-018	518-019	518-020	N/A
Locks Along Entire Lead Lumen	Yes	Yes	Yes	Yes	Yes	No; locks only small distal segment
Proven Ability to Unlock and Reposition	Yes	Yes	Yes	Yes	Yes	No
Average Tensile Strength	19 lbs.	19 lbs.	12 lbs.	24 lbs.	45 lbs.	Not published in IFU
Low-Profile Loop Handles	Yes	No	No	No	No	N/A
Locking Range (Diameter)	0.015"/0.38 mm to 0.02"/0.58 mm	0.015"/0.38 mm to 0.023"/0.58 mm	0.01"/0.33 mm to 0.01"/0.41 mm	0.01"/0.43 mm to 0.02"/0.66 mm	0.02"/0.69 mm to 0.03"/0.81 mm	0.01"/0.41 mm to 0.03"/0.81 mm
Working Length	65 cm	85 cm	65 cm	65 cm	65 cm	70 cm
Packaged with Clearing Stylet	Yes – 0.01"/ 0.30-mm diameter	Yes – 0.01"/ 0.30-mm diameter	Yes – 0.01"/ 0.30-mm diameter	Yes – 0.01"/ 0.38-mm diameter	Yes – 0.01"/ 0.38-mm diameter	No
Target Lead	Atrial and ventricular lead	Coronary sinus lead	Fractured lead	Fineline lead		

(Cook Medical; Figure 4.1, **Video 4.1**) has a similar function to transmit traction force to the lead tip during the traction. Unlike the LLD series, in which the entire lead inner coil is locked, the Liberator style locks only the distal lead tip.

LEAD AND LOCKING STYLET COMPRESSOR

The One-Tie Compression Coil (Cook Medical) is used to bind the proximal components of the lead to an engaged locking stylet. **Figure 4.2** shows the middle point of One-Tie (Panel A) crossing the proximal lead cutting end (Panel B) at 45 degrees. The tie is twisted around and compressed on the lead on one end, while the other end is rotated on the locking stylet (Panel C). Then, the plastic handles on the coil ends are released (Panel D). Some operators may tie a securing suture such as Prolene sutures (Johnson & Johnson Medical) or nylon sutures to the lead outer insulation, compressing the insulation and conductance coils together to keep forces uniform on the lead components. For an ICD lead, an additional securing suture applied to the shocking conductance coils is necessary to equalize the pulling force to all internal wires. The uniform traction force helps avoid sleeve bunching or externalizing the wires shown in **Videos 4.2, 4.3,** and **4.4**. Together, the holding sutures, along with the locking stylet, increases the traction force transmission. The lead insulation may break down during the traction, while the locking stylet and the Prolene suture may still hold the lead inner elements for pulling.

LEAD EXTENDER

The Bulldog lead extender (Cook Medical) is commonly used for locking lumenless leads and leads that cannot take a locking stylet due to lead damage. Bulldog extends the lead so it can be pulled into an extraction sheath. After the loop is slipped over the lead or cable conductors' end, the metal sleeve is advanced over the loop to firmly grasp the lead and facilitate removal. **Figure 4.3** illustrates how the Bulldog lead extender works.

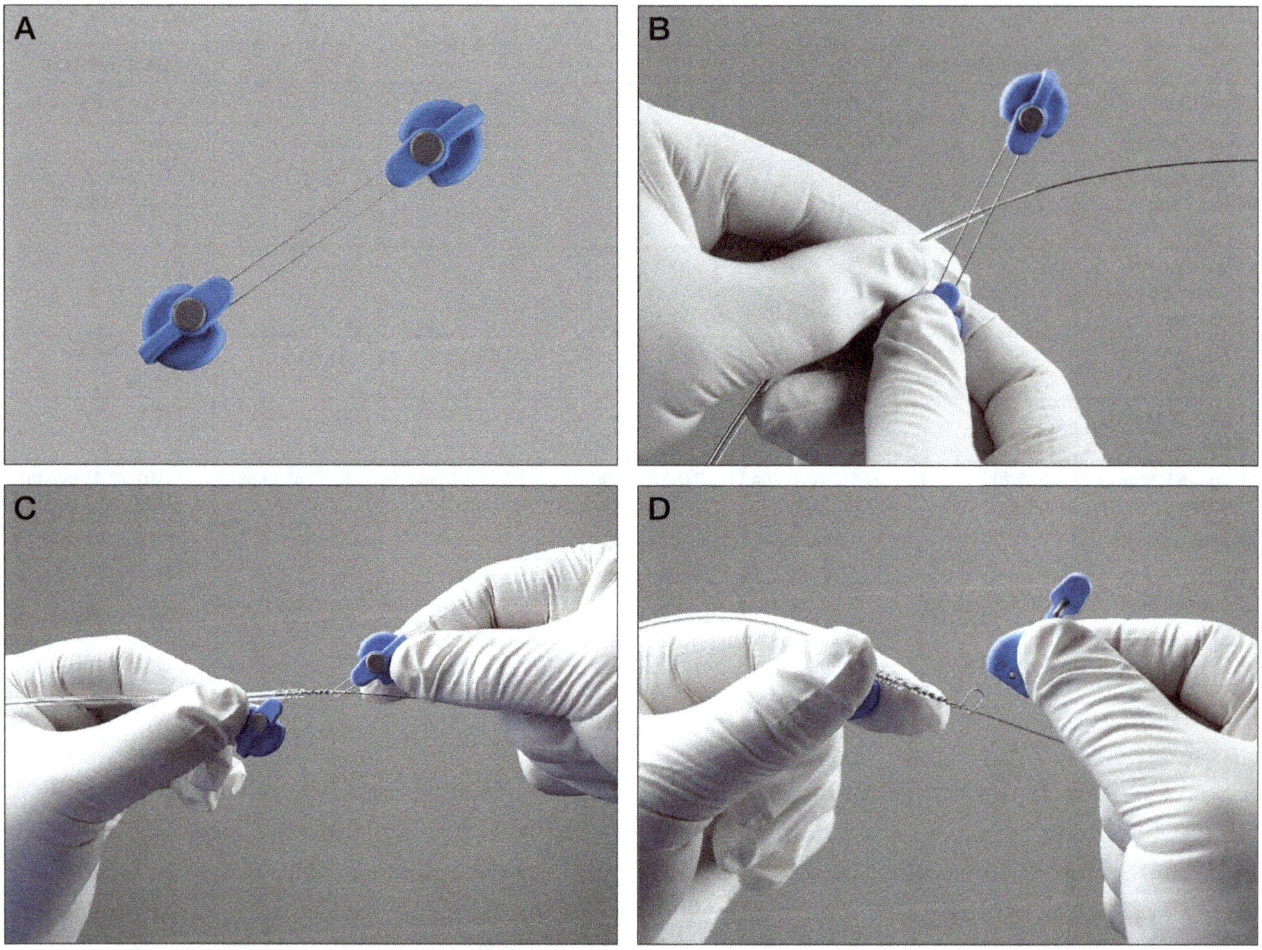

Figure 4.2 The middle point of One-Tie (**Panel A**) crosses to the proximal lead cutting end (**Panel B**) in a 45-degree angle. The tie is twisted around and compressed on the lead on one end, while the other end is rotated on the locking stylet (**Panel C**). Then, the plastic handles on the coil ends are released (**Panel D**).

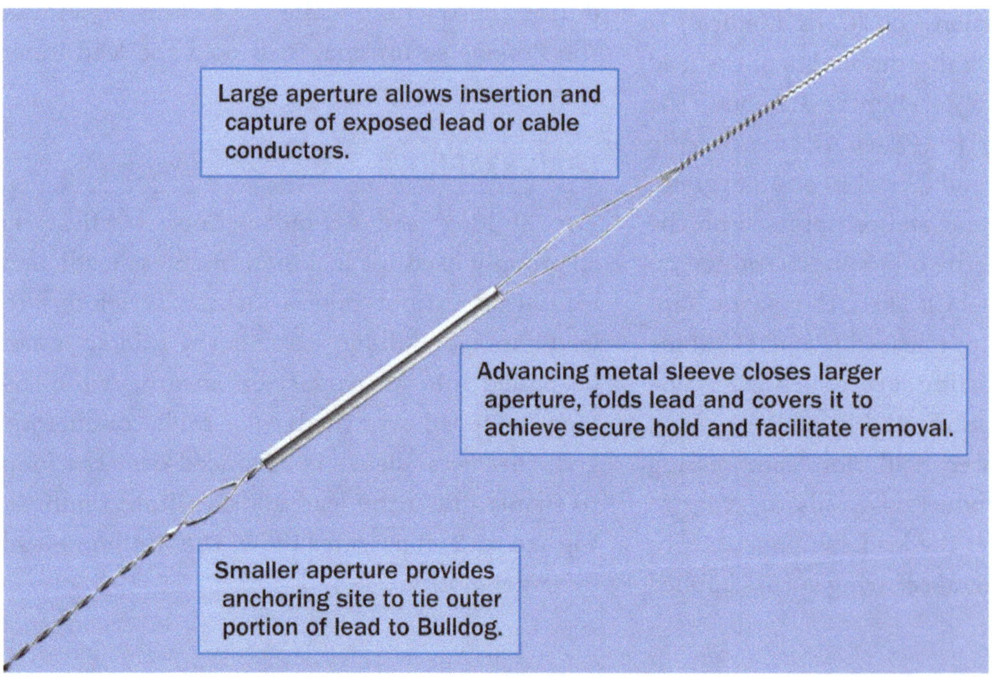

Figure 4.3 The Bulldog lead extender.

POWERED MECHANICAL SHEATHS

Powered sheaths have tips that can cut through fibrous tissue using laser power or mechanical cutting. Extraction using powered sheaths have resulted in a greater success rate and fewer lead breakages. There are a few options on powered mechanical sheaths.

Laser Sheath

The GlideLight laser sheath (Philips Medical) has circumferential fiber-optic cables delivering pulses of wavelength 308 nm in the ultraviolet spectrum for 10 seconds and off for 5 seconds. At 80 Hz, the GlideLight laser sheath requires up to 55% less advancement force and advances up to 62% more efficiently through challenging binding sites than the SLS II laser sheath (40 Hz). Vaporization of water leads to photoablation of fibrous adhesions with tissue penetration of 50 μm (▶ **Video 4.5**). The sheath needs to be calibrated before use to assess its proper function. All staff in the room and the patient should wear protective glasses to shield their eyes from laser light. The circumferential nature of the energy delivery allows separating the binding fibrosis around the lead. While advancing a sheath, the traction maintains the sheath in a coaxial alignment over the lead and separating the lead from the fibrotic adhesions. A misalignment could radiate the photo light through the vascular wall, leading to a vascular tear. An available outer sheath can be used to support the laser sheath advancement or serving for countertraction (▶ **Video 4.6**). Caution must be undertaken (▶ **Video 4.7**) when the laser sheath turns the corner from the innominate vein to the SVC (using lower force, pulling the lead from below to let the lead off the SVC lateral wall). The SVC rupture is the most common location of the vascular tear. A laser sheath may not be considered the first option or used with great caution in the SVC location.[4] When multiple leads are present, it is imperative to realize the lead-to-lead adhesions or binding sites. Alternating laser application to different leads may help break up the binding sites (▶ **Video 4.8**). The use of laser energy should be ceased approximately 1 cm from the endocardial surface to prevent perforation. When there is "snowplowing" from a large amount of fibrotic tissue accumulated at the tip of the laser sheath, the outer sheath helps go over the tissue debris towards the lead tip for countertraction.

The GlideLight laser sheath comes in three different sizes; 12-Fr, 14-Fr, or 16-Fr outer diameters. Each sheath permits the removal of lead with a maximum outer diameter of 7.5 Fr, 9.5 Fr, and 11.5 Fr, correspondingly. The 12-Fr laser sheath has an inner diameter of 8.4 Fr (2.8 mm) and an outer diameter of 12.4 Fr (4.1 mm). **Figure 4.4** shows a comparison of laser sheaths, TightRail sheaths, and Evolution extraction sheath diameters.

The PLEXES study showed a laser sheath had a greater success rate of complete lead removal (94% vs. 64%) and shorter extraction time than a mechanical sheath.[2] The large cohort study on laser sheath extraction demonstrated a complete lead removal rate of 90%.[8]

TightRail Mechanical Rotating Dilator Sheath

TightRail Mechanical rotating dilator sheath has a flexible shaft to keep the sheath coaxial to the lead (**Figure 4.5**). The dilating blade is shielded within the sheath's tip until it is activated by the operator's hand squeezing the handle. The sheath has a bidirectional rotating mechanism designed to dilate fibrotic lesions by rotating 574 degrees (287 degrees clockwise from 0 and 287 degrees counterclockwise from 0), while the blade extends just 0.5 mm by each trigger. However, caution should be undertaken when the sheath is in an angulation, such as advancing from the right innominate vein to SVC or from the venipuncture entrance to the subclavian vein (lack of linear alignment between the vessel and the sheath). The lead can be transected, shown in **Figure 4.6**. As the blade edge is

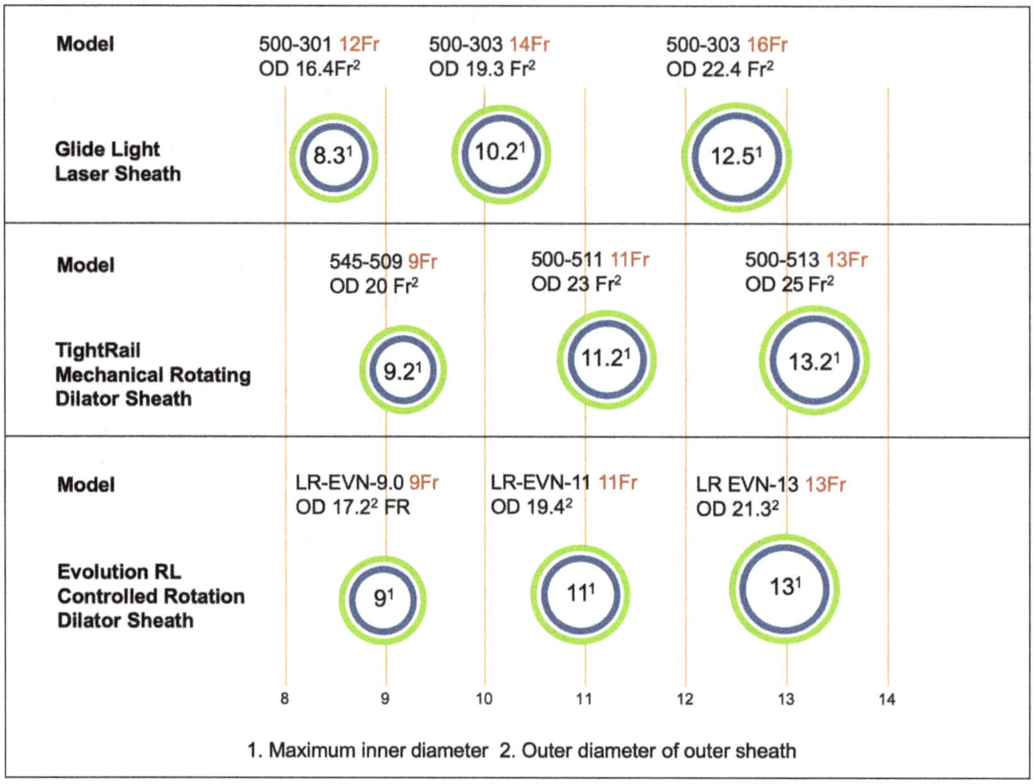

Figure 4.4 The inner diameter reference available for GlideLight laser sheath, TightRail mechanical rotating dilator sheath, and Evolution RL controlled-rotation dilator sheath.

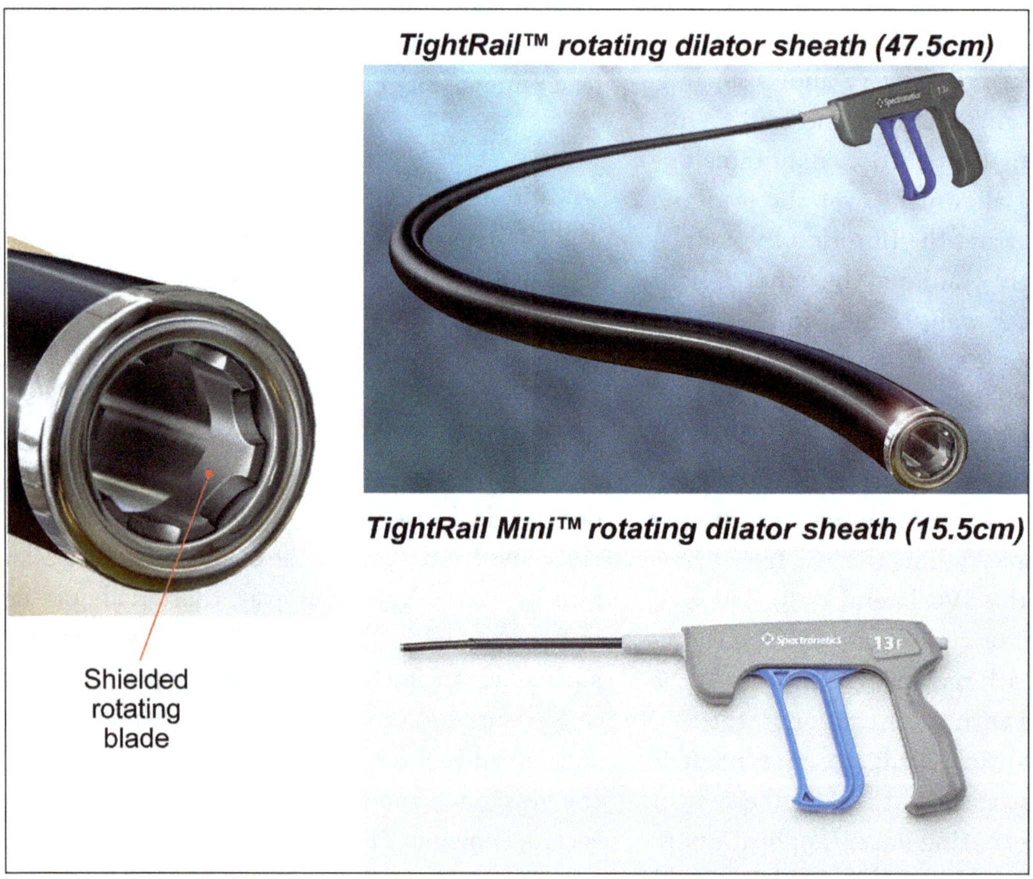

Figure 4.5 The TightRail rotating dilator sheath. The rotating blade is shielded inside the tip of the sheath to minimize damage to the nearby leads or vasculature. TightRail Mini sheath is designed for use in the axillary subclavian region. (Courtesy of Royal Philips.)

shielded, it allows countertraction at the distal tip of the targeted lead. The outer shaft does not rotate with the blade and has a function of support and countertraction. The outer sheath is optional, based on the operator's preference.

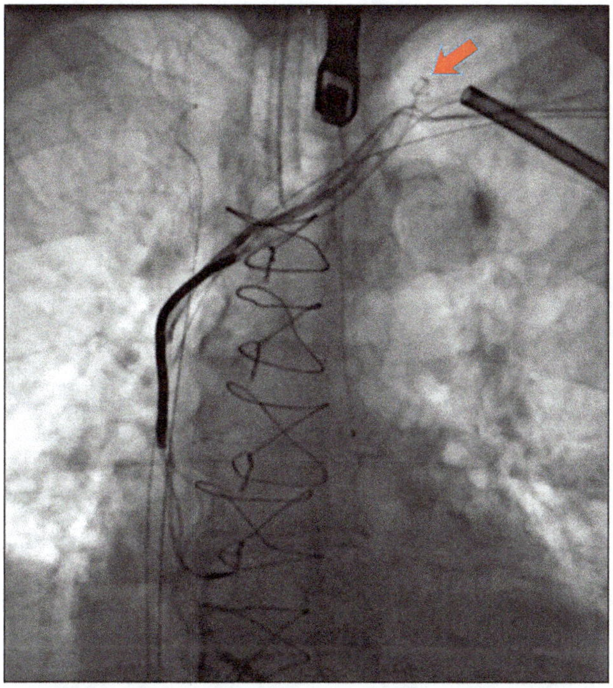

Figure 4.6 Partial lead transection by the mechanical sheath at left subclavian vein (**red arrow**).

The TightRail rotating dilator sheath has three sizes in 9-Fr, 11-Fr, and 13-Fr (inner diameter), corresponding to the outer diameters in 15.9-Fr, 18-Fr, and 20-Fr, respectively. Please see **Table 4.4** for the details. The length of the sheath is 47.5 cm. TightRail mini rotating dilator sheath (see Figure 4.5) is shorter in 15.5 cm, designed for entering the vasculature.

Evolution RL Controlled-Rotation Dilator Sheath

Evolution Right Left (RL) controlled-rotation dilator sheath set is designed for percutaneous dilation of tissue surrounding indwelling leads. The device is a hand-controlled mechanical sheath; the amount of sheath rotation is proportional to the length of the trigger pull. The operators control the sheath direction, alignment with the lead, and the speed of rotation. The sheath can be rotated in both directions and is flexible. The ten-sided tip, designed to disrupt tissue directly in contact with the sheath tip with no forward extending blades, peels the scar tissue off the leads (**Figure 4.7**). The Evolution RL sheath is 40.6 cm in length and has 3 sizes, 9-Fr, 11-Fr, and 13-Fr inner diameter (**Table 4.5**). Correspondingly, the outer sheaths are in 17.2 Fr, 19.4 Fr, and 21.3 Fr outer diameter, with a function of support and countertraction. The Evolution Shortie RL is 13.6 cm in length and has 9-Fr and 11-Fr, designed for entering the vasculature. SteadySheath (outer sheath) offers a textured radiopaque tip providing better visibility for the outer sheath's distal end. The textured tip provides additional support by holding the tissue in place while the inner sheath rotates and frees the lead.

Table 4.4 TightRail mechanical rotating dilator sheath

TightRail Rotating Dilator Sheath					
Model Number	**Size**	**Device Inner Diameter Fr/in./mm**	**Device Outer Diameter Fr/in./mm**	**Outer Sheath Outer Diameter Fr/in./mm**	**Working Length in./cm**
545-509	9 Fr	9.2 / 0.119 / 3.0	15.9 / 0.207 / 5.3	20.0 / 0.266 / 6.8	18.7 / 47.5
545-511	11 Fr	11.2 / 0.145 / 3.7	18.0 / 0.234 / 5.9	23.0 / 0.293 / 7.4	18.7 / 47.5
545-513	13 Fr	13.2 / 0.171 / 4.3	20.0 / 0.260 / 6.6	25.0 / 0.319 / 8.1	18.7 / 47.5
TightRail Mini Rotating Dilator Sheath					
Model Number	**Size**	**Device Inner Diameter Fr/in./mm**	**Device Outer Diameter Fr/in./mm**	**Outer Sheath Outer Diameter Fr/in./mm**	**Working Length in./cm**
540-009	9 Fr	9.2 / 0.119 / 3.0	15.9 / 0.207 / 5.3	20.0 / 0.266 / 6.8	6.1 / 15.5
540-011	11 Fr	11.2 / 0.145 / 3.7	18.0 / 0.234 / 5.9	23.0 / 0.293 / 7.4	6.1 / 15.5

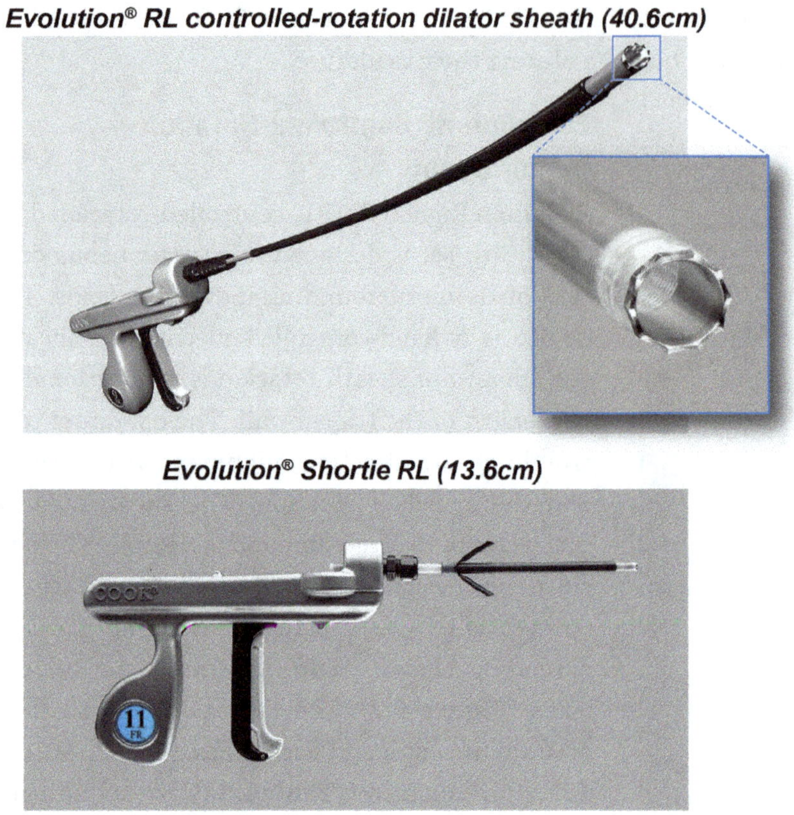

Figure 4.7 The Evolution RL dilator sheath has an exposed rotating blade. The Evolution Shortie RL is designed for use in the axillary subclavian region

Table 4.5 Evolution RL controlled-rotation dilator sheath

Reference Part Number	Inner Sheath Inner Diameter Fr	Outer Sheath Outer Diameter Fr	Inner Sheath Length cm
LR-EVN-9.0-RL	9.0	17.2	40.6
LR-EVN-11.0-RL	11.0	19.4	40.6
LR-EVN-13.0-RL	13.0	21.3	40.6

Clinical studies using Evolution mechanical extraction sheaths have shown that 98.4% of leads with an implant duration of > 10 years were removed with complete success.[9] A multi-center investigation compiled and analyzed data from an estimated 50,545 lead extraction cases from 2011–2016. It was found that lead extraction with laser sheaths appears to be associated with a higher risk of mortality than rotating sheaths.[10] The procedural and clinical success rates utilizing both the Evolution and TightRail rotational extraction sheaths were high, with a low complication rate in chronically implanted leads.[11]

EXTRACTION SNARES

The ONE Snare Endovascular Snare System (Merit Medical) is a single-loop snare. It can be used to retrieve the indwelling lead, inferior vena cava (IVC) filters, reposition indwelling venous catheters, and strip fibrin sheath formation. Gold-plated tungsten is wrapped around the nitinol loop for excellent visualization under fluoroscopy. The ONE Snare is available in 10 loop diameter sizes ranging from 2 mm to 35 mm (**Figure 4.8**, Panel A). 15 mm–25 mm size is commonly used for lead extraction. The snare from the femoral station can capture the end of the lead or transected lead and pull the lead down to IVC. It facilitates the mechanical extraction sheath from above to rail down and remove the lead. A multi-loop snare is available for a lead catch (Figure 4.8, Panel A). Amplatz Goose Neck snare (Medtronic) has a 90-degree loop, and nitinol design allows optimal wall apposition and ideal capture ability (Figure 4.8, Panel B and Panel C, red arrow). The snare sizes are from 5 mm to 35 mm, incremental

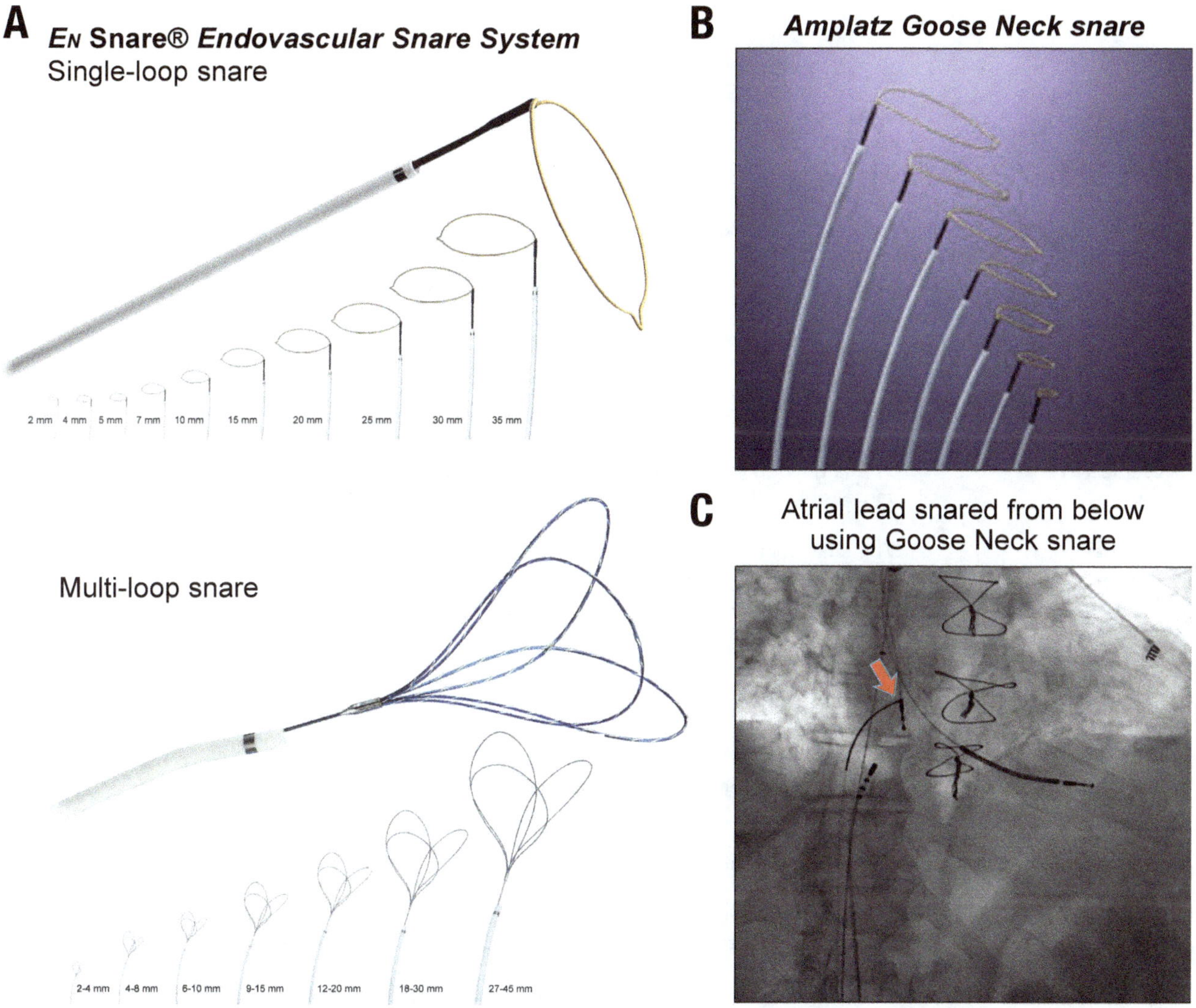

Figure 4.8 Extraction snares.

by 5 mm. **Video 4.9** demonstrates a successfully snared pacing lead is pulling down toward the IVC, facilitating the mechanical sheath to rail down the lead from above.

The Needle's Eye Snare (Cook Medical) is a transvenous grasping device that forms a basket-like snare around the targeted cardiac lead. It is delivered to the lead's vicinity through a long, flexible 12-Fr sheath placed coaxially within a larger outer 16-Fr (outer diameter) sheath with a hemostasis valve at its proximal end (**Figure 4.9**). Advancing the inner sheath closes the snare in a controlled manner and ensures a firm grasp of the target object. Inner and outer sheaths may be used to disrupt fibrous binding tissue.

BRIDGE OCCLUSION BALLOON

A tear in the SVC during a lead extraction procedure is rare, occurring in just 0.5% of cases. But when a tear does occur, the Bridge Occlusion Balloon (Philips Medical) can be quickly deployed to stem blood loss and allow time for transition to surgical repair (**Figure 4.10**). The Bridge Occlusion Balloon can be deployed in less than 2 minutes via a preplaced guidewire.[2] Radiopaque markers guide proper placement. Bridge Occlusion Balloon is designed to cover the entire length and diameter of the SVC in 90% of patients. Once deployed, the Bridge Occlusion Balloon can dramatically reduce blood loss by up to 90% on average in tears up to

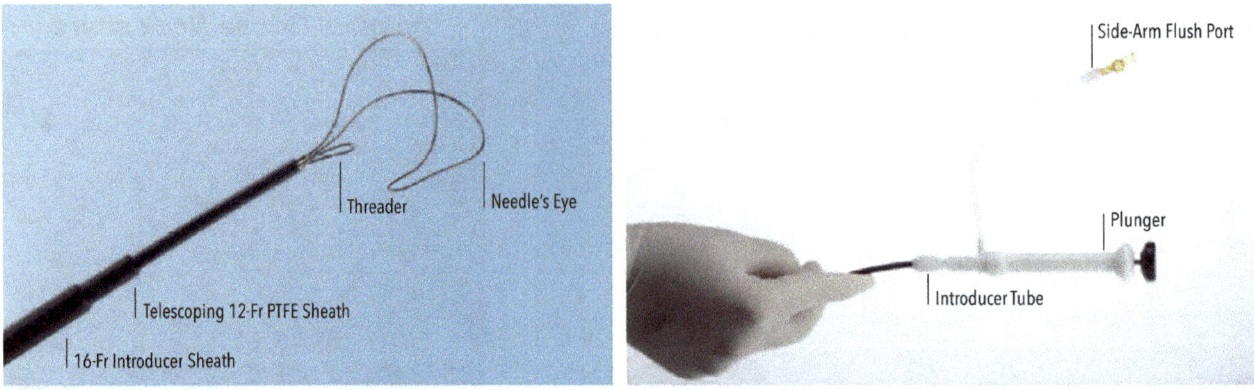

Needle's Eye	This large loop is made of a nitinol alloy that allows it to retain its shape and hook the target object during deployment. Loop profile diameters are available in 13 and 20 mm.
Threader	This smaller nitinol loop passes through the first to fully encircle the target object.
Handle	The design allows the threader to be engaged with one hand.
Plunger	Depressing the plunger advances the threader; retracting it releases the snare.
Side-Arm Flush Port	The side-arm flush port may be used for fluid infusion or to prefill the snare's innermost lumen with saline.
Telescoping 12-Fr PTFE Sheath	Advancing the sheath tightens the snare to firmly grasp the target object.
16-Fr Introducer Sheath	Advancing the sheath over the snared and folded target object prepares it for removal.
Introducer Tube	The introducer tube can slide forward to compress the snare and ease its reinsertion if replacing the telescoping 12-Fr PTFE sheath with the 12-Fr curved femoral sheath.
Luer Connector	Rotating the connector releases the introducer tube from its storage position atop the handle.

Figure 4.9 Needle's Eye Snare device explanation.

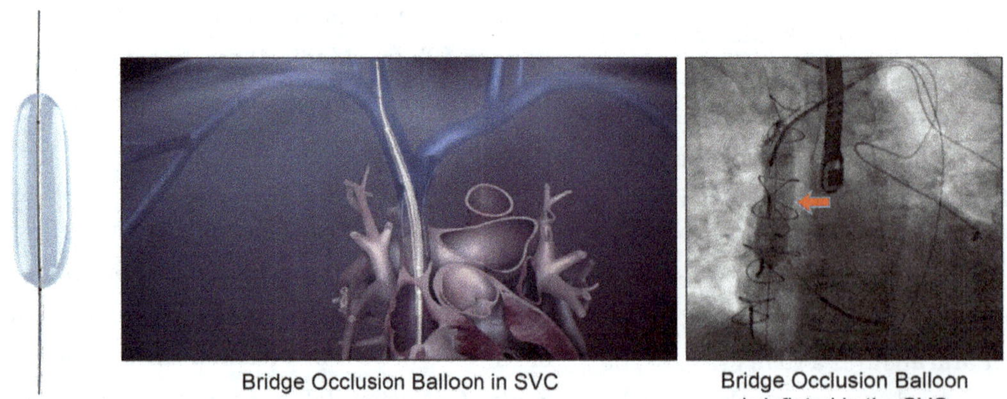

Figure 4.10 Bridge Occlusion Balloon application for SVC tear. (Courtesy of Royal Philips.)

3.5 cm. Proper Bridge Occlusion Balloon utilization has improved SVC tear survival from 56.4% to 91.7%.[12]

OTHER TOOLS

Large-Bore Sheaths

Extraction operators have used large-bore sheaths such as Micra outer sheath (Medtronic). The sheath has a 27-Fr outer diameter and 23-Fr inner diameter. The lubricious hydrophilic coating facilitates smooth vessel entry. The larger inner diameter accommodates sheath-in-sheath catheters, and snare operation. Cryoballoon FlexCath Steerable sheath (Medtronic) is 12 Fr in size. The sheath has steerability with a hemostatic valve to introduce, withdraw, and exchange smaller-size catheters, snares, and wires.

Radial Jaw 4 Biopsy Forceps

Radial Jaw 4 Biopsy Forceps (Boston Scientific) is intended to collect tissue for histologic examination. This surgical stainless steel jaw can be used for capturing the lead from below. The Jumbo Jaw catheter (**Figure 4.11**) is 160 cm in length with an outer jaw diameter of 2.8 mm. **Video 4.10** shows the right atrial lead is captured by a Jumbo Jaw biopsy forceps via an Agilis sheath and pulled down towards IVC. The mechanical sheath is railing down close to the Jumbo Jaw.

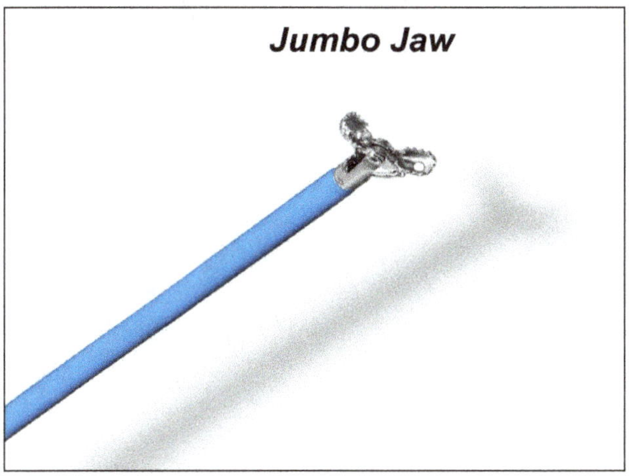

Figure 4.11 Endoscopy biopsy forceps (Jumbo Jaws, Boston Scientific) can be used to used to grab lead tip for fragments.

REFERENCES

1. Voigt A, Shalaby A, Saba S. Rising rates of cardiac rhythm management device infections in the United States: 1996 through 2003. *J Am Coll Cardiol.* 2006;48(3):590–591.
2. Wilkoff BL, Byrd CL, Love CJ, et al. Pacemaker lead extraction with the laser sheath: Results of the pacing lead extraction with the Excimer sheath (PLEXES) trial. *J Am Coll Cardiol.* 1999;33(6):1671–1676.
3. Smith MC, Love CJ. Extraction of transvenous pacing and ICD leads. *Pacing Clin Electrophysiol.* 2008;31(6):736–752.
4. Bongiorni MG, Kennergren C, Butter C, et al. The European Lead Extraction ConTRolled (ELECTRa) study: A European Heart Rhythm Association (EHRA) Registry of Transvenous Lead Extraction Outcomes. *Eur Heart J.* 2017;38(40):2995–3005.
5. Kusumoto FM, Schoenfeld MH, Wilkoff BL, et al. 2017 HRS expert consensus statement on cardiovascular implantable electronic device lead management and extraction. *Heart Rhythm.* 2017;14(12):e503–e551.
6. Fu HX, Huang XM, Zhong LI, et al. Outcomes and complications of lead removal: Can we establish a risk stratification schema for a collaborative and effective approach? *Pacing Clin Electrophysiol.* 2015;38(12):1439–1447.
7. Wasserlauf J, Esheim T, Jarett NM, et al. Avoiding damage to transvenous leads—A comparison of electrocautery techniques and two insulated electrocautery blades. *Pacing Clin Electrophysiol.* 2018;41(12):1593–1599.
8. Byrd CL, Wilkoff BL, Love CJ, Sellers TD, Reiser C. Clinical study of the laser sheath for lead extraction: The total experience in the United States. *Pacing Clin Electrophysiol.* 2002;25(5): 804–808.
9. Mazzone P, Migliore F, Bertaglia E, et al. Safety and efficacy of the new bidirectional rotational Evolution mechanical lead extraction sheath: Results from a multicentre Italian registry. *EP Europace.* 2018;20(5):829–834.
10. Diaz CL, Guo X, Whitman IR, et al. Reported mortality with rotating sheaths vs. laser sheaths

for transvenous lead extraction. *EP Europace*. 2019;21(11):1703–1709.

11. Cay S, Ozeke O, Ozcan F, Topaloglu S, Aras D. Transvenous lead extraction, only once or repeatable? *Pacing Clin Electrophysiol*. 2019;42(2):298.

12. Carrillo R. Increased safety in lead extraction: New evidence. EHRA 2018; Barcelona. 2018.

VIDEO LEGENDS

Video 4.1 This video shows the mechanism of Liberator Locking Stylet and its application. (Permission for use granted by Cook Medical, Bloomington, Indiana.) [00:43]

Video 4.2 The lead (pace-sense) inner lumen is locked, but not the conductance coils. Pulling the lead inner lumen alone results in insulation breach and conductor cable externalization. A multi-lumen ICD lead is used to illustrate the concepts. [00:20]

Video 4.3 Pulling the lead inner lumen and high-voltage conductor cables together (tied by separate sutures) is illustrated in a multi-lumen ICD lead prepared with the locking stylet. Note that as pulling force is not applied to the insulation, bunching can occur. Bunching of the insulation, in turn, leads to difficulty in advancing the extraction sheath. [00:25]

Video 4.4 Uniform force transmission on the components of a multi-lumen ICD lead is illustrated. The pace-sense lumen is locked with a locking stylet. Separate sutures on placed on the high-voltage cables and the outer insulation. All the components are pulled together for more straightforward advancement of the inner extraction sheath and the outer sheath. [00:23]

Video 4.5 Laser sheath with circumferential fiber-optic cables delivering pulses of wavelength 308 nm in the ultraviolet spectrum (green) and photo-ablating the fibrous adhesions. In the animation, we illustrate the use of laser energy to pass through adhesions. When greater lateral forces are noted, the sheaths are pulled back, and only the inner laser sheath is advanced. The combination of inner and our sheaths results in a stiffer system over the lead. It may be easier to advance the outer sheath when the inner sheath is in the low right atrium. Countertraction using the inner sheath is used to free the lead tip. [01:03]

Video 4.6 Laser sheath (blue) is advanced over the lead, separating the lead from the surrounding fibrosis. The outer sheath (orange) is pushed forward for support and countertraction. [00:36]

Video 4.7 When the laser sheath is advancing from innominate vein to SVC, caution is undertaken to align the sheath with the lead in a straight downward force and avoid focusing the energy to the lateral SVC wall. [00:22]

Video 4.8 When lead-to-lead binding is significant, alternating the laser sheath to a different lead helps to free the lead from the binding site. [02:06]

Video 4.9 A pacing lead is captured by the Goose Neck snare, pulled down, and creates a straight line for the mechanical sheath railing down. [00:01]

Video 4.10 The right atrial lead is captured by a Jumbo Jaw biopsy forceps (Boston Scientific) through a deflectable sheath and pulled down towards IVC. The mechanical sheath is railing down close to the Jumbo Jaw. [00:01]

EXTRA VIDEO LEGENDS

Below are videos demonstrating procedural techniques that were not covered elsewhere in the book.

Video 4.11 How to use a Bull Dog device (Cook Medical). [03:15]

Video 4.12 How to use a One-Tie device (Cook Medical). [01:47]

Video 4.13 Lead preparation for extraction. [10:14]

Video 4.14 Principles of using a Needle's Eye Snare (Cook Medical). [03:21]

Video 4.15 How to use a fish hook tool to pull a prepared lead through the extraction sheath. [01:26]

5 Anesthetic Considerations and Preparation for Lead Extraction

Shane M. Gillespie, MS, DO; William J. Mauermann, MD

INTRODUCTION

Lead extraction is defined as the removal of a lead that has been implanted for more than 1 year or requires specialized extraction tools (locking stylets, telescoping sheaths, femoral extraction tools, etc.).[1] Lead removal can be simple or complex depending on the age, number, type of lead(s), patient comorbidities, and the reason for extraction. Cardiovascular implantable electronic device (CIED) lead extractions are increasing in the United States, and this increase is accompanied by more CIED-related complications.[2] Retrospective studies and the 2017 HRS expert consensus statement on CIED lead management and extraction have reported major complication rates of approximately 2%, but complications are often higher in patients with device-related infections, decompensated heart failure, and/or severe left ventricular (LV) dysfunction.[2–6] Detailed planning and communication between the anesthesia, interventional cardiology, and cardiovascular surgical teams are paramount to a successful outcome and minimizing complications.

PLAN FOR ANESTHESIA

The preoperative role of the anesthesiologist includes understanding the indications for lead extraction, age of the leads, number and location of leads, and type of device that was originally implanted. A comprehensive review of the patient's preexisting comorbidities, cardiac function, and identifying any high-risk characteristics to the preexisting leads are necessary for appropriate preanesthetic planning.[7] General anesthesia is typically used to provide optimal procedural and surgical conditions and provide the ability to use continuous transesophageal echocardiography (TEE). This can be accomplished with any number of induction agents (often based on cardiac function and comorbidities), a short-acting narcotic, and a muscle relaxant. Anesthesia is typically maintained with either volatile anesthesia or a propofol infusion. Monitored anesthesia care may be used in select cases assuming there are no patient comorbidities that would preclude monitored anesthesia care and also based on risk stratification for lead extraction. This is typically accomplished with short-acting narcotics and benzodiazepines. Low-dose propofol is often frequently utilized and well tolerated.

PROCEDURAL RISK STRATIFICATION

At our institution, patients are risk stratified in low, intermediate, or high-risk cohorts based on a retrospective review of more than 650 patients (see Chapter 4, Table 4.1). Any implantable cardioverter-defibrillator (ICD) or permanent pacemaker lead(s) that have been in place less than 1 year are extracted under conscious sedation. ICD leads placed between 1 to 5 years ago and permanent pacemaker leads placed between 1 to 10 years ago are considered an intermediate risk. This patient cohort typically undergoes general anesthesia, but with appropriate patient selection and good communication between the teams, conscious sedation can be safely used in select situations. Any ICD leads older than 5 years or permanent pacemaker leads older than 10

 Cardiotext Publishing. ISBN: 978-1-942909-54-5

years are considered high risk. Patients are also considered high risk if they have complex congenital heart disease. All high risk lead extractions are performed under general anesthesia. Patients would be in the intermediate-risk group in relation to the time of lead placement and are on hemodialysis or have coronary artery disease, NYHA class IV heart failure, or a calcified superior vena cava (SVC) or myocardium.

PROCEDURAL PREPARATION

Equipment

The site of intermediate or high-risk lead extraction should take place in a hybrid operating room or procedural suite able to accommodate a cardiopulmonary bypass (CPB) machine. Other essential equipment needed include sternotomy equipment (sternal saw, retractors, etc.) and SVC occlusion balloons. Intermediate and high-risk patients require large-bore intravascular access, invasive monitoring, and alternative ways to pace or cardiovert/defibrillate the heart. Temporary pacing boxes for transvenous pacing need to be available in the operating room, and defibrillator/pacing pads need to be placed appropriately on the patient prior to the start of the procedure.

Arterial and Venous Accesses

Invasive monitoring consists of an upper extremity arterial catheter for continuous blood pressure monitoring and laboratory draws. Large-bore intravascular access (9 Fr) is typically placed in one of the femoral veins rather than the SVC or internal jugular due to concerns of SVC or right atrial disruption. Rapid infusion through a superior access venous catheter in case of venous tear/injury often does not reach the central circulation and ends up in the pleural or pericardial space. Inferior venous access through the femoral vein provides a reliable way to deliver medications or blood products to the central circulation in the event of venous tear. The contralateral femoral vein and artery should be readily accessible for rapid cannulation by the cardiovascular surgical team if rescue CPB is required. The contralateral femoral artery and vein can also be utilized for peripheral extracorporeal membrane oxygenation (ECMO) cannulation postprocedure or postCPB in patients with worsening cardiac function and end organ failure. A central venous catheter placed through the internal jugular vein is often used to monitor central venous pressure (CVP). Loss of "y" descent and increase in CVP is noted in patients with pericardial tamponade. Abrupt drop in pressure with loss of CVP waveforms indicate vascular tear and potential bleed into the pleural space.

Transesophageal Echocardiogram

TEE is typically utilized as it allows for rapid assessment and continuous monitoring of hemodynamic perturbations, new or enlarging pericardial effusions/tamponade, right ventricular rupture or inversion, and migration of vegetations or thrombus from the CIED leads, as well as assessing tricuspid valve function after right ventricular lead(s) removal.

Transfusion

There should be an active type and screen with blood readily available or in the procedure room. Rapid transfusing equipment and cell saver for blood conservation need to be immediately available. Many centers have massive transfusion protocols in case of a venous tear resulting hemodynamic collapse.

Post-Anesthesia Recovery

Normally, minimal narcotics are required secondary to the peripheral approach and the use of local anesthetics by the procedural team. Assuming the lead extraction is uneventful and there are no ongoing hemodynamic perturbations, the patient can be extubated in the procedural suite and monitored in the post-anesthesia care unit. Patients that required emergent surgical interventions, had procedural complications, or require ongoing resuscitation should remain intubated and further managed in the intensive care unit.

SUMMARY

In summary, the preoperative role of the anesthesiologist is to understand the indications for lead extraction and risk stratify the patients to plan for the safest anesthetic. This includes a comprehensive review of the patient's comorbidities, reviewing all available laboratory and imaging data, and most importantly, ensuring open communication in and out the operating suite between all teams to ensure the best possible patient outcome.

SUMMARY POINTS

- Large-bore access needs to be placed below the diaphragm in case of SVC or right atrial disruption.
- Continuous monitoring with TEE is very helpful in diagnosing the cause of hypotension.
- Preoperative briefing regarding approach and anticipated difficulties is essential, as is ongoing communication throughout the procedure
- Utilization of a hybrid procedural suite in high-risk patients is necessary to facilitate emergent cardiopulmonary bypass or ECMO.

REFERENCES

1. Bhatia M, Safavi-Naeini P, Razavi M, Collard CD, Tolpin DA, Anton JM. Anesthetic management of laser lead extraction for cardiovascular implantable electronic devices. *Semin Cardiothorac Vasc Anesth.* 2017;21:302–311.
2. Kusumoto FM, Schoenfeld MH, Wilkoff BL, et al. 2017 HRS expert consensus statement on cardiovascular implantable electronic device lead management and extraction. *Heart Rhythm.* 2017;14:e503–e551.
3. Rodriguez Y, Mesa J, Arguelles E, Carrillo RG. Tricuspid insufficiency after laser lead extraction. *Pacing Clin Electrophysiol.* 2013;36:939–944.
4. Roux JF, Page P, Dubuc M, et al. Laser lead extraction: Predictors of success and complications. *Pacing Clin Electrophysiol.* 2007;30: 214–220.
5. Byrd CL, Wilkoff BL, Love CJ, Sellers TD, Reiser C. Clinical study of the laser sheath for lead extraction: The total experience in the United States. *Pacing Clin Electrophysiol.* 2002;25: 804–808.
6. Tarakji KG, Chan EJ, Cantillon DJ, et al. Cardiac implantable electronic device infections: Presentation, management, and patient outcomes. *Heart Rhythm.* 2010;7:1043–1047.
7. Practice Advisory for the Perioperative Management of Patients with Cardiac Implantable Electronic Devices: Pacemakers and Implantable Cardioverter–Defibrillators 2020: An Updated Report by the American Society of Anesthesiologists Task Force on Perioperative Management of Patients with Cardiac Implantable Electronic Devices*. *Anesthesiology: J Am Soc Anesthesiol.* 2020;132:225–252.

6 | Room and Equipment Preparation

Kevin J. Mulligan, RCIS

INTRODUCTION

Lead extraction is one of the complex, technically challenging procedures performed in the cardiac electrophysiology procedure suites. Allied health staff (AHS) play a critical role in coordinating the case setup, arranging supplies, preparing the room and the patient during these procedures. Several tips and tricks on preprocedural, intraprocedural, and postprocedure setups will be discussed throughout the next few sections. Our role as AHS involved in lead extraction procedures is vitally important and will aid in the procedure's overall success.

PREPROCEDURAL PLANNING

Allied Health Staff and Team Huddle

Before bringing the patient to the procedure suite, the extraction team should consider performing a preprocedure huddle. The huddle includes discussing the planned extraction approach, equipment necessary for the procedure, and a management plan for potential major complications. Gathering information about the patient and specifics nuances of the procedure will aid in AHS planning. An extraction checklist used by the AHS at the Mayo Clinic, Rochester, MN, is included at the end of this chapter (**Table 6.1**)

Depending on each lab's specific protocols, there may be times when additional input for patient preparation is sought from other specialties (e.g., interventional radiology, echocardiography team, cardiovascular surgery, and general surgery). At Mayo Clinic, all lead extraction procedures require surgical backup from a cardiothoracic surgical team. As an AHS member, it is best to identify all specialties involved in every individual procedure. Open lines of communication should exist among team members. Often a direct communication line to the additional teams may come from the charge nurse, lead technologists, or staff in the procedural suite. However, the delegation of roles within the communication chain will minimize miscommunication errors. It is good practice to list all involved personnel with their contact numbers.

The AHS can take on various roles and responsibilities within the extraction procedure. The AHS team members can be represented from the operating room, electrophysiology practice, anesthesia service, and perfusion medicine. A list of essential roles and responsibilities is outlined in **Table 6.2**.

Room Setup

When AHS begins to set up for a lead extraction procedure, identifying where the equipment should be placed is critical for easy access to required tools. A hybrid operating room (OR) generally offers a larger footprint, but the equipment needed is usually confined near the operating table in the most complex cases. Sterile instrument table, laser machine, echo machine, anesthesia machine, and device programmers are all within close proximity to the operating field (**Figure 6.1**). In this regard, AHS should consider preprocedural planning to ensure the best space utilization for equipment setup. Once established, standardization of such a layout will aid in overall equipment positioning and avoid troubleshooting space utility during the procedure.

Certain procedures may require specific equipment, and the setup is carried out before starting the procedure by multi-specialty teams (**Table 6.3**). Proper equipment setup minimizes inefficiencies during the procedure. Transesophageal

Cardiac Lead Extraction: A Case-Based Contemporary Approach.
 ISBN: 978-1-942909-54-5

Table 6.1 Lead extraction checklist for the allied health staff

Patient Information	
Name:	
MRN:	
DOB:	
Age:	
M/F:	
Side of Implant:	
Date of Extraction:	
Indication:	
Location (Pacing Lab/Hybrid OR):	
Pacemaker Dependency:	
Informed Consent Date:	

Extraction Staff
Referring Physician:
Extracting Physician:
Fellow:
Nurse:
Techs:

Additional Teams Involved				
	Name		**Contact-Phone #**	
CV Surgery				
General Surgery				
Echo Lab				
Wound Vac				
Industry Rep				
Device				
Manufacturer				
ICD/Pacemaker				
Location/Side				
Year Implanted				
Model #				
Serial #				
Leads				
Lead #	**1**	**2**	**3**	**4**
Lead Location				
Manufacturer				
ICD/Pacemaker				
Date Implanted				
Model #				
Serial #				
Lead Length				

(continued)

Table 6.1 Lead extraction checklist for the allied health staff *(continued)*

Leads *(continued)*				
Active or Passive				
Laser Sheath Size				
TightRail Size				

Additional Teams Involved				
	Name		**Contact-Phone #**	
CV Surgery				
General Surgery				
Echo Lab				
Wound Vac				
Industry Rep				
Device				
Manufacturer				
ICD/Pacemaker				
Location/Side				
Year Implanted				
Model #				
Serial #				
Leads				
Lead #	**1**	**2**	**3**	**4**
Lead Location				
Manufacturer				
ICD/Pacemaker				
Date Implanted				
Model #				
Serial #				
Lead Length				
Active or Passive				
Laser Sheath Size				
TightRail Size				

Procedural Considerations
Temporary pacemaker needed?
SVC wire placed during procedure?
SVC balloon prepped?
TEE vs. ICE – Echo needed?
Drape the internal jugular site in the field?
Vascular access sites needed?
Reimplanting after extraction?

Access Sites

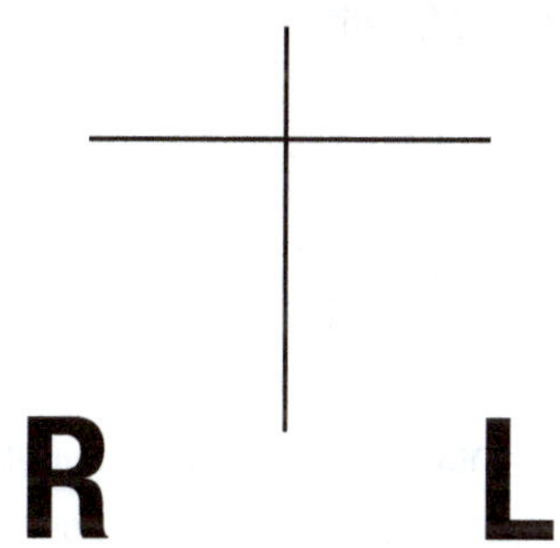

Table 6.2 Roles taken on by allied health staff members

Allied Health Staff for Lead Extractions	
Registered Nurse	Device programming (device nurse), procedural charting and orders, circulating (OR nurse), and temporary pacemaker programming
Cardiovascular Technologist	Scrubbing, circulating, table and room setup, coordination of extraction supplies, and quality control of equipment
Radiologic Technologist	Operation of fluoroscopic equipment, positioning, image review, store, and archiving of imaging data
Perfusionists	Standby for hemodynamic circulatory support and bypass
Monitor/Anesthesia Staff	Anesthesia operation, transesophageal echocardiography, assist in OR-specific supplies, arterial line, and vital sign monitor setup
Surgical Assistants	Patient positioning, preparation, surgical team standby, and assistance
Surgical Technologist	OR instrumentation setup, draping, surgical counts, and surgical team standby

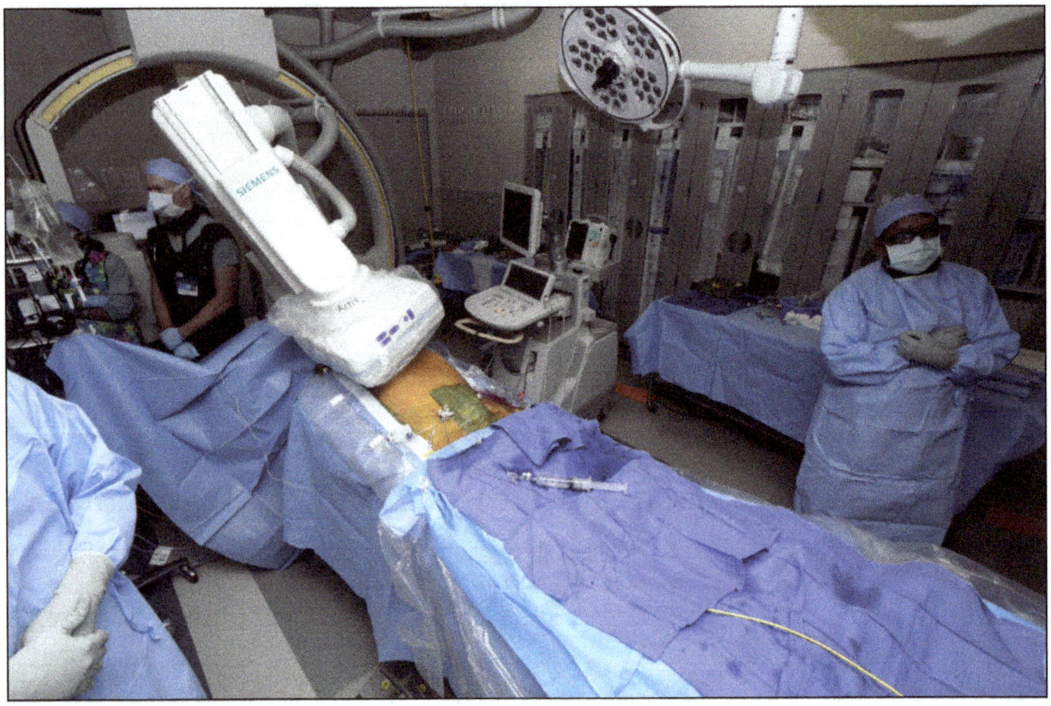

Figure 6.1 Extraction room preparation in the hybrid OR. Consideration of instrumentation and equipment placement is completed during the preextraction procedure huddle.

Table 6.3 Specific equipment considered for lead extraction

Imaging Modalities
• Ultrasound for vascular access • TEE or intracardiac echo machine • Thoracotomy/thoracoscopy
Extraction Specific
• Laser machine console • Cautery (PlasmaBlade) console
Additional Equipment for Patient Management
• Cell saver (standby and used during perforation or centesis) • Wound vac console and supplies • Suction supplies

echocardiography (TEE) or intracardiac echocardiography (ICE) is standard on all lead extractions performed in the hybrid OR. AHS will communicate with the anesthesia team and OR techs to ensure a TEE probe and machine are available in the room. The laser system should be calibrated to ensure proper function. The laser sheath's tip is directed at the machine's calibration port, and calibration is performed after taking all laser precautions (**Figure 6.2**). AHS should be familiar with the control panel. Some physicians may alter the pulse repetition frequency when applying laser energy at specific areas like the superior vena cava (SVC).

In the hybrid OR, separate tables may be used to set up lead extraction and cardiac surgical instruments. Our practice has allowed the cardiovascular surgical team to prepare and set up their surgical instruments. A back table is often set aside specifically for cardiovascular surgical instruments. The orderly arrangement of instruments aids in performing an emergency sternotomy and initiation of cardiopulmonary bypass. AHS from the pacemaker service and surgical teams should discuss the instrument setup and work collaboratively on these logistical issues.

Extraction Supplies

AHS must provide careful attention to supply planning, quantity assessment, and the availability of specialty instruments needed for the procedure. Verbal communication with the multifaceted teams will help AHS be prepared for multiple scenarios (such as extraction from below, snaring, or internal jugular venous approach). We commonly review the number of leads planned for extraction,

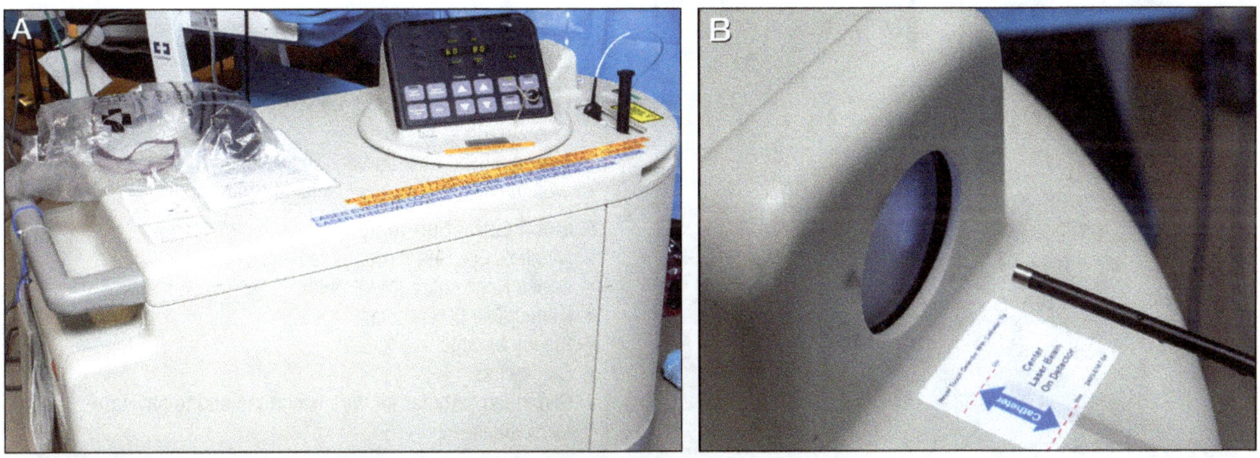

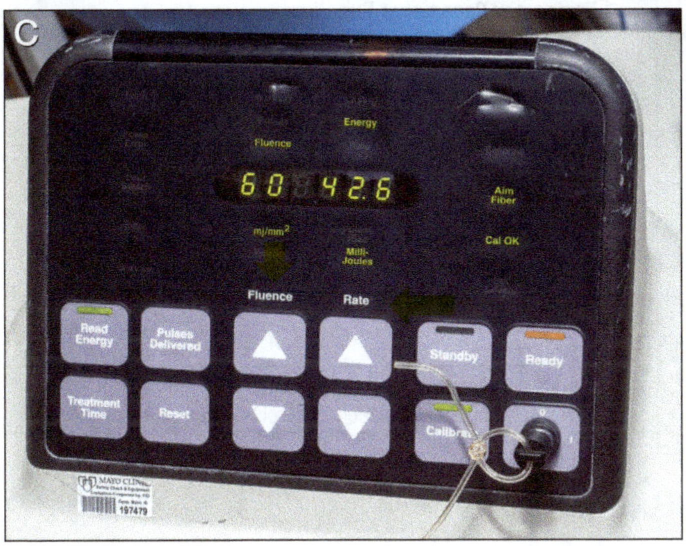

Figure 6.2 **Panel A** illustrates the laser machine (CVX-300, Excimer laser system) used during the extraction procedures. The catheter is pointed towards the calibration port and is tested prior to loading on the prepared leads (**Panel B**). **Panel C** shows the control panel of the laser machine. Fluence refers to the laser energy delivery per unit area (**yellow arrow**). The rate refers to repetition rate of laser (**green arrow**). It is can be programmed up to 80 Hz. Some operators may prefer to reduce the rate when passing through critical areas such as the SVC.

as well as the design details and caliber of the leads (https://www.usa.philips.com/healthcare/education-resources/lead-lookup). Based on this information, AHS will fill out the checklist to ensure the availability of vascular access tools, locking stylets, and the correct size extraction sheaths. The utilization of such a checklist (see Table 6.1) can easily be integrated into a preprocedural timeout or procedural pause to ensure all members agree with the planned approach.

A designated lead extraction supply cart can aid in easy availability, efficient retrieval, and utilization of extraction-specific supplies (**Figure 6.3**). This cart is mobile and can be easily transported to the pacing lab or the hybrid OR. The supply cart should be of adequate size to accommodate supplies used in lead extraction procedures (**Table 6.4**). This includes various sizes of laser extraction sheaths and snares. Pericardiocentesis supplies such as access needles, sheaths, and wires should be readily available for emergency pericardial tap during the extraction procedure. Critical factors for a useful extraction cart include standardization, clear labeling, and uncluttered organization of stocked supplies.

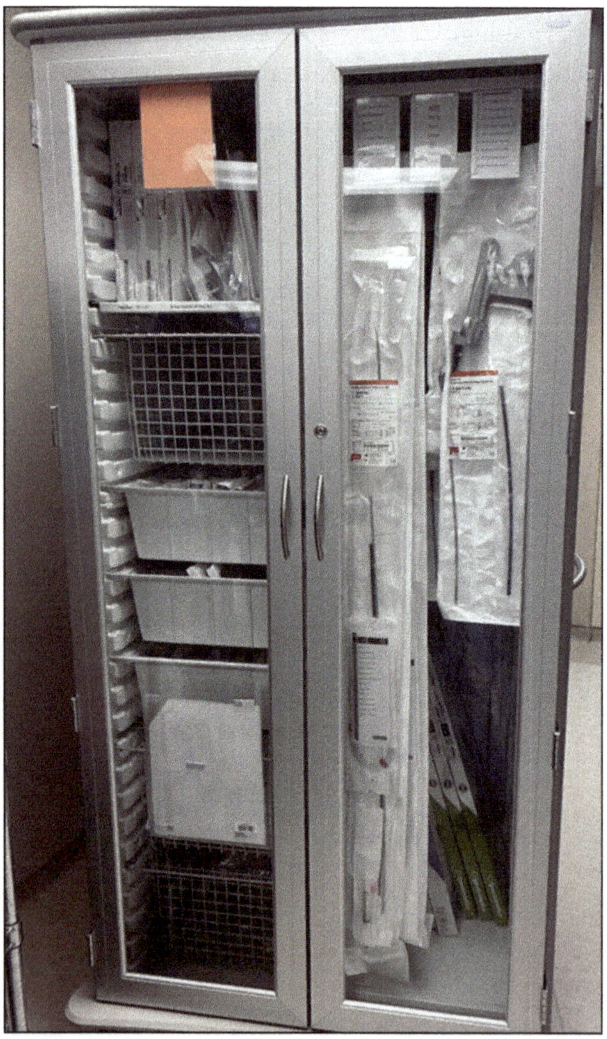

Figure 6.3 Example of lead extraction supply cart holding specialty supplies for lead extraction. This cart can be easily transported to the hybrid OR.

Table 6.4 Extraction procedural supplies

Extraction procedural supplies
Vascular Access Sheaths • 4-Fr to 10-Fr sheaths
Basic Device Supplies • Lead stylets • Clip-on tool for helix retraction • Setscrew wrench
Lead Extraction Tools • Locking stylets • Laser sheaths (12 Fr, 14 Fr, 16 Fr) • Mechanical sheaths (9 Fr, 11 Fr, 13 Fr) • Lead extenders (Bulldog, Cook Medical) • One-Tie (Cook Medical) • Suture (absorbable and nonabsorbable) • Wound closure supplies (Jackson Pratt drain)
Femoral Extraction Tools • Needle's Eye Snare (Cook Medical) • Goose Neck snare (Medtronic) • Deflectable EP catheter • Biopsy forceps • Guidewires • Glidehead catheter for wire exchange and to navigate tortuosities
Temporary Pacemaker Supplies • Pacing box • Catheter, lead • Cables • Dressings (postprocedure)
SVC Bridge Occlusion Balloon • Balloon prep kit
Pericardial Centesis Kit • Needles (MD specific) • Wires • Sheaths • Pigtail
Device and Lead Reimplant Supplies • All standard supplies needed to reimplant new system
VAC Kit • Sponge and dressing • VAC console

PROCEDURAL COURSE

Patient Preparation and Sterile Draping

The patient is brought to the OR suite and monitoring patches are placed. Defibrillation pads are positioned to ensure adequate shocking vector while also minimizing intrusion into the sterile prep site. General anesthesia is used for most procedures. After induction, a radial arterial line is placed for hemodynamic monitoring. A urinary catheter is often inserted for monitoring urine output. A clipper is used to remove hair in the groin region. The chest hair is also clipped among male patients. Unless contraindicated, the patient's surgical sites are prepared with iodine povacrylex (DuraPrep, 3M Healthcare), and proper dry time is allowed. All pressure points are padded, and the arms are placed in a thumbs-up position (**Figure 6.4**). Pillows may be placed to slightly flex the knees to minimize strain on the lower back. Bed sheets are used to tuck the arms at the side of the patient. A bed sheet is typically placed below the back and brought above and underneath the arm and tucked back under the patient's body. Arm boards use restricts access to the central chest in the event of an emergency.

Following the aseptic and sterile technique, the patient is then draped, allowing full exposure of the chest and vascular access sites (**Figure 6.5**). Care should be taken to ensure the internal jugular and groin sites are included in the sterile field. This inclusion allows access to these sites for

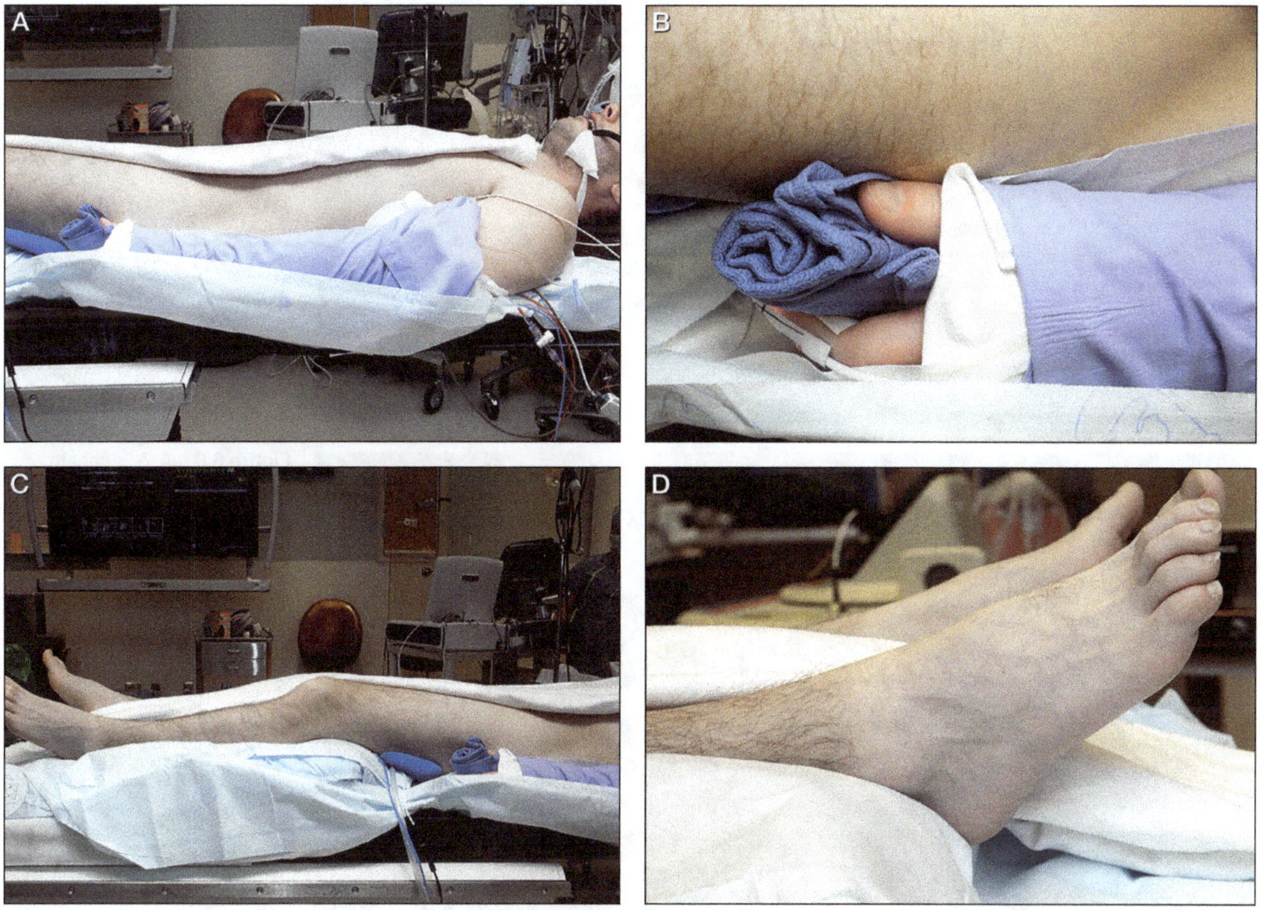

Figure 6.4 Patient positioning on the operating room table. **Panel A** shows use of sheets to secure patient's arms by wrapping around and tucking the sheets behind the back. This preparation allows the operator to get closer to the center of the chest by avoiding the use of arm boards. Notice the Bair Hugger warming blanket (3M) system is used to maintain normothermia. **Panel B** shows appropriate hand padding and positioning (thumbs up) to avoid injury. **Panel C** shows a pillow placed under the legs to create knee flexion and to relieve pressure over the lower back (DVT prevention pneumatic compression wrappings are not shown in the picture). **Panel D** illustrates appropriate support below the heels.

alternate extraction routes during the procedure (**Figure 6.6**). A formal instrument, sharps, and sponge count is completed and documented before skin incision.

Following a procedural timeout, vascular access is obtained before opening the device pocket. Ultrasound guidance is used for vascular access, and the cardiovascular technologist will ensure the ultrasound probe is prepped in a sterile fashion and ready for use. Vascular access is achieved by a modified Seldinger technique. A micropuncture access kit is utilized in some patients. Multiple venous access sites may be required when performing complicated lead extractions (**Figure 6.7**). Specific venous access sites are identified and noted during the preprocedural huddle. Outer gloves are often changed upon completion of vascular access in the femoral region. It is an added precaution to minimize the transfer of microbes from the inferior access site to the superior operating field and the device pocket.

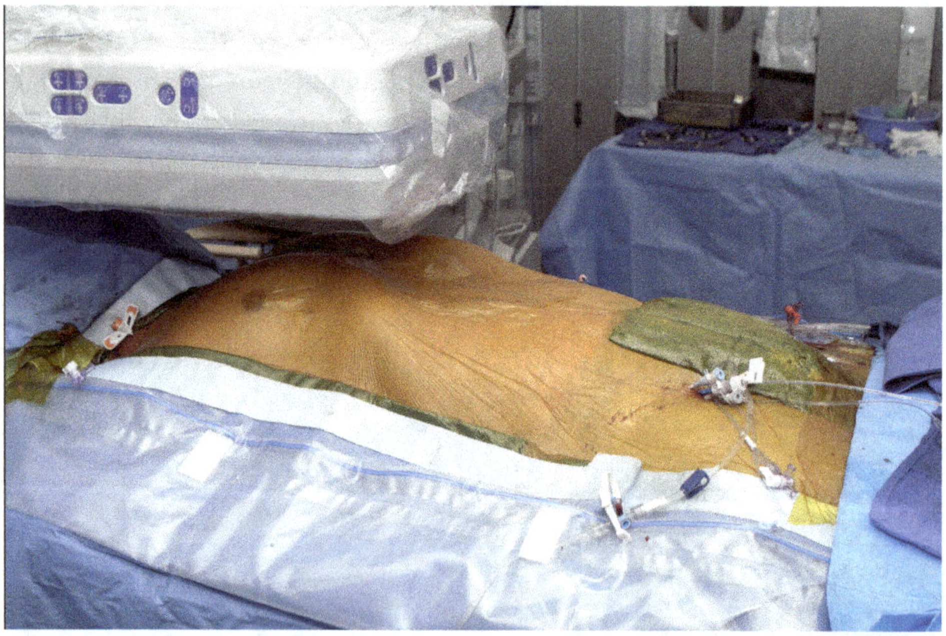

Figure 6.5 Patient prepped and draped for lead extraction. Exposure of full chest and venous access sites is standard practice on all lead extractions.

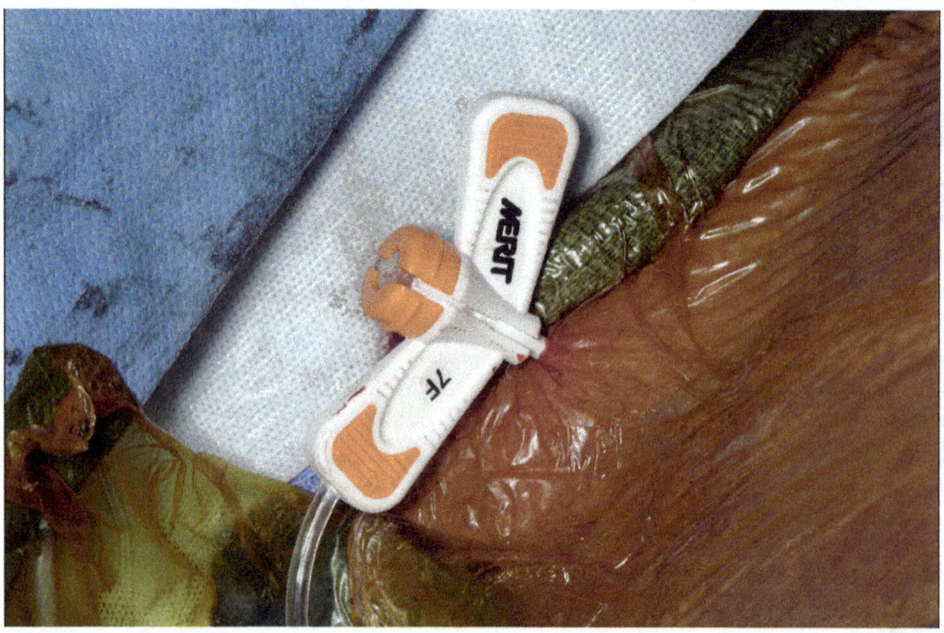

Figure 6.6 A 7-Fr sheath is placed in the right internal jugular vein for temporary permanent lead placement. The access site is prepped into the sterile field and can be used during the extraction procedure, thereby keeping the sterile field intact.

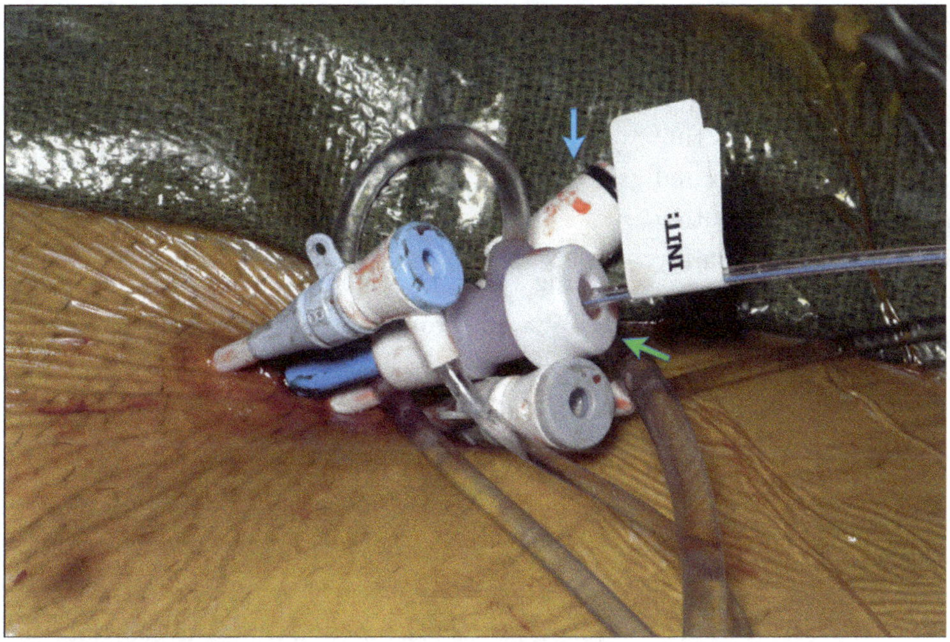

Figure 6.7 Venous sheaths of various sizes placed in the femoral vein. A 12-Fr sheath is used for SVC occlusion balloon (**green arrow**) catheter placement. Please note that a marker is placed on the shaft of the balloon catheter during optimal balloon deployment. In an emergency, the balloon catheter can be pushed to the marker over the wire for rapid deployment. The large-bore sheath is for anesthesia fluid administration (**blue arrow**) the 8-Fr sheath for extraction tools from below (**blue hub**); and the additional sheath is used for intracardiac echocardiography imaging or temporary pacing (**gray hub**).

Equipment/Tools and Instrumentation Handling

If the patient is pacemaker dependent or demonstrates the need for pacing support, a temporary pacemaker is placed at this time. The temporary use of a permanent pacemaker may be considered if the patient will require prolonged pacing, whereby a permanent lead is placed and connected to an external pacing device. Our practice is to place a 12-Fr venous sheath for a Bridge Occlusion Balloon (Philips) placement in all high-risk extraction cases. A SVC Bridge Occlusion Balloon is placed over a stiff 0.035-in. wire for rapid deployment in a vascular tear event. The 60-cc syringe with diluted contrast and the balloon are prepared for deployment. AHS will aid in the preparation and the deployment of the SVC occlusion balloon.

The device pocket is opened using electrosurgical cautery. In most cases, the patient is intubated with no open oxygen source. If there is an open oxygen source, FiO_2 is turned down to minimize the fire risk while performing electrosurgery around the device pocket. Careful attention should be paid to the use of electrosurgery around the leads. A PlasmaBlade (Medtronic) cautery pen is used on our lead extractions when pocket fibrosis is evident. It helps free up leads while minimizing the risk of lead damage. Some operators prefer to reduce the power settings to reduce heat-related damage to the insulation material.

The leads are dissected down to the suture sleeve within the device pocket, often close to the point of vessel entry. The device is disconnected, and leads are prepared for extraction. Scrub AHS should have standard stylets, device wrench, and clip-on tools handy during the lead preparation part of the procedure. An attempt to retract the helix of an active fixation lead is made with close observation of the lead tip under fluoroscopy. Gentle traction may be used on the lead to identify areas of lead binding within the vasculature. In cases without any significant binding sites, the lead may come out with simple traction.

Lead scissors are used to cut through the lead, exposing the inner lumen. The suture sleeve is then removed. An appropriately sized locking stylet is placed in each lead and is advanced to the lead tip. The stylet's locking mechanism is deployed, and a prolene suture is attached to secure the outer insulation to the body of the lead. At this point, either mechanical extraction tools or laser sheath is requested. The technologists in the room will identify the size of laser or mechanical sheaths to accommodate each lead being extracted.

The laser machine is often tested at the beginning of the procedure. Proper signage indicating the use of class IV laser is in progress is required and posted on all entrances into the operating room. Staff and the patient will wear laser safety goggles that protect from the appropriate laser spectrum for a 308-nm XeCl Excimer laser. The laser sheath is calibrated before loading onto the prepared lead.

The cardiovascular surgical team is made aware before the application of laser energy. Also, AHS will have cell saver and pericardial tap supplies nearby. Throughout the extraction, our role as AHS can be critical in preparing and handling the extraction tools and equipment.

Case Completion

After all the leads have been successfully removed during the final stages of lead extraction, pocket debridement, capsule excision, and application of drain or vacuum-assisted device may be performed in selected patients. Care should be taken when X-ray detectable sponges (Ray-Tec), lap pads, or other foreign bodies are inserted into the pocket. Accounting for those abovementioned items will ensure there is no retained material within the pocket upon wound closure (**Figure 6.8**). A formal sharps, instruments, and sponge count is performed before and after wound closure. The scrub tech and circulator will confirm these surgical counts and document accordingly.

Following lead extractions procedures, AHS will consider the following: sheath status, wound closure, temporary pacing, or permanent device programming. The device nurse gives a handoff report to the receiving unit caring for the patient after the procedure. When the extraction is performed for infection indication, explanted devices and lead tips are sent for culture. Leads that are taken out for failure are sent to the company for return product analysis. Pocket swabs and tissue cultures are sent in patients with device infection. Care is taken to ensure clear and accurate labeling of the contents sent to the laboratory. The analysis results are ultimately reported to the performing physician who collaborates with infectious disease experts on formulating a final treatment plan.

Imaging from echocardiography and fluoroscopy systems are sent to the image archiving server upon completing the case. X-ray dosage data are signed and forwarded after procedure closure. AHS will ensure the images are assigned to the correct patient and procedure before transfer. Cine loops taken during the procedure are easily accessible for reviewing the case later on image archiving systems.

POSTPROCEDURAL CONSIDERATIONS

Restocking Supplies

Surgical instruments undergo sterile processing upon completion. Any additional instruments opened during this time are noted and are packaged separately for postsurgical sterile processing. The surgical staff may complete this process if the procedure is performed in the hybrid operating room. If the extraction occurs within the pacemaker lab, the AHS will clean the instruments and prepare them for sterilization through the central service. If pocket debridement requires general surgery expertise, they may often bring their own specialized sterile instrument trays. These trays are returned to them for sterilization upon case closure.

AHS should replace items used after each procedure and create a supply restocking list to ensure items are not missed from the extraction cart. Additional extraction supplies and specialty equipment should be stocked within an area of the supply room core specific to lead extraction.

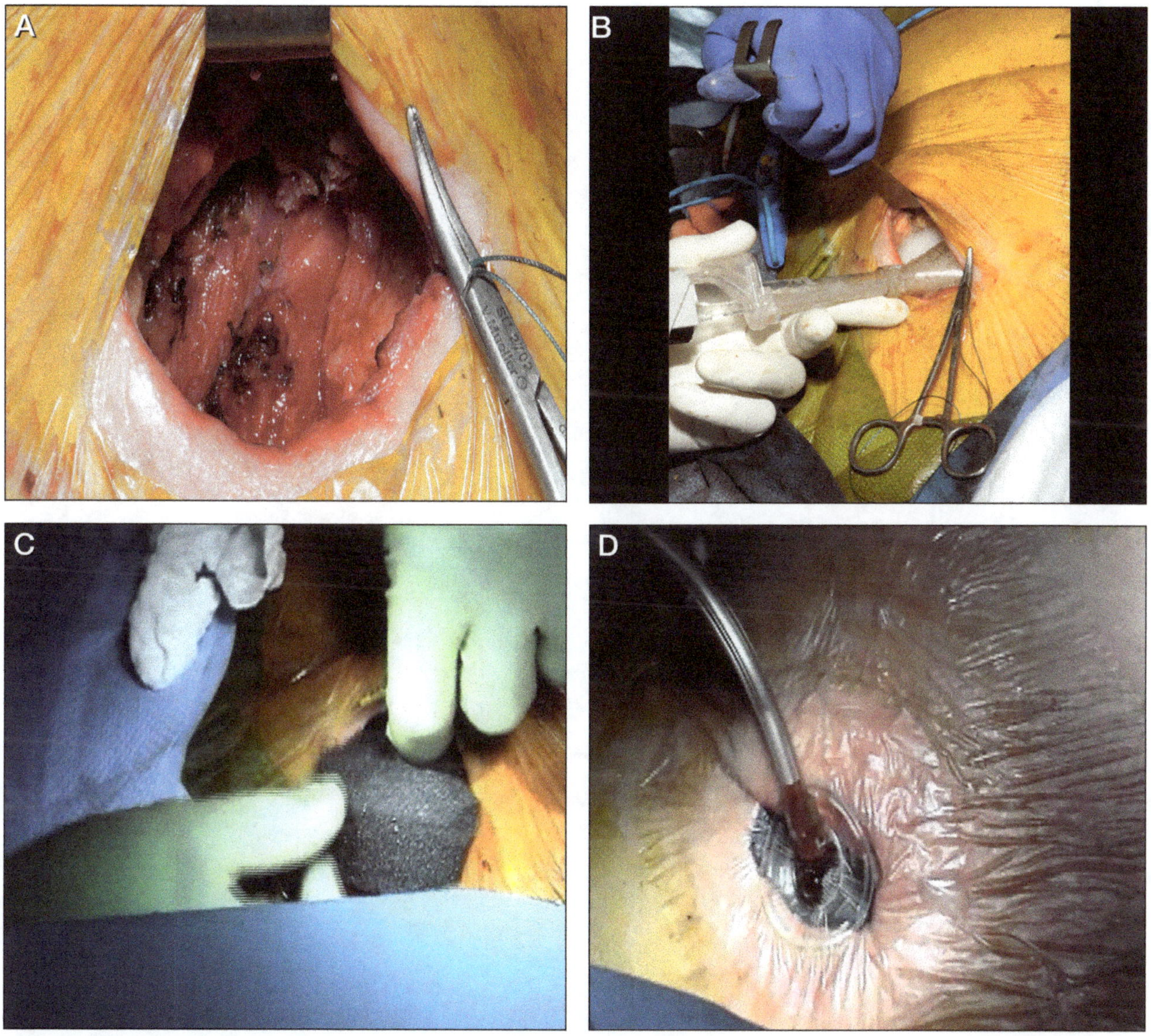

Figure 6.8 **Panel A:** A device pocket after debridement and capsulectomy. **Panel B:** Pulse irrigation used for clearing debris after extraction. **Panel C:** Sponge inserted into a pocket for negative-pressure wound therapy. **Panel D:** Vacuum-assisted suction device applied to CIED pocket.

Procedural Debriefing

A formalized debrief is carried out after every lead extraction. The purpose of the debrief is to:

- Review the overall procedure
- Highlight the positives
- Identify improvements for the future
- Help standardize workflow for pre-, intra-, and postprocedure logistics
- Allows everyone to have a voice
- Helps build the team

AHS play a crucial role in lead extraction procedures. With careful planning and desire to improve current extraction practices, we should feel comfortable sharing ideas and aim to work collaboratively to achieve the best overall outcomes for the patients undergoing lead extraction procedures.

7 | Team Collaboration and Decision Making During Lead Extraction Procedures

Siva K. Mulpuru, MD, MPH; Yong-Mei Cha, MD

CLINICAL VIGNETTE

A 70-year-old female with ischemic cardiomyopathy, obstructive sleep apnea, chronotropic incompetence, and hypertension underwent a dual-chamber dual-coil implantable cardioverter-defibrillator (ICD) implantation in 2004 for secondary prevention. She was NYHA class II functional status and was on guideline-directed medical therapy. The ICD lead was Medtronic model 6949 (Medtronic). In June 2019, the device clinic received several alerts due to high impedance and noise on the right ventricular ICD lead. Fortunately, the patient did not receive any shocks, and she presented to the clinic to discuss various management options. The patient was seen by a cardiac electrophysiologist who is 4 years out of training. The physician has a keen interest in developing the lead extraction program at the presenting hospital.

The patient was aware that the ICD lead was on advisory, and the option of extraction versus capping the old lead with the implantation of a new lead was offered to the patient. The risk of a current lead extraction procedure versus abandoning the lead, with the potential for future difficulty in extracting the abandoned lead, was carefully discussed with the patient. Eventually, the patient decided to proceed with a lead extraction procedure. A senior experienced cardiac electrophysiologist offered to help with any technical issues during the procedure.

Surgical consultation for surgical backup during the lead extraction procedure was requested. The senior cardiac surgeon on consult service suggested that he has a big surgical backlog and recommended speaking with a junior colleague. The junior cardiac surgeon reluctantly agreed to provide backup during the procedure. Due to scheduling conflicts, the patient's procedure was scheduled at 3 P.M. in the hybrid operating suite. The extraction operator had a complex ablation case before the extraction. She was brought to the operating room. After a preprocedure pause, appropriate lines were inserted for hemodynamic monitoring and fluid resuscitation. The surgical setup and the equipment were handled by the operating room technicians and not regular electrophysiology lab staff, and the team was not thrilled about doing a late case. Some degree of friction was noted between the operating room team and the electrophysiology team. The pocket was opened, and the leads were prepared with locking stylets.

A stiff wire was placed through the femoral vein in the superior vena cava (SVC) to place an SVC occlusion balloon. A transesophageal echocardiography (TEE) probe was placed for monitoring during the procedure. After confirming the surgeon and the perfusionist's presence, a 14-Fr laser sheath was placed on the prepared ICD lead. Significant adhesions were noted in the subclavian region, requiring the use of laser energy. The sheath was slowly advanced to the SVC coil. The operating charge nurse informs that there will be a shift change at 6 P.M., and she has requested the on-call team to stay to the end of the case. As the laser sheath was advanced over the proximal portion of the SVC coil, blood pressure drops. A large pericardial effusion was noted on TEE imaging.

The SVC balloon, which was on the table, was placed on the stiff wire. However, during the balloon catheter advancement, the wire was pulled back to the right atrium and could not be advanced back. Resuscitation was started immediately after recognition of hypotension, and a pericardiocentesis was attempted. The surgeon was called immediately into the room. The surgeon scrubbed in and performed an urgent sternotomy. A major tear was noted in the SVC. A massive transfusion protocol was initiated, and the patient was started on a central cardiopulmonary bypass. However, the SVC area was fragile, and the tear kept on extending. The surgeon requested additional help and the senior surgical colleague joined him for the procedure. Multiple units of packed red cells, coagulation factors were transfused during the procedure. Adequate control of bleeding was eventually achieved. The ICD lead was removed under direct visualization. The SVC region was reconstructed with pericardial graft tissue. The chest was packed due to massive tissue edema, and the patient was transferred to the ICU for monitoring. The patient did not make any neurological recovery, and a CT scan of the brain showed extensive ischemic injury. The family decided to withdraw care consistent with the patient's wishes.

DISCUSSION

This case illustrates several key points associated with decision making and planning of lead extraction procedures.

Patient Decision Making

Patients make critical decisions during their clinical care. In the clinical vignette, the patient was presented with lead extraction, or capping the old lead, and placing a new lead. After careful contemplation, she chose to proceed with the extraction procedure. A reasonable nonmedical observer may find her decision irrational given the low risks of abandoning the dysfunctional lead and placing a new lead. However, not all patient choices are based on rational reasoning. New insights from behavioral economics and psychology can help us understand how patients decide in their day-to-day medical care.

Humans utilize dual-process cognition to make decisions in their daily lives. System 1 uses a fast, high-capacity, intuitive, and less accurate cognition system, while system 2 is a slow, deliberate, precise, and quickly overwhelmed system of cognition.[1] While using system 2 (slow system) is ideal for making decisions is ideal, several systematic biases may lead an individual to make less rational decisions. Some of the pertinent biases related to patient decision making are discussed below.

- ***Present bias or hyperbolic discounting:*** Individuals place a higher value on the benefits of a decision at present compared with a decision associated with a more considerable benefit in the future.[2] The patient presented in the vignette had to make a tradeoff between the procedural risks and benefits of a current extraction procedure (certainly a low, albeit serious, present risk) versus a potential extraction procedure in the future for an indication such as device infection (uncertain occurrence with a higher but future risk). Many patients like ours may choose to undergo a lead extraction procedure due to present bias or hyperbolic discounting (**Figure 7.1**).
- ***Hot-cold empathy gap:*** This is a form of cognitive bias in which patients underestimate the analytical reasoning behind their decisions based on their emotional states (**Figure 7.2**).[3] Many patients are presented with a lead extraction option after they had noise detected on their leads, remote monitoring alerts of impending shocks, or delivery of inappropriate therapies (emotionally charged or "hot" state). Their decisions could be potentially different when they can think through their options in an emotionally neutral or "cold" state.

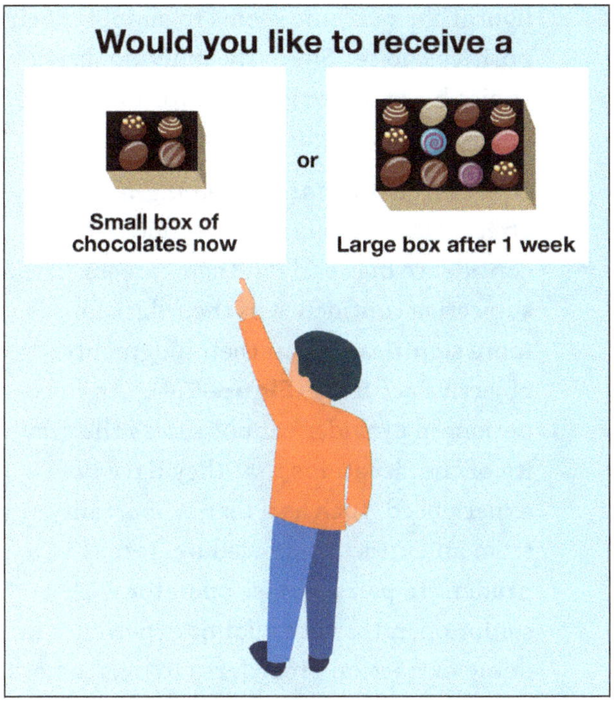

Figure 7.1 Present bias or hyperbolic discounting: When an individual is given a choice of current benefit compared to more considerable future benefit, many tend to choose the current benefit.

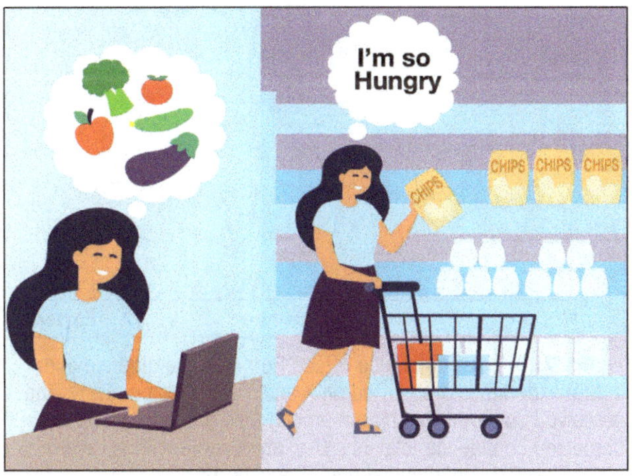

Figure 7.2 Hot-cold empathy gap: The decisions we make depend on the background emotional state. Individuals may aspire (cold state) to eat healthy choices, but they may end up buying unhealthy options when they are hungry (hot state).

- ***Loss aversion:*** Individuals tend to make decisions that focus on avoiding losses than making potential gains.[4] Twice as much weight is given to avoiding losses compared to potential gains. The lead extraction providers most likely frame the clinical procedures in terms of risks than potential benefits as it is easy to comprehend the risks associated with the extraction of a lead with an extended dwell time compared to an intangible (less quantifiable) benefit of extracting the lead now to minimize the risk associated with a future risky procedure.
- ***Bounded theory and decision fatigue:*** Patients with defibrillators have chronic conditions, and they often experience decision fatigue (**Figure 7.3**) after deciding on their medical management. Bounded rationality proposes that people have limited cognitive resources, and they do not usually review all the available information before making their decisions.[5] They often use rules of thumb or mental shortcuts (heuristics) to accept the presented option as satisfactory. Decision fatigue (friction between teams and nurses informing the operator about shift change) can also impair the operator's cognition during the procedure.

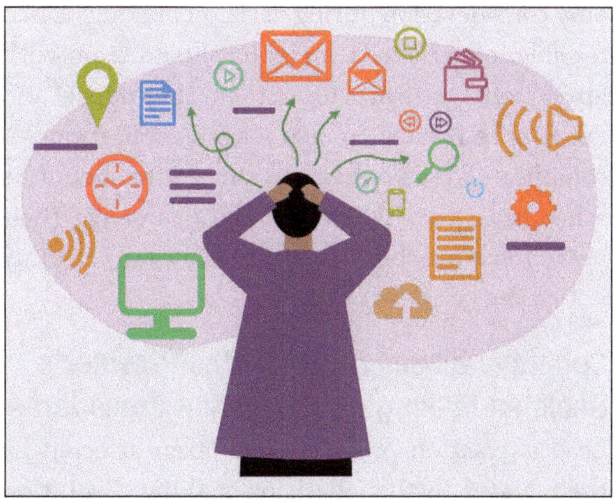

Figure 7.3 Decision fatigue: Patients and the providers are often provided with lots of choices. When the cognition systems are overwhelmed, individuals make decisions by rules of thumb.

As providers, we must be aware of these psychological processes for decision making and their potential biases and educate and counsel patients to make decisions that align with their values accurately.

Team Preparedness for the Extraction Procedure

Lead extraction procedures are often scheduled in the hybrid operating room with the surgical team as backup. Many surgeons consider that a complication or mortality from lead extraction may adversely affect their reported mortality rates and are less willing to provide surgical backup.[6] In particular, high-volume surgeons are reluctant to provide surgical backup because there is no additional reimbursement for the surgical team's time devoted to the procedure, and the procedures are sometimes scheduled later in the day, as seen in our patient. The task is thus often relegated to a junior surgical colleague, who may not have experience in repairing a significant vascular tear.

It is imperative to have coherent teams (dedicated cardiovascular surgeon, extraction operator, and allied health staff (AHS) working together) to have optimal outcomes from lead extraction procedures. Discussions should happen at the leadership level to create seamless workflows that keep the patient's interests as the only consideration during decision making. When feasible, experienced surgeons should team with junior colleagues providing them the counsel and experience needed to deal with complications. A complicated lead extraction procedure should be scheduled when the team's abilities are at their best, which may be earlier in the day and certainly not as the last case of the day.

Cognitive Biases Affecting the Provider's Decision Making for Extraction Procedures

Lead extraction providers are often affected by their biases in their decision making. Cognition biases are defined as a systematic deviation from rational or ideal cognition.

- ***Choice-supportive bias:*** In the previously described vignette, the provider was interested in developing a lead extraction program at the presenting hospital. Providers are likely to frame a procedure in a positive light if the outcome seems to support their positive choice.[7] Similarly, individuals with choice bias tend to ignore information that opposes their firmly held viewpoints.
- ***Overconfidence bias or Dunning-Kruger effect:*** Many providers are prone to overconfidence bias early in their careers. Their subjective confidence in their decisions is more significant than their judgments' objective accuracy (**Figure 7.4**).[8] An inexperienced provider cannot assess the gravity of the situations that they have not experienced, such as a tear or mortality from an extraction procedure. It may be prudent to pair a novice operator with a senior operator with a lot of experience in doing extraction procedures to overcome this particular bias.

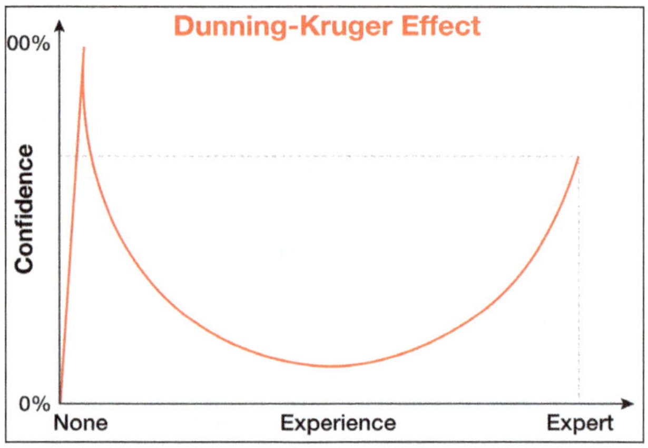

Figure 7.4 Overconfidence effect: Perceived confidence and actual experience are plotted on X and Y axes, respectively. The perceived confidence is higher among new proceduralists. The perceived confidence follows a U-shaped curve with an eventual higher level of confidence among the experts.

Teamwork

The quality of the care involving teamwork can be understood by the framework proposed by Avedis Donabedian[9] (**Figure 7.5**). The framework assesses how care was delivered (structure), what was done during care (process), and what happened during care (outcomes). The process part of the model encompasses the team care model and communication dynamics between the team members. The enduring principles of well-functioning teams include shared goals, clear values, mutual trust, effective communication, and measurable processes and outcomes.[10] Structured tools such as Team Strategies & Tools to Enhance Performance & Patient Safety (TeamSTEPPS) can be effectively used to improve teamwork and communication skills.[11]

Mental Skills Training for the Proceduralist

Daniel Spoon and colleagues presented a mental skills training framework drawing from sports psychology for providers performing invasive cardiology procedures (**Figure 7.6**).[12] We believe that such a framework is pertinent for high-risk procedures such as lead extraction. The following are components of building blocks in their framework.

- ***Mental toughness.*** The authors propose four constructs:
  - Control: Handle many critical tasks during an emergency. The operator was unable to advance the SVC occlusion balloon over the wire in the presented vignette.
  - Commitment: Pursuit of excellence and constant push to improve patient outcomes.
  - Challenge: Consider problems as opportunities for growth.
  - Confidence: Belief in one's skills despite setbacks.

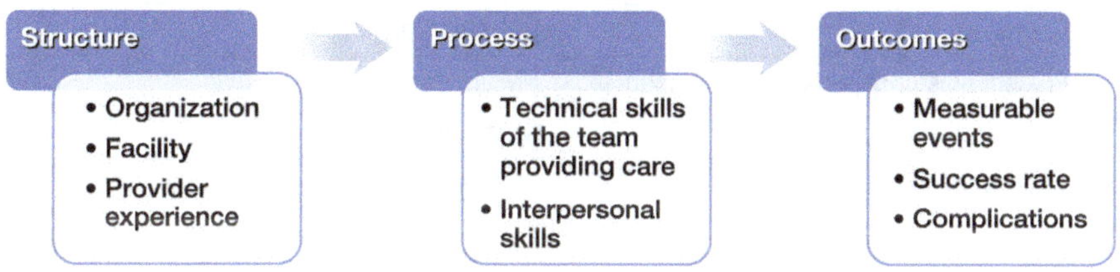

Figure 7.5 Quality of care for lead extraction procedures.

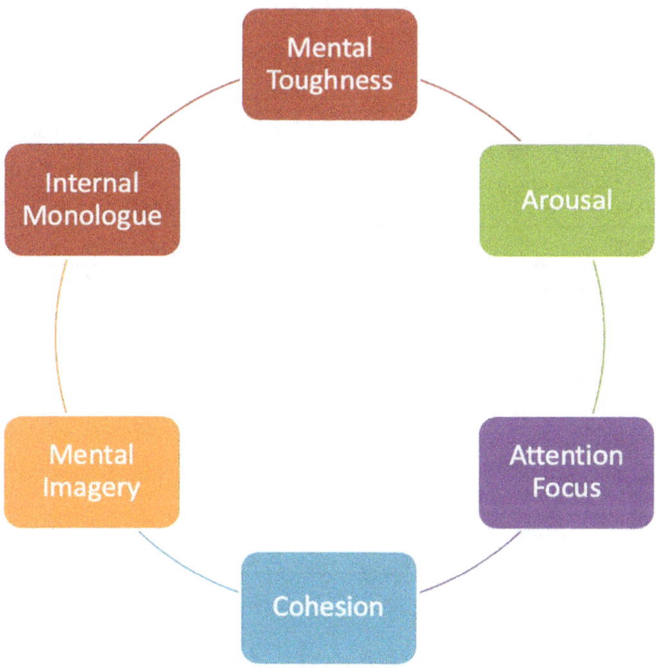

Figure 7.6 Building blocks of mental skills training for lead extraction proceduralists.

- ***Arousal.*** Moderate arousal may lead to optimal outcomes, while high levels of stress may impair provider performance during the procedure.
- ***Attention and focus.*** The ability to concentrate on the task at hand involves minimizing distractions. The vignette presented several interruptions due to friction between the team members and a shift change message from the nursing team.
- ***Internal monologue.*** The ability to maintain or verbalize positive thoughts during stressful events is associated with less anxiety, better performance, and higher self-confidence levels.
- ***Mental imagery (mental simulation).*** Picturing oneself during a challenging situation and devising plans to solve issues at hand effectively.
- ***Cohesion.*** Interpersonal connectedness between team members sharing a common goal. The clinical vignette presented has illustrated team dynamics (junior surgeon assigned to the case) and effective communication (friction between team members).

Lead extraction procedures are one of the highest-risk procedures performed in cardiac electrophysiology. Understanding the importance of patient and provider decision making as well as team expertise, dynamics, and interpersonal communication is crucial for good patient outcomes (**Table 7.1**).

Table 7.1 Summary of learning points from the case

Factor	Problem	Mitigation
Patient decision making	Present bias or hyperbolic discounting	Make patient aware of bias
	Hot-cold empathy gap	May give additional time
	Loss aversion bias	Make the patient aware of bias
	Bounded theory/decision fatigue	Convey information in stages
Scheduling conflicts	Suboptimal scheduling (later in the day/ fewer resources)	Assess for signs of overload
		Perform complex cases earlier in day
		Stronger norms of reciprocity
		Enhance team collaboration
Cognitive bias affecting the proceduralists	Choice bias	Aim to provide an unbiased position
	Overconfidence bias	Team up with experienced collegue
Teamwork	Shared goals	Better outcomes should be the goal
	Clear roles	Simulation/role play
	Mutual trust	Team-building activities
	Effective communication	Continous refinement of skills
	Measurable processes and outcomes	Continous performance improvement
Mental skill-building blocks for the proceduralist	Mental toughness	Adequate stress management
	Arousal	
	Attention focus	
	Cohesion	
	Mental imagery	
	Internal monologue	

REFERENCES

1. Kahneman D. *Thinking, fast and slow*. Macmillan; 2011.
2. Rice T. The behavioral economics of health and health care. *Annu Rev Public Health*. 2013;34: 431–447.
3. Loewenstein G. Hot-cold empathy gaps and medical decision making. *Health Psychol.* 2005;24(4, Suppl): S49–S56.
4. Kahneman D, Tversky A. Prospect theory: An analysis of decision under risk. In: *Handbook of the Fundamentals of Financial Decision Making: Part I.* World Scientific. 2013:99–127.
5. Tierney J. Do you suffer from decision fatigue. *The New York Times.* 2011.
6. Shahian DM, Jacobs JP, Badhwar V, D'Agostino RS, Bavaria JE, Prager RL. Risk aversion and public reporting. part 1: Observations from cardiac surgery and interventional cardiology. *Ann Thorac Surg.* 2017;104(6):2093–2101.
7. Blumenthal-Barby JS, Krieger H. Cognitive biases and heuristics in medical decision making: A critical review using a systematic search strategy. *Med Decis Making.* 2015;35(4): 539–557.
8. Berner ES, Graber ML. Overconfidence as a cause of diagnostic error in medicine. *Am J Med.* 2008;121(5): S2–S23.
9. Donabedian A. Evaluating the quality of medical care. *Millbank Q.* 2005;83(4):691.
10. Mitchell P, Golden R. *Core Principles & Values of Effective Team-Based Health Care.* National Academy of Sciences; 2012.
11. King HB, Battles J, Baker DP, et al. TeamSTEPPS™: Team strategies and tools to enhance performance and patient safety. In: *Advances in Patient Safety: New Directions and Alternative Approaches (Vol. 3: Performance and Tools).* Agency For Healthcare Research and Quality (US); 2008.
12. Spoon DB, Vickers KS, Alkhouli M. Mental skills training in cardiology. *J Am Coll Cardiol.* 2020;76(16):1905–1909.

8 Surgical Management of Bleeding Complications Associated with Transvenous Lead Extraction

Bradley Genovese, MD; Travis Pollema, DO

INTRODUCTION

Transvenous lead extraction (TLE) has become an increasingly common procedure as part of the treatment algorithm for cardiac implantable electronic devices and lead management. Although it is performed with increasing frequency, it can still portend a significant morbidity or mortality risk for patients who experience vascular or cardiac injuries. The injuries can range from minor bleeding and hematomas to life-threatening, catastrophic tears or perforations of the great vessels or heart leading to tamponade and death. For this reason, it is the recommendation from the 2017 HRS expert consensus on lead management that a cardiothoracic surgeon be immediately available for surgical intervention if the principal operator is not a surgeon.[1] Vascular and cardiac injuries have been previously categorized by their size and also by their hemodynamic presentation.[2] This is clinically important for centrally located injuries, but little has been described about injuries and their management along the course of the entire lead. This chapter will describe potential injuries and their surgical repair during lead extraction cases from the lead post to the lead tip. Anatomic locations include the subclavian vein, innominate vein, superior vena cava (SVC), right atrium, tricuspid valve, right ventricle, and the coronary sinus.

POCKET/SUBCLAVIAN VEIN

Vascular injuries during the creation or exploration of the deltopectoral pocket are infrequent. They may arise from the lead tract's aggressive dissection under the clavicle or removal of a suture sleeve placed near the subclavian vein. The most common and unavoidable vascular injury at the pocket or subclavian vein level is the entrance site for the extraction tool. Both laser and mechanical tools create a venotomy of 12 Fr to 16 Fr. This tract can be easily controlled with a vicryl purse-string that can be gently tied down following the completion of the lead removal or reimplantation (**Figure 8.1**).

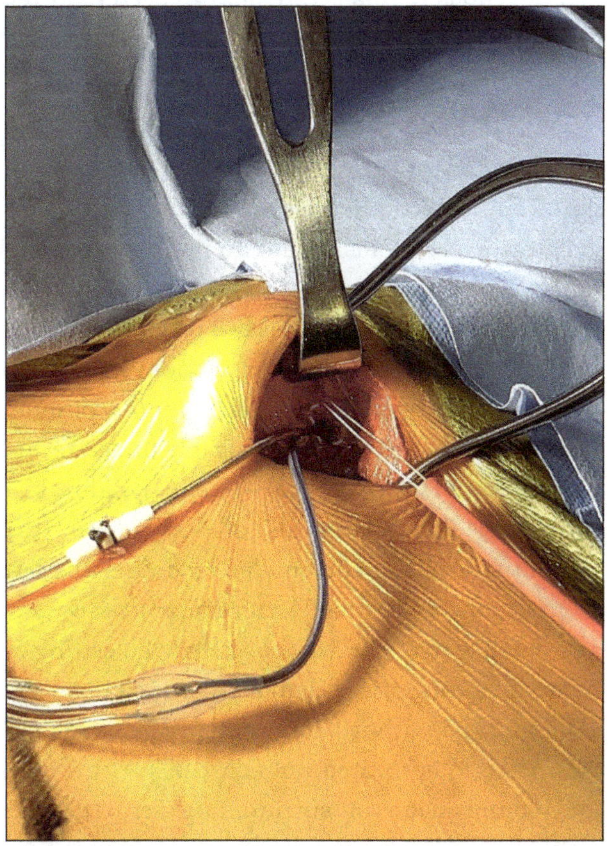

Figure 8.1 Vicryl purse-string suture around the lead track and entry site for a powered sheath.

If the subclavian vein has been inadvertently exposed, mobilization and primary repair of the anterior vessel wall may need to be performed.

Cardiac Lead Extraction: A Case-Based Contemporary Approach.
 ISBN: 978-1-942909-54-5

This can usually be accomplished with 5-0 or 6-0 prolene sutures in a running two-layered fashion. If the injury defect is large (> 50% of vessel circumference) and primary repair is likely to cause stenosis, a patch repair can be performed with bovine pericardium or an extracellular matrix. An injury to the subclavian vein's posterior wall is uncommon but can occur during the use of a laser-powered or mechanical sheath. The patient may develop sudden hypovolemia and hypotension with new left pleural effusion on echocardiogram or fluoroscopy. Distal subclavian vein injuries are best approached through supraclavicular or infraclavicular exposure, while more proximal subclavian vein injuries can be approached via median sternotomy. Isolated injury to the subclavian artery or arteriovenous fistula is rare but has been reported and been managed with an endovascular approach.[3]

INNOMINATE VEIN

In many patients presenting for TLE, the innominate vein is found to have significant stenosis or even complete occlusion due to multiple indwelling leads or previous catheter/device interventions. These situations usually require larger caliber tools for successful extraction. Injuries to the innominate vein are likely more common than one would expect but probably under-recognized due to lack of clinical or hemodynamic significance. For nearly all of its course, the innominate vein is surrounded by soft tissue left from thymic involution. This remnant tissue acts as a defense to minimize the extent of bleeding or hematoma formation. Hemodynamic changes are also minimal with isolated innominate vein injuries since it is located outside the pericardium, and compression of surrounding structures is unlikely. Incidental innominate vein injuries are often identified during a left-arm venogram if performed following TLE. Contrast extravasation is usually present but contained. In more extensive injuries, it is not uncommon to see contrast extravasation tracked along the course of the vein toward the SVC and terminate outside the pericardium (**Figure 8.2**).

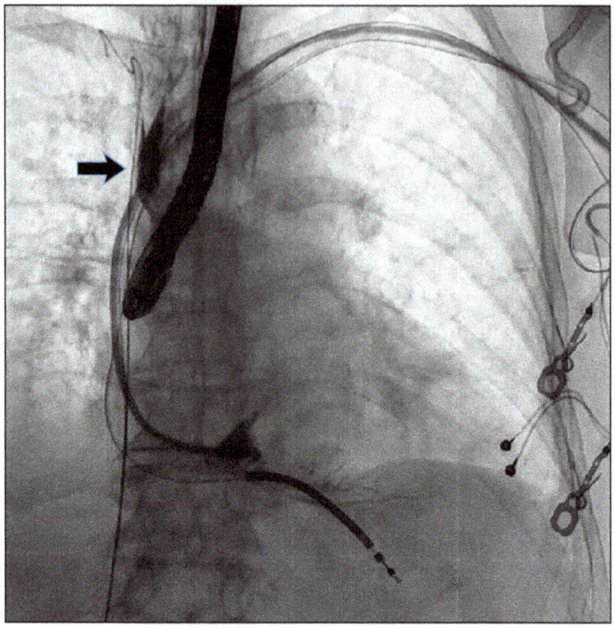

Figure 8.2 Contrast extravasation (**black arrow**) tracking along innominate vein from injury and stopped by pericardial reflection.

Isolated innominate vein injuries can be managed conservatively and are not likely to cause harm to the patient. In patients with prior stenosis or occlusion, a network of venous collaterals is expected to be present, which will minimize left arm swelling complications.

Should the patient have a concomitant venous or cardiac injury during the same TLE procedure requiring emergent sternotomy, or if an innominate vein injury is unknown or not expected, it is important to avoid opening the superior extent of the thymic remnant. Aggressive dissection in the mediastinum's superior portion can expose a self-contained hematoma that will now bleed freely. During a sternotomy for cardiac tamponade, opening the pericardium just enough to have a possible cannulation site for cardiopulmonary bypass (CPB) will avoid unwanted innominate vein bleeding. If an injury is exposed, the type of repair depends on the amount of vessel wall involved or complete disruption. Smaller partial wall injuries can be repaired by primary repair with prolene sutures in two layers. Larger partial wall defects involving half of the vessel are best treated with patch repair similar to the subclavian vein, provided the remainder of the vessel wall's integrity is amenable to suturing. The surrounding tissue can often be used to buttress the sutures and repair them to give another layer of coverage and strength. For vessels that are entirely disrupted, an end-to-end interposition graft with ringed PTFE may be necessary (**Figure 8.3**).

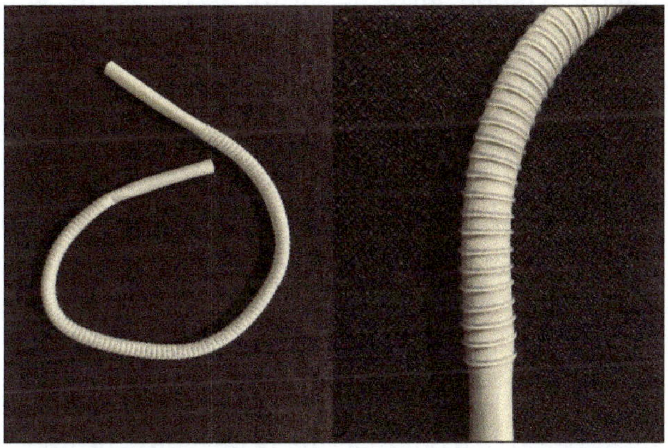

Figure 8.3 Ringed PTFE graft for vessel bypass or interposition.

The graft size is typically between 12–14 mm. A ringed graft is chosen here as excess length may lead to kinking, especially since the repair is performed with an open chest, and space will decrease during reapproximation of the sternotomy. This repair depends on finding the uninjured proximal and distal portions of the injury and controlling them to prevent ongoing bleeding. If suitable ends for graft are not present, the final option for managing this injury is vessel interruption by oversewing the ends and leaving the vein in discontinuity.

Every attempt should be made to manage innominate vein injuries conservatively, and if a sternotomy is performed, limiting dissection in the thymic remnant will help avoid uncovering a potential injury.

SUPERIOR VENA CAVA

The most common injury during TLE, and the best-described, is the SVC injury. The lethal nature of this injury has prompted the development of an endovascular Bridge Occlusion Balloon (Philips Medical) to help temporize the patient in hopes of a more controlled repair and decreased associated mortality (**Figure 8.4**).[4] It is an 80-mm conformable balloon with a diameter of 20 mm when inflated. It is typically staged in the SVC-right atrial junction from the common femoral vein through a 12-Fr sheath over a stiff 0.035-in wire. It has a maximum inflation volume of 60 mL but typically requires 20 mL to provide venous occlusion in an average-sized patient.

The presentation of a SVC injury is based on the location of the injury. The distal two-thirds portion of the SVC is extrapericardial, and the lateral wall's injury can cause bleeding into the right pleural space. Hypovolemia and hypotension will ensue, and a new right pleural effusion will be present. The proximal SVC is

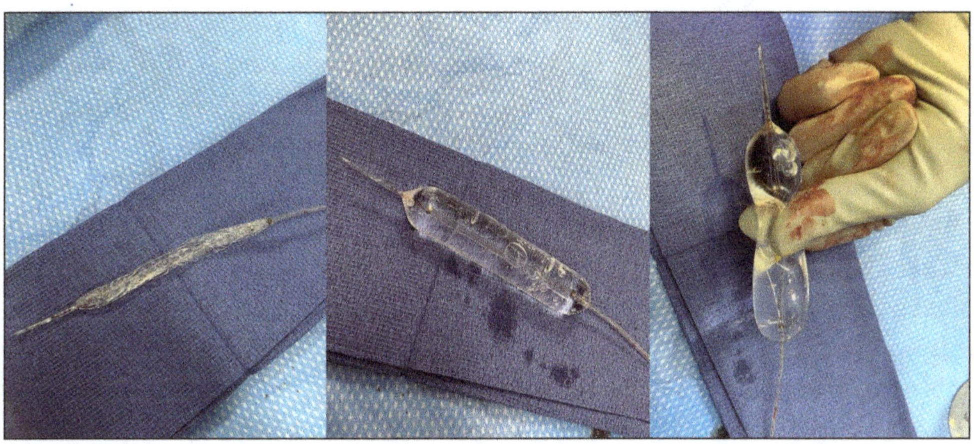

Figure 8.4 **Left Panel:** Deflated occlusion balloon. **Middle Panel:** A balloon filled with contrast. **Right Panel:** Balloon conformability.

intrapericardial, and an injury here will present with tamponade, the quickness of which is determined by the injury size.

Hypotension and new pericardial effusion can be rapid. The first step in management is suspecting or recognizing the injury. Confirming the findings of hypotension by transesophageal echocardiogram (TEE) findings should be quick and followed immediately by the deployment of the endovascular occlusion balloon and resuscitative measures by anesthesiology. If the patient can be stabilized, a pericardial window or pericardiocentesis can be considered to alleviate the impending tamponade. If the patient is unstable despite balloon deployment and resuscitative efforts, an immediate sternotomy is required. A cell saver collection system is ideal since a large amount of blood loss is likely, but sternotomy should not be delayed to obtain one. After sternotomy, the pericardium will appear blue and tense. Entrance will likely reveal a large amount of blood under pressure and impair the ability to identify the exact location or size of the injury. If the occlusion balloon is deployed correctly, evacuation of the pericardial effusion should restore hemodynamics. If the injury is extensive and the balloon cannot occlude the site, ongoing bleeding will be present and immediate packing of the SVC region should be performed. Packing may slow the blood loss, at which time the injury can be controlled with vascular clamps. Large and complex injuries that cannot be controlled can be dealt with using cardiopulmonary bypass for hemodynamic support and better blood salvage. Patients are typically cannulated centrally if no previous cardiac surgery has been performed and peripherally in the common femoral artery and vein if the patient has had a previous sternotomy.

Injuries to the SVC during TLE are usually linear and range from small subcentimeter perforations to large, complex linear disruptions with extensive tissue loss. For bleeding to escalate to a large pericardial effusion and cardiac tamponade, a full-thickness injury within the pericardium must be present. Since the venous injuries can vary so much, repair of the SVC depends on the extent and location of the injury and the amount of vessel involved. If hemodynamic stability can be achieved, primary or patch repair can be performed with the endovascular occlusion balloon in place, provided there is minimal or no ongoing blood loss. Care must be taken to avoid puncturing the balloon with the suture needle as this will cause loss of control of the injury. If proximal and distal control of the injury can be obtained, the balloon can be removed. Sometimes the injury originates from above the pericardial reflection. The superior portion of the pericardium needs to be opened to complete the repair to the extrapericardial SVC. A repair performed with the endovascular occlusion balloon in place or with the vessel controlled with vascular clamps or snares must be carried out in a timely fashion. The upper extremities and head will not have venous drainage during this time. This will lead to elevated venous pressures upstream from the site of occlusion. Patients with chronic occlusions of the innominate vein may already have a network of venous collaterals in place, but they may still drain to the azygous vein, which would still be upstream from the injury site. Patients without venous occlusions are unlikely to have a venous collateral system. Significant elevations in the central venous pressure (CVP), and in turn, the cerebral venous system can lead to brain edema and further neurological insult. Diuretics are useful postoperatively to counter this change in physiology, and some have argued for continued anticoagulation following surgery.[5]

If control of the injury cannot be obtained, a repair with the vessel open can be performed after instituting CPB and using cardiotomy suction to salvage ongoing blood loss. In a series by Bashir et al., almost all large injuries (> 20 mm) required CPB to complete repair.[2] An open repair using cardiotomy suction allows for decompression of the upper extremities and cerebral venous system as no clamp or snare is placed on the SVC distal to the injury. If the ongoing bleeding is too much for the cardiotomy suction to control, a vent can be placed into the SVC through the injury and snared for control. Alternatively, if there is room on the SVC distal to the injury, a small, right-angled cannula can be placed directly into the SVC and snared for control as in any cardiac operation requiring bi-caval cannulation. The SVC proximal to the injury may need to be controlled to prevent air from entraining into the right atrial cannula and causing an airlock to the CPB circuit. This can also be alleviated by percutaneous femoral venous cannulation and snaring the inferior vena cava (IVC)–right atrial junction or having the perfusionist place the venous drainage cannula on vacuum suction temporarily.

In extremely devastating injuries to the SVC that usually involve large amounts of the vessel wall, extend for great distances, involve the innominate–SVC or azygous–SVC junctions, satisfactory repairs may not be possible without the use of deep hypothermic circulatory arrest. In these situations, cannulation or distal control of the injury is not achievable, or circumferential repair with an interposition graft may be required. SVC replacement with an interposition graft is typically performed with a non-ringed PTFE graft ranging in caliber between 18–20 mm. Historically, a spiral graft has also been used as a conduit for central venous replacement. This involves the harvest of the greater saphenous vein and opening it completely in a longitudinal fashion. It is then sewn into a cylinder around a chest tube or syringe using 5-0 prolene sutures. This is a time-consuming creation and also requires the legs to have been prepped into the sterile field.

As the range of presentation and severity of SVC injuries can be wide, so are the techniques and options available to treat the most minor and even the most severe problems.

RIGHT ATRIUM AND RIGHT VENTRICLE

Implanted leads can be found to have adhesions to the free wall of the right atrium as they course towards the right atrial appendage or right ventricle. Excessive lead slack is likely a contributor as the leads are more likely to follow their course's greater curvature. This is especially true for leads that appear to hug the lateral atrial wall or loop down toward the IVC on chest X-ray (CXR). This configuration often leads to another point of adhesion development where the leads are in contact with tissue, which would not be the case with a lead in the middle of a vessel or chamber.

Leads can also be attached to the tricuspid valve leaflets or sometimes unknowingly placed through the subvalvular apparatus. By design, the leads will have some degree of adhesion to the right ventricle myocardium as this is necessary for their proper function, particularly with passive fixation leads. The RV lead may be placed at the free wall, although the intended destination is the septum.

Injuries to the right atrial wall will present as a new and possibly expanding pericardial effusion. The degree of hemodynamic compromise will depend on the size of the injury. Smaller injuries in patients with new pericardial effusion but stable hemodynamics can be managed first by pericardiocentesis or subxiphoid pericardial window and drain placement. The patient can then be monitored for ongoing bleeding by tracking the drain output. The continued output from the pericardial drain is best addressed through a median sternotomy. A right anterolateral thoracotomy is also an option but may limit visualization and repair depending on the location of the injury. Injury to the right atrial wall is often controllable with packing or direct pressure. With bleeding controlled, a repair can usually be performed without CPB. A primary repair in two layers with 5-0 prolene sutures should be satisfactory for small injuries. Injuries of moderate size or with very thin atrial walls may need to be reinforced with pericardium or pledget material. Larger injuries can be treated with a patch repair technique using pericardium or an extracellular matrix, but this will likely require CPB.

Injuries to the right atrial appendage occur when there is difficulty in removing the right atrial lead tip. Atrial appendage injury should be suspected when a pericardial effusion develops after freeing the lead tip, certainly, in situations where a powered sheath was necessary to dislodge the lead at its distal end. These injuries are often smaller and easy to control since the atrial appendage can be clamped with no consequence, but unfortunately, a median sternotomy is usually required for repair. CPB should not be needed to control and repair an atrial appendage injury unless a more complex injury has occurred along the lead course.

An injury to the right ventricle myocardium typically involves the free wall and is related to some degree of lead perforation. This can range from an unknown micro-perforation or lead tip protruding into epicardial fat to a known grossly perforated lead in the pericardial space. The right ventricle wall is thicker than the right atrial wall, and therefore, more likely to self-seal a small perforation or lead tract. Injury to the right ventricle free wall can also be related to using powered sheaths to remove deeply imbedded lead tips, in which case the injury is caused by the sheath or by traction during lead removal. These injuries are likely to be larger than lead perforations and may not self-seal. In this case, a pericardial effusion will likely develop. Identification and monitoring of the effusion by TEE are necessary. An intervention can be started with pericardiocentesis or pericardial window and escalated if necessary in the event of an expanding effusion and evidence of tamponade. Usually, bleeding from a right ventricle injury is not as profuse as an SVC or atrial injury. It can be monitored for ongoing bleeding if a window or drain is present. Some injuries to the right ventricle can be visualized and repaired through a subxiphoid incision by proper retraction of the distal sternal body. Simple suture repair without pledget material is often enough to close a right ventricle perforation or injury. If the injury cannot be visualized through the subxiphoid incision or a pericardiocentesis drain was used, monitoring the output for a period of time can be done prior to the decision for sternotomy. If sternotomy is required for a right ventricle injury, cardiopulmonary bypass is typically not needed for control and repair. Direct pressure to the injury can be used to control bleeding while a suture repair using a 4-0 or 5-0 prolene suture is performed. If the surrounding tissue is weak or friable, pledget material can be used to buttress the repair, or a topical hemostatic patch can be applied for reinforcement.

Right ventricular leads can also present with known gross perforation of the lead with or without existing pericardial effusion. A CXR can raise suspicion of a lead perforation, but a computed tomography scan or echocardiogram can be confirmatory.

Perforated leads can often be extracted safely without untoward patient consequences. However, they can also lead to bleeding and tamponade. The extractor must be prepared for this scenario and plan for drainage and surgical repair if necessary. When no pericardial effusion is present, perforated leads can be extracted as usual. If the primary extractor is not a cardiothoracic surgeon, one should be immediately available to support the case in the event of bleeding. A TEE should be utilized during the procedure to monitor for new and enlarging pericardial effusion. If present, pericardiocentesis drain placement or subxiphoid window and evacuation should be performed. Ongoing bleeding can be monitored in a stable patient to determine the need for surgical repair. Some perforation injuries can be repaired through a subxiphoid window incision, while others may require a sternotomy.

Perforated leads present with a pericardial effusion should be treated with drainage of the pericardial space prior to proceeding with TLE. If a perforated lead is removed in the presence of a pericardial effusion, new or ongoing bleeding is hard to quantify even by echocardiogram. Also, there is less room for expansion before reaching tamponade physiology and hemodynamic compromise. A subxiphoid window and pericardial drain placement with a 24-Fr 4-channel drain in the window or 7-Fr pigtail catheter retained in the pericardium can be performed prior to TLE. The fluid quality can be assessed and, if bloody in nature, should raise suspicion for more bleeding following lead removal. Through the subxiphoid incision, the right ventricle can be visualized and inspected for the perforated lead. Identifying the lead prior to TLE can allow for repair prior to lead removal. This can be performed with 4-0 or 5-0 prolene suture in purse-string or figure-eight fashion. The pericardial space can be irrigated following lead removal and repair and then monitored for ongoing bleeding.

TRICUSPID VALVE

Tricuspid valve injury leading to tricuspid regurgitation (TR) at the time of lead extraction is a complication that merits further discussion. The majority of tricuspid injuries at the time of lead extraction are silent. However, the operator and team must be able to recognize changes in valvular function. Intervention to the tricuspid valve at the time of TLE is typically not warranted unless a concomitant venous injury requires sternotomy. With TEE imaging, the incidence of TR after lead extraction may be as high as 9%.[6] Injury to the tricuspid valve is due to disruption of the fibrotic adhesions between the lead(s) and tricuspid valve apparatus. This can lead to leaflet perforation/avulsion, prolapse, or chordal or papillary rupture. The risks for postoperative TR are as follows: leads due to pacemaker system rather than defibrillator, the advanced age of right ventricular lead and a combined age of right ventricular leads, extraction of more than 3 right ventricular lead or use of more than 2 extraction tools.[7] The majority of postprocedural TR is graded trace to mild, with a small subset reaching moderate to severe TR. Although most cases are observed with serial echocardiograms, medical management is reserved for patients with elevated right-sided pressures leading to symptoms. Surgical management is indicated in severe TR with right ventricular failure not able to be medically managed.

Approaching the tricuspid valve for urgent or emergent repair is best performed through a median sternotomy. Bi-caval cannulation and arresting the heart with cardioplegia is performed to optimize visualization. A right atriotomy is then performed. The valve is inspected. The septal and posterior leaflets are more susceptible to injury given their anatomic position. The goal should be to reconstruct the valve rather than replacement whenever possible. The three fundamental principles of tricuspid valve reconstruction are to restore or preserve full leaflet mobility, provide a large surface of leaflet coaptation, and remodel and stabilize the annulus. Our armamentarium of techniques to repair the tricuspid valve comes from our experience with mitral valve repair. As meant by Carpentier,[8] the various findings on inspection of the surgical technique employed leading to severe TR are as follows:

- ***Leaflet perforation or tear:*** A tear or perforation of the leaflet first involves resection of nonviable tissue, leaving at least a 2-mm ridge of normal tissue. Primary repair may be attempted if distortion is limited; otherwise, the leaflet is patched using glutaraldehyde-treated autologous pericardium or extracellular matrix. A ring annuloplasty is usually indicated as an adjunct procedure to stabilize the valve apparatus. If the posterior leaflet is severely damaged and cannot be salvaged, a bicuspidization technique can be performed. This is a palliative technique that plicates the posterior segment of the annulus and the corresponding posterior leaflet.
- ***Limited chordae rupture or chordae elongation:*** Triangular resection can be performed if it involves less than 10% of the surface

area; otherwise, patching is necessary to avoid distortion.

- ***Extensive prolapse:*** Resection of damaged leaflet tissue and restoration of leaflet continuity by annular plication and leaflet reapproximation or patching as discussed above.
- ***Chordae rupture:*** Chordae transposition using adjacent leaflet or artificial chordae for stabilization.
- ***Papillary muscle rupture:*** Reimplantation of the papillary muscle can be performed by reapproximating the viable fibrous cuff attached to chordae into an adjacent muscle or the septum.

CORONARY SINUS

Injury to the coronary sinus during TLE is rare despite the delicate nature and small caliber of the vessel. Major injury requiring surgical repair has been reported in a case report to extract an active fixation coronary sinus lead.[6] Repair of an injury to the coronary sinus is complicated by its location in the atrioventricular groove. Its location is on the posterior aspect of the heart near the base. Performing a repair in this location requires the heart to be elevated out of the chest, leading to hemodynamic compromise. If the ongoing bleeding is controlled, an off-pump suction device can be used to elevate the heart without compromising hemodynamics. A repair can be performed with 5-0 or 6-0 prolene sutures. If ongoing bleeding is too much or the patient is hemodynamically unstable, CPB should be instituted to support the patient and aid in blood salvage and repair.

Injuries during a TLE can vary widely in terms of location, presentation, approach, and management. Intervention can range from observation to emergent sternotomy and the use of CPB for repair. **Table 8.1** gives a summary of common injury locations and their management.

Table 8.1 Summary of injury location, presentation, and repair approach

	Injury	Presentation	Response	Approach	Repair
Pocket/subclavian vein	Sheath entry	Not HD significant		Via pocket	Purse-string
	Posterior wall injury	Hypovolemia/left pleural effusion	Volume, transfusion	Infraclavicular or supraclavicular, sternotomy	Primary or patch repair
Innominate vein	Laser or mechanical sheath exposed during sternotomy	Not HD significant			Primary or patch repair, interposition graft
		Significant bleeding in superior mediastinum	CPB if unable to control	Sternotomy	
Superior vena cava	Extra-pericardial	Hypovolemic shock/new right pleural effusion	Volume, transfusion, occlusion balloon	Sternotomy	Primary or patch repair
	Intra-pericardial	Cardiac tamponade	Volume, transfusion, pressor, occlusion balloon	Sternotomy +/– CPB	Primary or patch repair, interposition graft
Right atrium	Small or lead perforation	New stable or enlarging pericardial effusion	Volume monitor echo	Pericardiocentesis or window	Primary or patch repair
	Large lead perforation	Cardiac tamponade	Volume, transfusion, pressor	Sternotomy +/– CPB	Primary or patch repair
Right ventricle/ tricuspid valve	Lead perforation	None to new effusion	Volume, monitor echo	Subxiphoid window	Primary repair
	Leaflet/chord rupture	New regurgitation	Repair if opening for other injury	Sternotomy, CPB	Reconstruction preferred
Coronary sinus	Perforation or tear	None to new effusion	Volume, monitor echo	Pericardial window Sternotomy +/–	Primary repair

SUMMARY POINTS

TLE has been proven to be a safe and effective method with low morbidity. However, recognition and management of complications are vital. Injuries to venous and cardiac structures during TLE can vary widely from silent injuries that pose no ongoing harm to the patient to complex, devastating injuries that can be life-threatening if not treated immediately.

- A multidisciplinary team of anesthesia, cardiothoracic surgery, perfusion, and electrophysiology is essential to patient safety and procedural success.
- Preoperative imaging can identify problematic areas that may arise during TLE.
- Arterial waveform and echocardiography are imperative to early identification of injuries.
- An endovascular occlusion balloon should be utilized in all moderate to high-risk cases.
- Injury management should be guided by the events immediately preceding effusion or hemodynamic change.
- New and expanding pericardial effusions need to be drained and monitored to determine need for surgical escalation.
- Many injuries can be controlled and repaired without CPB.
- CPB may be necessary to repair complex injuries, salvage blood loss when injuries are not controllable, or patients need hemodynamic support.

REFERENCES

1. Kusumoto FM, Schoenfeld MH, Wilkoff BL, et al. 2017 HRS expert consensus statement on cardiovascular implantable electronic device lead management and extraction. *Heart Rhythm.* 2017;14(12):e503–e551. doi:10.1016/j.hrthm.2017.09.001
2. Bashir J, Fedoruk LM, Ofiesh J, Karim SS, Tyers GF. Classification and surgical repair of injuries sustained during transvenous lead extraction. *Circ Arrhythm Electrophysiol.* 2016;9(9):e003741. doi:10.1161/CIRCEP.115.003741
3. Brunner MP, Cronin EM, Wazni O, et al. Outcomes of patients requiring emergent surgical or endovascular intervention for catastrophic complications during transvenous lead extraction. *Heart Rhythm.* 2014;11(3):419–425. doi:10.1016/j.hrthm.2013.12.004
4. Azarrafiy R, Tsang DC, Wilkoff BL, Carrillo RG. Endovascular occlusion balloon for treatment of superior vena cava tears during transvenous lead extraction: A multiyear analysis and an update to best practice protocol. *Circ Arrhythm Electrophysiol.* 2019;12(8):e007266. doi:10.1161/CIRCEP.119.007266
5. Ventura F, Rendina E, Coloni G. Surgery of the superior vena cava: Resection and reconstruction. CTSNet.org. Published October 18, 2009. Accessed on April 5, 2021.
6. Franceschi F, Thuny F, Giorgi R, et al. Incidence, risk factors, and outcome of traumatic tricuspid regurgitation after percutaneous ventricular lead removal. *J Am Coll Cardiol.* 2009;53(23):2168–2174.
7. Birgersdotter-green U, Dawood FZ. Transvenous extraction of pacemaker and defibrillator leads and the risk of tricuspid valve regurgitation: Making a case for thoughtful lead management. *JACC Clin Electrophysiol.* 2018;4(11):1429–1430.
8. Filsoufi F, Adams DH, Carpentier A, Williams M. *Carpentier's Reconstructive Valve Surgery: From Valve Analysis to Valve Reconstruction (Reconstructive Valve Surgery).* Elsevier Health Sciences. 2010.

9. Green MS, Wu D, Patel V, Tariq R. A case of arterial and venous tear during single lead extraction. *Case Rep Cardiol.* 2016;2016:3836754. doi:10.1155/2016/3836754

10. Doty JR, Flores JH, Doty DB. Superior vena cava obstruction: Bypass using spiral vein graft. *Ann Thor Surg.* 1999;67(4):111–1116. doi.org/10.1016/S0003-4975(99)00145-9

1 | Device Extraction from Superior Venous Access

Siva K. Mulpuru MD, MPH

CLINICAL VIGNETTE

A 75-year-old male patient presented with copious orange-colored discharge from the pacemaker site. He underwent dual-chamber pacemaker implantation for sinus node dysfunction in 2008. Subsequently, he underwent a generator change after his device reached the elective replacement indicator. Five weeks after the generator change, he noticed that the pacemaker pocket's lateral edge did not heal well, and he started noticing swelling of the pocket site with discharge (**Figure 1.1**).

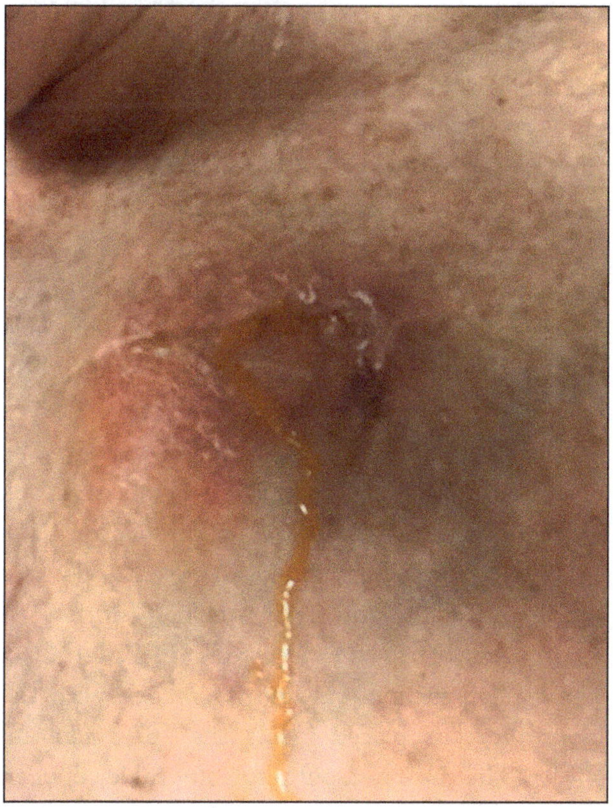

Figure 1.1 Redness around the incision site, swelling, orange color discharge from the pocket is noted three weeks after device surgery. Please note the scaly lateral part of the incision, which the patient subjectively felt, did not heal well.

He denied fevers, chills, and rigors. His pertinent past medical history included obesity, hypothyroidism, permanent atrial fibrillation, thyroid cancer status post-thyroidectomy, bipolar disorder, and prostate enlargement. He had a history of symptomatic left subclavian vein thrombosis after his initial pacemaker implantation procedure and was on anticoagulation for six months. The most recent device details are as follows:

Device Details

Device Component	Manufacturer/ Model	Date of Implant
Pulse generator	St. Jude Medical Assurity	04/2017
Right atrial lead	St. Jude Medical 1646 T	01/2008
Left ventricular lead	St. Jude Medical 1646 T	01/2008

The patient was in atrial fibrillation and was pacing about 71% from the right ventricle. Laboratory workup was unremarkable, and his echocardiogram revealed a structurally normal heart with an ejection fraction of 55%. There were no valvular or pacemaker lead vegetations noted on the transesophageal echocardiogram (TEE). Blood cultures remained persistently negative.

PREPROCEDURAL PLANNING

The patient was evaluated by cardiac surgery and electrophysiology teams before the procedure. Anticoagulation with rivaroxaban was stopped 2 days before the procedure. A preprocedural CT scan was also performed to understand venous anatomy for the procedure. The device was programmed to VVI at a lower rate of 50 bpm, and

 Cardiotext Publishing. ISBN: 978-1-942909-54-5

the pacemaker paced less than 1% of the time 48 hours before the extraction procedure.

PROCEDURAL DETAILS

A preprocedural huddle was performed with all teams in attendance. The patient was taken to the hybrid operating room and was prepped from the neck to the groin in a sterile manner. General anesthesia was administered, and a TEE probe was placed for monitoring during the procedure. Four units of blood cross-matched, packed red cells were available in the room for the procedure. Venous and arterial accesses were obtained using ultrasound guidance and modified Seldinger's technique. Dedicated arterial and venous sheaths were placed in the left femoral venous site for rapid initiation of peripheral cardiopulmonary bypass in the event of a complication. Multiple sheaths were also placed in the right common femoral vein. A 9-Fr sheath was placed in the right common femoral vein for high-volume crystalloid or blood product infusion. An 8-Fr SRO sheath (Fast Cath, Abbott) was placed in the right femoral vein over a wire with the sheath's tip in the right atrium (RA). A 12-Fr sheath was also placed in the left common femoral vein to place a stiff 0.035-inch wire. A Bridge Occlusion Balloon (Philips Medical) was placed over the stiff wire. An appropriate position was confirmed after contrast injection. A marker was placed on the shaft of the catheter. The balloon was deflated, and the catheter was pulled down to the inferior vena cava (IVC). A 7-Fr sheath was also placed in the right internal jugular vein for CVP measurement. The pocket was opened, and the leads were freed till the suture sleeves. A lot of pus and active inflammation was noted in the pocket. The sutures were cut, and the sleeves were pulled back. The leads were prepared using locking stylets (Lead Locking Device, size 1, Philips Medical). The locking stylet could not be advanced to the tip of the atrial lead (▶ **Video 1.1**). An 11-Fr mechanical extraction sheath (TightRail, Philips Medical) was placed on the ventricular lead. It was advanced using the traction-countertraction technique, and the ventricular lead was eventually taken out of the vasculature.

The mechanical extraction sheath was also advanced on the atrial lead to the mid subclavian vein. Separation of the ring and tip electrodes was noted with traction on the pacemaker lead (▶ **Video 1.2**). An endoscopy biopsy forceps (Radial Jaw 4 Biopsy forceps, Boston Scientific) was placed through the SRO sheath to grab the lead proximal to the ring electrode and to apply downward traction (▶ **Video 1.3**). The biopsy forceps prevented transmission of the force beyond the ring electrode, thereby preventing the lead's transection. The snare provided a way to apply downward traction on the lead and serve as a rail to advance sheaths from a superior access site. The mechanical extraction sheath was advanced to the biopsy forceps. As the sheath could not be advanced further, a 12-Fr laser extraction sheath (GlideLight, Philips Medical) was used. However, the tip could not be freed, and an acute angulation is seen between the long axis of the extraction sheath and the tip electrode's axis (▶ **Video 1.4**).

As there were concerns about leaving the tip electrode in the body, we proceeded to the femoral route of extraction, which provides a favorable angle of approach to the tip electrode. The lead was cut at the pocket, and the lead was internalized in the vasculature using the biopsy forceps (▶ **Video 1.5**). The femoral venous access site was upgraded to a 16-Fr long introducer sheath (Cook Medical) over a guidewire. A 15-mm Goose Neck snare (GN 1500, Medtronic) was used to go over the tip of the lead and engage the body of the lead at the level of the ring electrode (▶ **Video 1.6**). The lead's proximal cut end is grabbed with the biopsy forceps placed inside the 16-Fr femoral sheath. The stretched-out conductor cable between the ring and tip electrodes can be appreciated on 3D echocardiography (▶ **Video 1.7**). The femoral sheath was slowly advanced with traction on the lead applied through the biopsy forceps and the

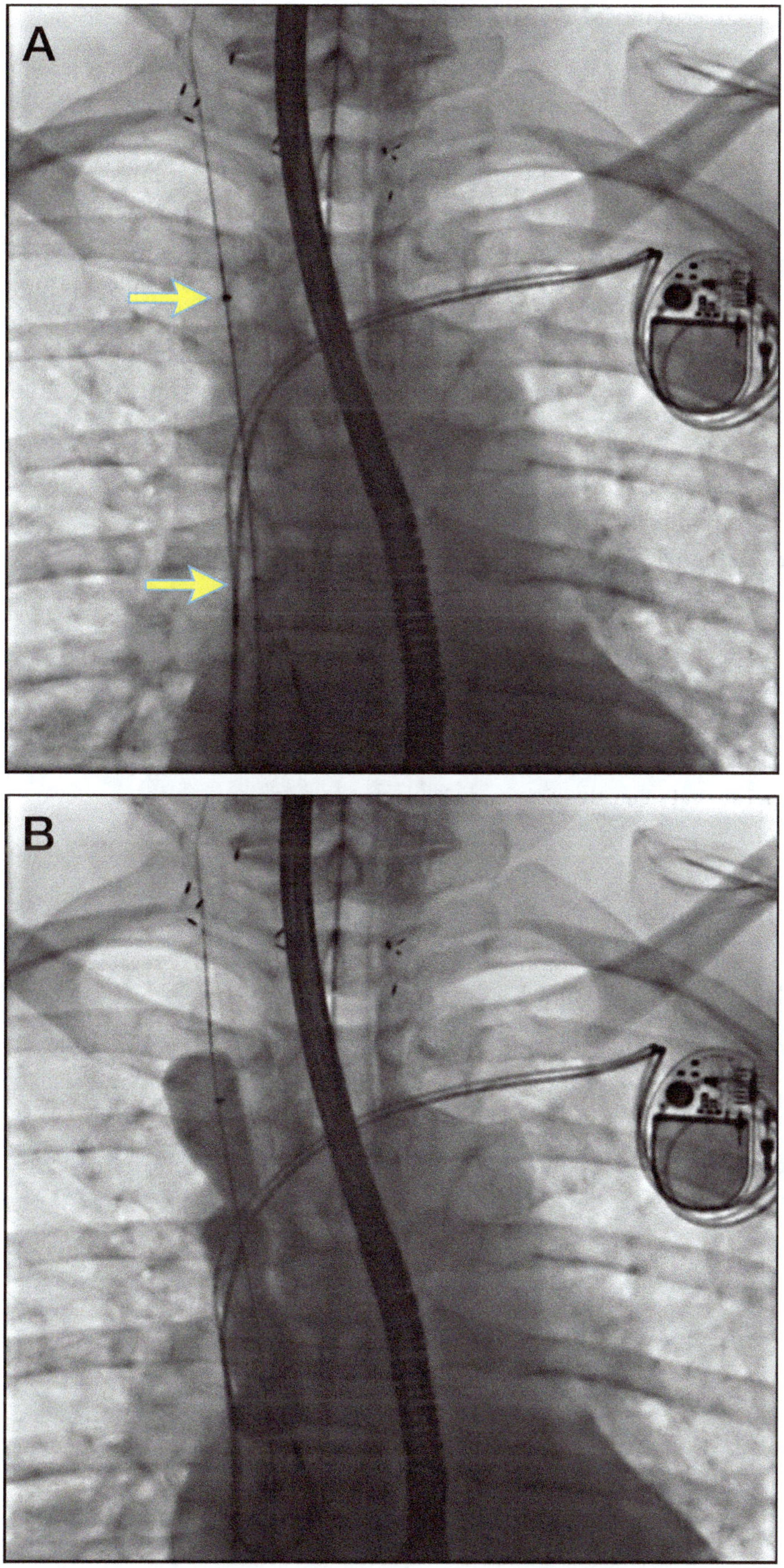

Figure 1.2 A Bridge Occlusion Balloon (Philips Medical) was placed over a stiff guidewire to cover the potential area of SVC lateral wall injury (**Panel A**). Diluted contrast is injected into the balloon to confirm adequate placement (**Panel B**). A marker (sticker) is then placed over the shaft of the catheter when the balloon is in an optimal position. The balloon is then deflated and is pulled down to the level of the IVC. The wire is left in place and serves as a rail to push the balloon up to the marker in an emergency.

snare (▶ **Video 1.8**). Once tissue contact is made with the femoral sheath, the Goose Neck snare is released and is pulled back on to the shaft of the femoral sheath. Traction with the biopsy forceps and countertraction with the femoral sheath is applied with careful monitoring on echocardiography. A pseudopericardial effusion can be appreciated as the RA wall is pulled away from the pericardial cavity (▶ **Video 1.9**). The lead tip was eventually freed and was taken out of the body.

All sheaths were eventually removed, and hemostasis was achieved by manual compression. TEE showed trivial pericardial effusion. As he required minimal pacing before the extraction procedure decision was made not to reimplant a pacemaker. The pocket was debrided, and a vacuum-assisted suction device was applied to the incision site.

POSTPROCEDURAL COURSE

The patient was extubated in the operating room and was transferred to the floor service. The vacuum suction device was removed on day 3, and the pocket was closed with non-absorbable sutures. As he was in permanent atrial fibrillation with controlled ventricular rates, the team opted not to reimplant the device. Pocket cultures grew mixed gram-positive organisms, and he received IV vancomycin for 2 weeks through a peripherally inserted central catheter line. Anticoagulation therapy was started with rivaroxaban after pocket closure. He was discharged from the hospital on day 5 after the extraction procedure and remained well during follow-up.

SUMMARY POINTS

- Understand the nuances of lead design and their relevance to the extraction procedure. Certain leads tend to separate between the ring and tip electrode.
- Appreciate the relationship between the lead axis and the long axis of the extraction sheath. Acute angulations can lead to unfavorable force transmission leading to increased risk of complications or lead transection.
- Familiarity with the femoral tools (snares, biopsy forceps, and deflectable catheters) is needed to seamlessly convert a superior route to femoral route of extraction.
- Pseudopericardial effusion is due to invagination of the atrial wall and creation of a false space in the pericardium. Prompt recognition prevents unnecessary interventions and also helps the operation reduce the traction on the lead.
- Device reimplantation decisions about should take into consideration of the continuing need for device therapy especially after device infection.

VIDEO LEGENDS

Video 1.1 A locking stylet was placed in the atrial lead. However, the tip of the stylet (yellow arrow) could not be passed to the lead's tip. [00:01]

Video 1.2 Separation of the ring (yellow arrow) and tip electrode (green arrow) can be appreciated when traction was applied on the lead. A conductor cable still connected the 2 electrodes. [00:01]

Video 1.3 An endoscopy biopsy forceps (Radial Jaw 4 Biopsy forceps, Boston Scientific) was used to grab the lead proximal to the ring electrode to prevent transection of the lead tip. [00:01]

Video 1.4 A 12-Fr laser sheath was advanced over the lead, and good separation between the ring electrode (yellow arrow) and the tip electrode (green arrow). Note the acute angulation between the long axis of the extraction sheath and the tip electrode's long axis. [00:02]

Video 1.5 The lead was cut in the pocket area. The body of the lead was grabbed using the biopsy forceps (pink arrow), and the proximal end (lead cut in the pocket) was internalized and was pulled down to the level of IVC. Notice the significant separation between the ring (yellow arrow) on the tip electrode (green arrow) connected by the conductor cable. [00:02]

Video 1.6 A Goose Neck snare was placed on the lead's body and was advanced to the ring electrode (yellow arrow). The cut end of the lead was grabbed by the biopsy forceps placed inside a 16-Fr sheath. The green arrow indicates the tip of the femoral sheath. The ring and the tip electrode are still connected by a conductor cable (blue arrows). [00:02]

Video 1.7 3D TEE delineates the conductor cable between the ring and tip electrode. Notice that the tip electrode was attached right below the superior vena cava (SVC)–RA junction. [00:01]

Video 1.8 The femoral sheath (yellow arrow) was slowly advanced until the tip electrode (green arrow). Notice that the angle between the femoral sheath's long axis and the pacemaker lead is favorable for preventing tip transection. The Goose Neck snare (pink arrow) is advanced as distally as possible to apply traction near the tip electrode. [00:01]

Video 1.9 As traction was applied on the lead using the biopsy forceps and countertraction was applied using the tip of the femoral sheath, an echo-free space (yellow arrow) can be appreciated on echocardiography. This echo-free space mimics the presence of a pericardial effusion (pseudopericardial effusion) and is caused by inversion of the atrial wall. An oval-shaped Goose Neck catheter (green arrow) pulled back on to the shaft of the femoral sheath can be appreciated in the video. [00:02]

2 | Extraction of Recalled Riata Lead

CASE 2

Yong-Mei Cha, MD

CLINICAL VIGNETTE

A 62-year-old male has dilated cardiomyopathy, for which he received a single-chamber defibrillator in 2005 for primary sudden death prevention. The device is a St. Jude Atlas model V-193 connected to St. Jude Riata lead, model 1581. He has had no ICD therapies, neither appropriate or inappropriate, after the implant. However, his overall NYHA functional status had gradually deteriorated. He has dyspnea on exertion on walking one block or climbing one flight of stairs. His other comorbidities include diabetes, depression, and hyperlipidemia.

On December 14, 2011, FDA issued Class 1 device recall on Riata ST silicone insulated leads (Models: 7000, 7001, 7002, 7010, 7011, 7040, 7041, 7042, St. Jude Medical). The recall was associated with all-cause insulation failure on the St. Jude Medical Riata, and Riata ST silicone endocardial defibrillation leads with specific emphasis on externalized conductors. Externalized conductors occur when an abrasion results in an outer insulation breach within the vascular or cardiac chambers allowing the normally contained conductors to become visible outside the lead body. Externalized conductors can be a result of relative motion of the conductor cables within the lead insulation lumen, referred to as "inside-out" abrasion, or from external sources of abrasion, e.g., lead-to-lead abrasion, where the outer insulation is breached and, as a result, the conductor cables are observed to be outside the lead body. The most common (approximately 75% of the confirmed cases) location of the externalization along the lead body is within 8 centimeters proximal to the RV shock coil, as the stress on that area of the lead may be higher than other areas of the lead due to lead movement associated with a patient's heartbeat. The externalized conductors may or may not be associated with electrical abnormalities; the electrical presentations included pacing or defibrillation impedance changes, noise, oversensing, inappropriate ICD therapy, and pacing threshold rise. A rare death event was reported. Examining the defibrillation lead by chest X-ray (CXR) and cine angiogram was recommended.

The patient underwent a CXR, as shown in **Figure 2.1**. There was evidence of internal conductor exteriorization in the vicinity of the distal shock coil. This was visualized in the PA view and the lateral view (red arrows). Device interrogation showed a normal lead sensing, lead impedance, and pacing function. A provocative test resulted in some noise reproduction by Valsalva-type maneuver (left arm reaches over to the right shoulder). The battery life had 11 months remaining.

Device Details

Device Component	Manufacturer/Model	Date of Implant
ICD generator	St. Jude Medical model V-193	2005
RV lead	St. Jude Medical Riata lead, model 1581	2005

PREPROCEDURAL PLANNING

The patient has developed NYHA class III symptoms. ECG showed an interval change of new LBBB with a QRS duration of 146 ms. An upgrade from the single-chamber ICD to a CRT-D is indicated based on the ACC/AHA/HRS 2008 guidelines for device-based therapy of cardiac rhythm

 ISBN: 978-1-942909-54-5

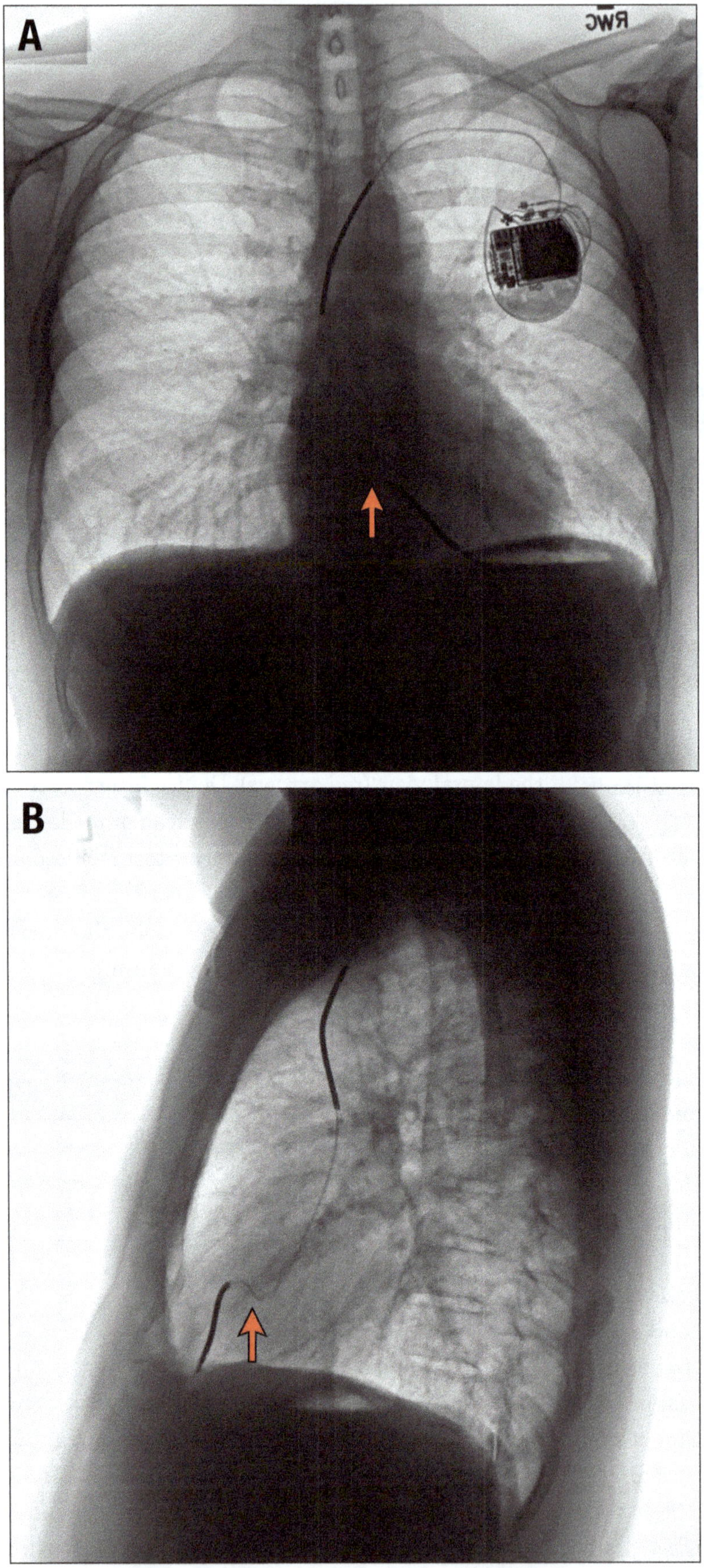

Figure 2.1 Revert CXR shows single-chamber ICD with dual coils. An interval conductor is separated from the lead, likely externalized in PA and lateral view (**red arrows**).

abnormalities and 2012 ACCF/AHA/HRS focused update incorporated into the ACCF/AHA/HRS 2008 guidelines for device-based therapy of cardiac rhythm abnormalities.[1,2] The patient consented to an ICD upgrade to a CRT-D device. At the time of upgrade, we considered the abandonment of the recalled Riata lead and reimplantation of a new ICD lead. Alternatively, the recalled abnormal Riata lead can be removed. Given the patient's relatively young age and the fact that there was only a single existing lead that had exposed lead conductors, the decision was made via shared decision making to extract the Riata lead.[3] According to our extraction risk stratification protocol, a procedure for extraction of a defibrillator lead that was implanted more than 5 years ago is classified as high risk, so the procedure was scheduled in the OR. The patient was scheduled for lead extraction, followed by a CRT-D implant.

PROCEDURAL DETAILS

- ***General anesthesia:*** The patient was intubated and ventilated throughout the procedure.
- ***Venous access:*** One venous access was obtained from the left femoral vein for fluid resuscitation and blood transfusion when needed. One venous access was obtained from the right femoral vein, ready for upsizing a 16-Fr workstation for extraction from below when required.
- A radial arterial line was obtained for BP monitoring throughout the entire procedure.
- Cardiovascular surgeon and the perfusionist were on standby and were readily available during the procedure.

The chest, abdomen, and bilateral groin areas were prepped and draped in a sterile fashion. The scar was re-incised, and dissection was carefully carried down to the pulse generator that was freed from the pocket. The right ventricular (RV) lead was disconnected from the generator. The sutures on the sleeve were removed. A stylet was placed into the RV lead lumen, and the lead active fixation screw was successfully retracted. However, the lead was unable to be removed by gentle extraction. The proximal lead was cut where a universal locking stylet (Philips Medical) was placed on the lead, and the lead was locked in place. A Prolene suture was used to tie the lead outer insulation to the inner coil to secure the force of traction. A second Prolene suture was tied to the conductor cables to strengthen the force of traction. This is an important technique that uses 2 Prolene sutures to hold the lead and separate defibrillation cables together, as shown in **Figure 2.2**, which illustrates the Riata lead design in a transect view. A 16-Fr Excimer laser sheath (Philips Medical) was selected and tested normal. The laser sheath was advanced over the lead and entered the left subclavian vein. When the laser sheath was well aligned to the RV lead, laser energy was delivered, enabling the sheath to be advanced to the innominate vein (**Video 2.1**). Next, the laser sheath passed the proximal coil to the superior vena cava (SVC) (**Video 2.2**).

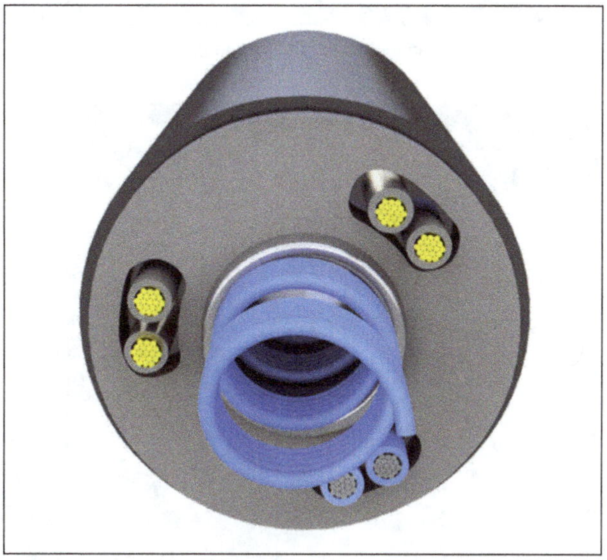

Figure 2.2 A lead design of Durata lead (Abbott). A conductor cable surrounds the central lumen to the tip electrode (**blue**). There were 3 pairs of wires surrounding the cable to the tip electrode. Two cables supply the SVC and RV coils (**yellow**), and the remaining pair supplies the RV ring electrode (**gray**). Each cable is covered by its own insulation. On top of that, the whole lead may be covered by an insulation layer (Optim).

Of note, the conductor externalization was seen between the proximal and distal coils (**Figure 2.3**). The laser sheath was moved forward in the SVC and entered the right atrium (RA) without lasing (▶ **Video 2.3**). The lead tip was freed from the RV apex by traction. At this point, the laser sheath had difficulty to be advanced further to pass the distal coil. "Snowplowing" due to tissue or externalized conductor cable bunching was suspected. The outer sheath was then advanced over the laser sheath toward the distal coil. The distal lead was successfully pulled back into the outer sheath and removed in its entity (▶ **Video 2.4**). **Figure 2.4** shows multiple sites of conductor externalization (red arrows). **Figure 2.5** is the lead photo showing 2 conductors between proximal and distal coils that were outside of lead insulation.

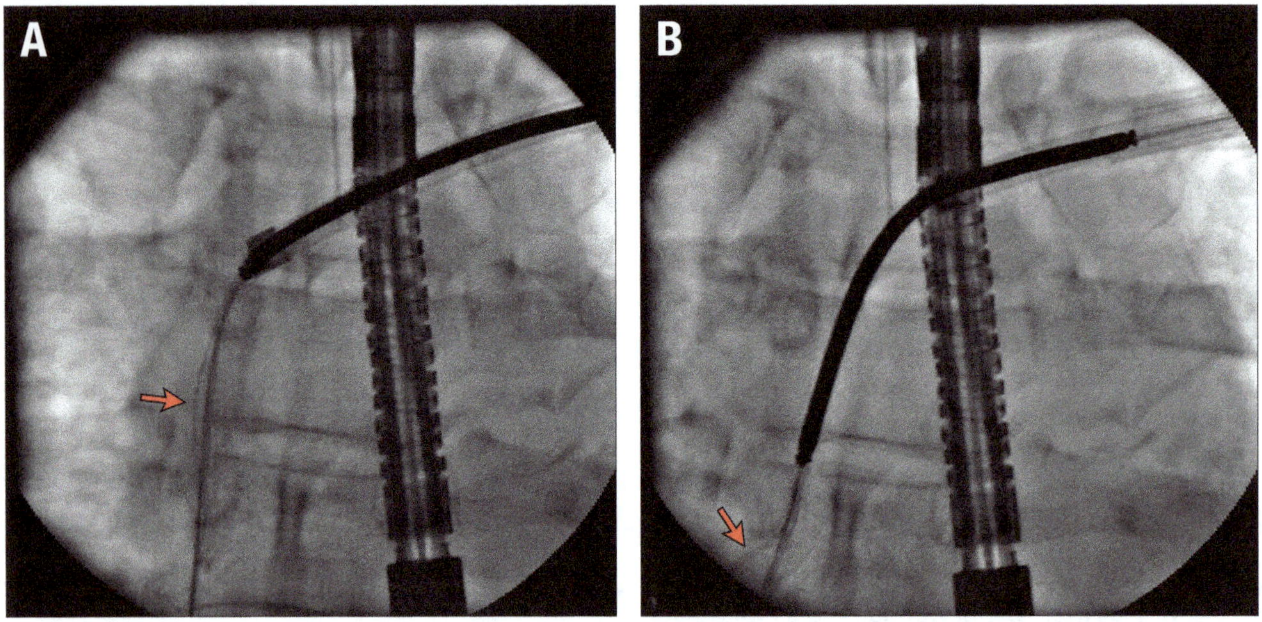

Figure 2.3 The conductor externalization distal to the proximal coil (**red arrows**).

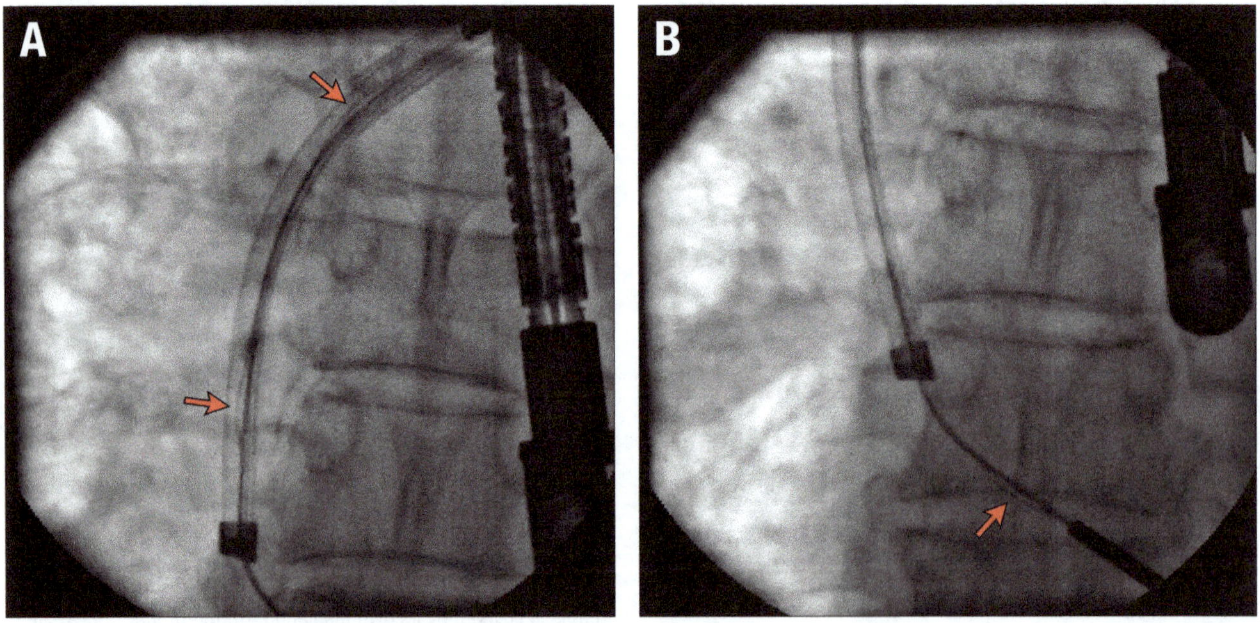

Figure 2.4 Cine frames show multiple sites of conductor externalization (**red arrows**).

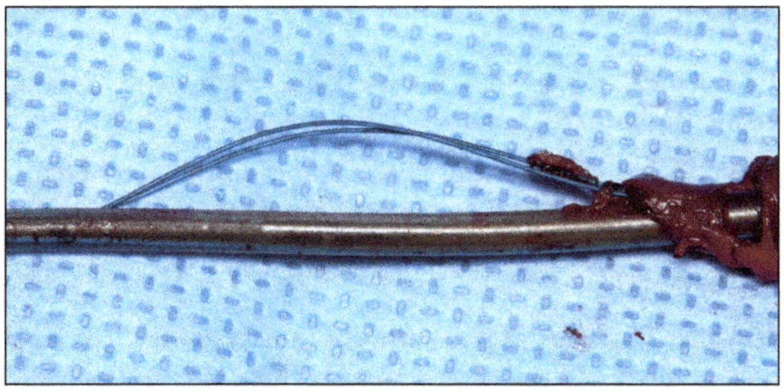

Figure 2.5 Two conductors between proximal and distal coils that were externalized from the lead insulation.

CRT-D IMPLANTATION

The left axillary vein was cannulated at 3 locations. First, the RV lead (Medtronic Sprint Quattro 6947-65) was placed in the RV septum via a safe sheath where R wave was 9.7 mV, impedance 605 ohms, and the pacing threshold 0.5 volts/0.5 ms. The lead was secured with the supplied sleeve adaptor and adaptor to the pectoral muscle. Then, a Worley sheath was placed in the RA over a long 0.035-in. wire. The long wire was able to be engaged in the coronary sinus, and the sheath was able to be advanced into the coronary sinus body. A coronary venogram showed a small lateral coronary vein (**Video 2.5**). The LV lead was selected Guidant EasyTrak 2, 4543-90) and advanced to this lateral vein's distal tributary. At this location, the R wave was 11.8 mV, impedance 973 ohms, and pacing threshold 0.5 volts/0.5 ms. There was no diaphragmatic stimulation at high output. Finally, the atrial lead (Medtronic Capsure Fix 5568-53) was placed in the right atrial appendage with P wave 2.7 mV, impedance 576 ohms, pacing threshold 0.9 volts/0.5 ms. The long sheath was successfully peeled away. The LV lead was secured with the supplied sleeve adaptor and adapted to the pectoral muscle. **Video 2.6** shows the implant positions of 3 leads in the left anterior oblique (LAO) view. All leads were connected to the pulse generator and tightly screwed. The incision was closed with 2 layers of subcutaneous 2-0 Vicryl and a single layer of 4-0 Monocryl.

SUMMARY POINTS

- Understand the rationale for the Class 1 lead recall for the St. Jude Medical Riata: conductor(s) externalized from the lead insulation breach with or without concomitant lead malfunction. Conductor externalization alone may be subjected to continued observation, while lead malfunction necessitates lead revision.
- When lead conductor externalization is evident, and a device upgrade or generator replacement is required, make an appropriate recommendation for considering recalled lead removal versus abandonment by assessing patient overall conditions and shared decision making.
- Lead extraction in this patient was considered high risk based on the ICD lead having been implanted more than 5 years ago, indicating that the procedure should be undertaken in the operating room.
- Externalized conductors should be secured to the entire lead using Prolene or One-Tie to maximize the traction force.
- The externalized conductors and the tissue debris may have a "snowplowing" effect preventing the laser sheath advancement. The outer sheath with a larger inner lumen may overcome the "snowplowing" to remove the lead.

REFERENCES

1. Epstein AE, DiMarco JP, Ellenbogen KA, et al. ACC/AHA/HRS 2008 guidelines for device-based therapy of cardiac rhythm abnormalities: A report of the American College of Cardiology/American Heart Association Task Force on Practice Guidelines (Writing Committee to Revise the ACC/AHA/NASPE 2002 Guideline Update for Implantation of Cardiac Pacemakers and Antiarrhythmia Devices). Developed in collaboration with the American Association for Thoracic Surgery and Society of Thoracic Surgeons. *J Am Coll Cardiol.* 2008;51:e1–e62.
2. Epstein AE, DiMarco JP, Ellenbogen KA, et al. 2012 ACCF/AHA/HRS focused update incorporated into the ACCF/AHA/HRS 2008 guidelines for device-based therapy of cardiac rhythm abnormalities: A report of the American College of Cardiology Foundation/American Heart Association Task Force on Practice Guidelines and the Heart Rhythm Society. *J Am Coll Cardiol.* 2013;61:e6–e75.
3. Kusumoto FM, Schoenfeld MH, Wilkoff BL, et al. 2017 HRS expert consensus statement on cardiovascular implantable electronic device lead management and extraction. *Heart Rhythm.* 2017;14(12):e503–e551.

VIDEO LEGENDS

Video 2.1 Laser sheath was advanced from subclavian to an innominate vein using laser energy. [00:13]

Video 2.2 Laser sheath was advanced from subclavian to an innominate vein using laser energy. The conductor externalization is shown between the proximal and distal coils. [00:05]

Video 2.3 The laser sheath was moved forward in the SVC and entered the right atrium without lasing. The lead tip was freed from the RV apex by traction. [00:31]

Video 2.4 The laser sheath had difficulty to be advanced further to pass the distal coil. "Snowplowing" (tissue or externalized conductors) was suspected. The outer sheath was then advanced over the laser sheath. The lead was successfully pulling back into the outer sheath. [00:13]

Video 2.5 This video shows a small lateral coronary vein by coronary venogram. [00:02]

Video 2.6 Right atrial, right ventricular, and left ventricular leads placement in LAO view. [00:01]

3 | Importance of Lead Countertraction

CASE 3

Yong-Mei Cha, MD

CLINICAL VIGNETTE

A 42-year-old female has familial hypertrophic cardiomyopathy. She underwent single-chamber implantable cardioverter-defibrillator (ICD) implantation in 2004 for primary sudden death prevention. In 2009, due to severe left ventricular outflow tract (LVOT) obstruction and debilitating dyspnea on exertion despite medical therapy, she underwent extended transapical ventricular septal myectomy. In 2014, she developed ventricular fibrillation, receiving 2 ICD shocks. Subsequently, she went into pulseless electrical activity and was successfully resuscitated. Due to sinus bradycardia, she had dual-chamber ICD upgrade. In 2019, the right ventricular (RV) lead's shock impedance was increased to 180 ohms with intermittent noise detection. The chest X-ray (CXR) is shown in **Figure 3.1**. The RV lead is located in the RV apex inferiorly. The decision was made to remove the malfunctioning RV lead and place a new lead given the patient's young age.

Device Details

Device Component	Manufacturer/Model	Date of Implant
ICD	Boston Scientific 163 Incepta DR	2014
RV lead	Boston Scientific 1084 Endotak Reliance G.	2004
RA lead	Cardiac Pacemakers Inc. 4470 Fineline II	2014

PROCEDURAL DETAILS

- The procedure was undertaken in the OR hybrid room given the right ventricular lead age of 15 years.
- The patient was intubated and ventilated throughout the procedure.
- A 0.035-inch guidewire was placed in the right internal jugular vein from the right femoral vein. The Bridge Occlusion Balloon catheter (Philips Medical) was advanced to the superior vena cava (SVC) and inflated. **Video 3.1** shows the RV lead is on the lateral wall of SVC (blue arrow) while the balloon is on the medial side in AP view. The balloon was then deflated and pulled back to the inferior vena cava (IVC), ready to be advanced to the SVC at any time.
- Left femoral vein access was obtained for fluid resuscitation.
- Radial arterial line was set for BP monitoring.

Lead Extraction

- The incision was made along the scar. Careful dissection was undertaken using a plasma blade (Plasmablad, Medtronic) to avoid Fineline atrial lead damage. RV lead active fixation was retracted.
- After a universal locking stylet (Lead Locking Device, size 1, Philips Medical) locked RV lead tip in place, an 11-Fr TightRail sheath (Philips Medical) was selected to free the lead. There was difficulty in advancing the sheath in the subclavian vein (**Video 3.2**), for which a 16-Fr Laser sheath (GlideLight, Philips Medical) with an outer sheath was replaced by the TightRail sheath. Note that the RV lead proximal coil was likely freed from the

Cardiac Lead Extraction: A Case-Based Contemporary Approach.
 Cardiotext Publishing. ISBN: 978-1-942909-54-5

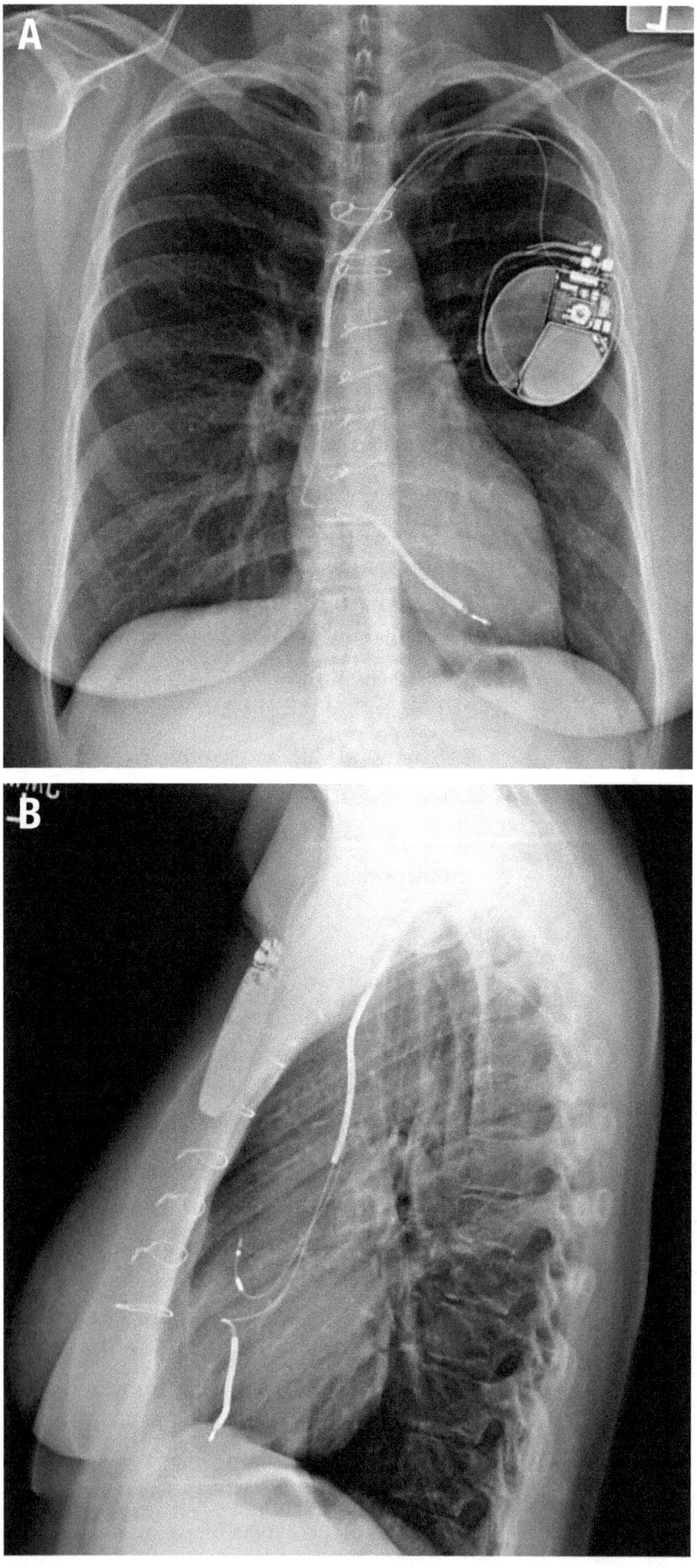

Figure 3.1 CXR PA and lateral view show the dual-coil RV lead is located in the RV apex inferiorly.

SVC lateral wall as the lead was pulled towards the medial side of SVC. The laser sheath was aligned with lead and was advanced to the innominate vein using laser energy (**Video 3.3**).

- The operator switched the laser sheath to the TightRail sheath to pass the SVC (avoiding laser energy at SVC if possible). The TightRail was advanced to the distal coil at the tricuspid annulus level, where a significant resistance was encountered. A large amount of fibrotic tissue ("snowplowing") at the tip of TightRail sheath was suspected (**Video 3.4**).
- The outer sheath was then advanced towards the lead tip alone and was able to contact RV endocardium. At this point, the critical maneuver was to apply for countertraction by using the outer sheath against the RV endocardium where the lead tip was embedded, as shown in **Video 3.5**. **Video 3.6** shows the RV lead was successfully extracted and pulled back into the outer sheath by countertraction (**Figure 3.2**).
- A new RV defibrillation lead was reimplanted after the lead extraction.

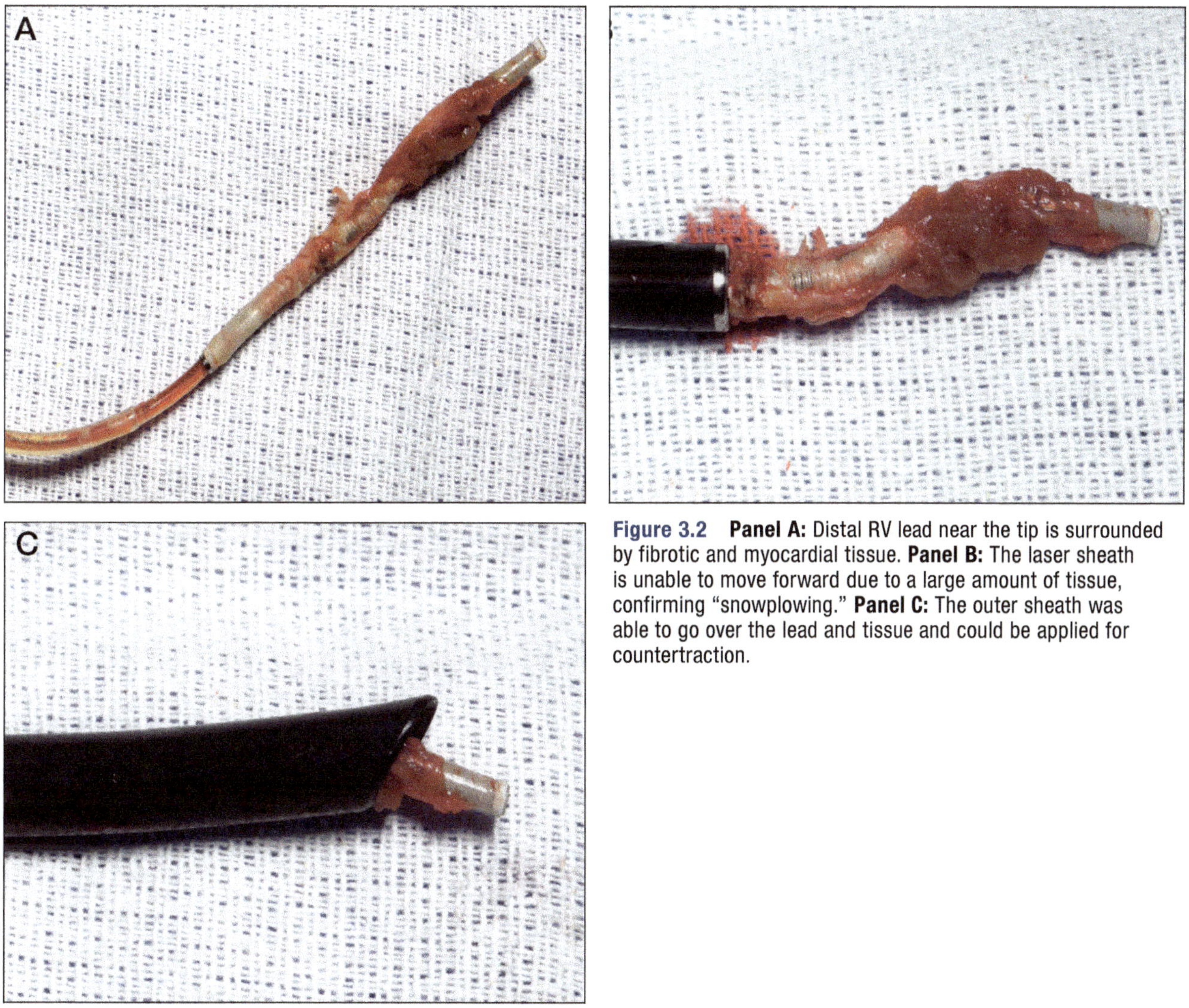

Figure 3.2 **Panel A:** Distal RV lead near the tip is surrounded by fibrotic and myocardial tissue. **Panel B:** The laser sheath is unable to move forward due to a large amount of tissue, confirming "snowplowing." **Panel C:** The outer sheath was able to go over the lead and tissue and could be applied for countertraction.

SUMMARY POINTS

- Alternating TightRail and Laser sheath to free the lead and avoid laser application at the SVC area.
- Countertraction using a mechanical sheath is safe and useful to remove the lead and minimize myocardial perforation.
- When "snowplowing" is suspected, use the outer sheath for countertraction.

VIDEO LEGENDS

Video 3.1 Bridge Occlusion Balloon catheter is inflated in the SVC. The RV lead proximal coil is on the lateral wall of SVC (blue arrow) in AP view. [00:01]

Video 3.2 The RV lead proximal coil is now on the medial side of SVC (solid blue arrow). The dashed blue arrow shows the original proximal coil location. [00:02]

Video 3.3 Laser sheath is advancing from the left subclavian to the innominate vein. [00:15]

Video 3.4 TightRail sheath is advanced to RV distal coil but met the resistance and cannot be advanced farther. [00:02]

Video 3.5 Using outer sheath apply for countertraction against RV endocardium where the lead tip was embedded in the myocardium (red arrow). [00:17]

Video 3.6 The RV lead was successfully removed back into the outer sheath. [00:02]

4 | Lead Extraction (Right-Sided ICD)

Fred M. Kusumoto, MD

CLINICAL VIGNETTE

A 59-year-old female with a history of chemotherapy-induced cardiomyopathy and implantable cardioverter-defibrillator (ICD) placement in the past has been admitted with a 2-day history of fever. She now has positive blood cultures for *Streptococcus agalactiae* (Group B *Streptococcus*). She has had no complaints of pain or redness anywhere on her body, including over her ICD generator pocket.

Her relevant cardiac history began 11 years ago when she had adriamycin cardiomyopathy with an left ventricular ejection fraction (LVEF) of 0.20. At that time, she underwent single-chamber ICD placement (Medtronic Maximo generator and a 6949 lead). She apparently had appropriate therapy for a ventricular arrhythmia 7 years ago. Five years ago, she had the placement of a new Medtronic 6947 lead, and the Medtronic 6949 lead was capped and abandoned. She underwent a generator change 2 years ago. This care was provided at another institution, and the details of the ventricular arrhythmia therapy and the reasons for the addition of a new ventricular lead are unknown.

Her past medical history is significant for diabetes mellitus. Six months ago, she underwent surgery for an open ulcer and osteomyelitis of the second toe on her right foot, which has now been clinically resolved after a course of antibiotics. Cultures from her wound were positive for *S. agalactae*.

She underwent transthoracic echocardiography (TTE) during her admission, which showed an LVEF of 0.52 with no significant valvular abnormalities. Her blood cultures were positive for *S. agalactae* with the same sensitivities from her prior admission, and she was started on ampicillin. A nuclear study showed no evidence of recurrent osteomyelitis in her toe or at other sites. Yesterday, she underwent transesophageal echocardiography (TEE), which revealed a mobile 1.5-cm mass on her right ventricular lead (**Video 4.1** and **Video 4.2**).

On physical examination, she has no evidence of heart failure or physical examination findings consistent with left-sided endocarditis. Her right-sided pocket shows no evidence of infection, and the site of her osteomyelitis surgery has healed well on examination. Her chest X-ray (CXR) is shown in **Figure 4.1**. Device interrogation reveals normal function with no ventricular arrhythmias identified on histograms.

PREPROCEDURAL PLANNING

In a patient with suspected cardiovascular implantable electronic device (CIED) infection, the 2017 HRS expert consensus statement on CIED lead management and extraction statement provides a IIa recommendation for performing TEE and does not make any specific recommendation for specific organism types.[1] In cases of bacteremia due to pathogens that generally do not cause lead-related endocarditis (gram-negative rods or gram-positive cocci other than *Staphylococcus aureus*, coagulase-negative staphylococci, or *Enterococcus faecalis*), clinical studies have suggested that it is reasonable not to perform routine TEE and focus on treating the primary source.[2] Lead-associated masses have been identified in 12%–15% of patients undergoing TTE and 2% of patients undergoing TTE.[3–5] All investigators emphasize the importance of the clinical context for differentiating between endocarditis

 ISBN: 978-1-942909-54-5

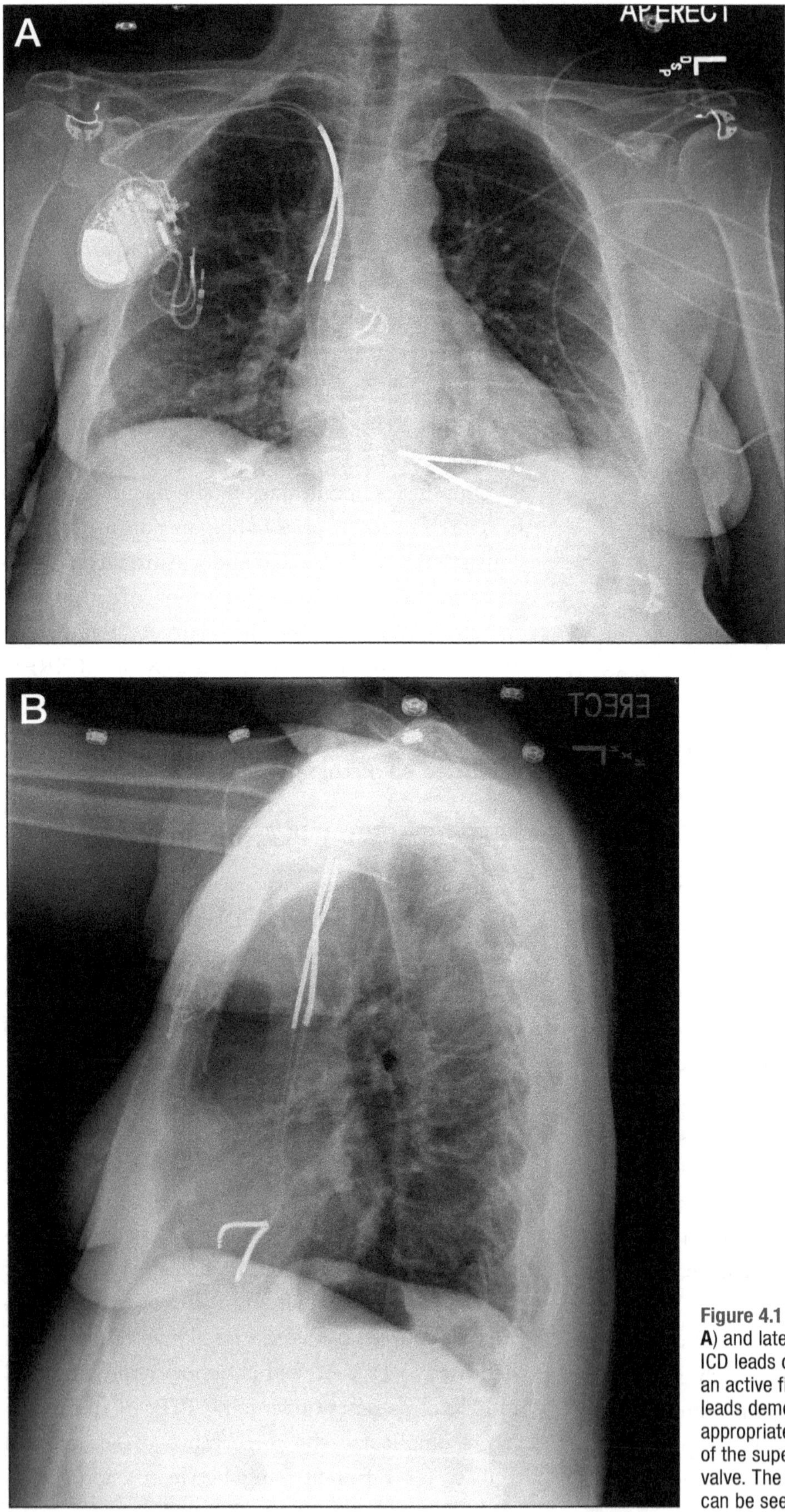

Figure 4.1 CXR showing posteroanterior (**Panel A**) and lateral (**Panel B**) projections. The two ICD leads can be seen, both with a dual-coil and an active fixation design. An inspection of both leads demonstrate no apparent flaws; both are appropriately placed and may "cross" at the level of the superior vena cava (SVC) and the tricuspid valve. The Silastic catheter in the innominate vein can be seen.

and thrombi. In this case, TEE has already been performed and reveals possible vegetations on the leads, and the infectious disease consultants have recommended lead extraction.

The patient has 2 right-sided, dual-coil ICD leads. Dual-coil leads are associated with higher risk during extraction and a 2.7-fold increased risk of 30-day mortality.[1,6] There has been a general trend over the past decade to use ICD leads that do not have a SVC coil.[7] The patient has an abandoned Medtronic 6949 lead (Medtronic Sprint Fidelis). A recent matched cohort analysis suggests that patients with abandoned leads and infection are more likely to present without systemic infection signs such as fever or leukocytosis.[8] In this case, the decision to abandon the lead rather than extract it 5 years ago now has important implications. The abandoned lead would have been easier to remove 5 years ago. Multiple studies have shown that leads that have been in place for more extended periods are more difficult to remove.[9–11] The decision to abandon a lead versus extract it can be complex and must be made on an individual basis. One analysis of the National Cardiovascular Data Registry (NCDR) found that although lead abandonment and lead extraction had similar long-term survival, extraction was associated with a lower risk of infection at 5 years.[12] Another study has reported a higher likelihood of significant tricuspid regurgitation (TR) with abandoned leads.[13] However, extraction procedures have risks, and studies have also reported that lead abandonment can be a clinically useful strategy.[14,15] Considerations for the decision-making strategy in an individual case are reviewed in the 2017 HRS expert consensus statement on CIED lead management and extraction, and a table with patient examples outlining the considerations is provided.[1] Generally, age is the primary consideration on whether to abandon or extract, and it is essential for the clinician to understand the ramifications of any decision over a patient's lifetime. Extraction complexity also increases if more leads require extraction, though the risk appears to increase when more than 3 leads are extracted.[1,9–11] Right-sided leads have historically been thought to be associated with higher risk during extraction.[16] However, recent large studies have not identified right-sided leads as being at higher risk for extraction, though this may in part be due to the relatively small number of leads extracted from the right side.[9–11] The author has found that although right-sided leads may have a relatively sharp initial bend at the junction of the subclavian vein and brachiocephalic vein that makes remaining coaxial to the lead more difficult, once this region has been negotiated, maintaining a coaxial orientation becomes easier for the remainder of the extraction than for left-sided leads. Even with the sharp bend, the forward force on the extraction tool tends to push the lead into the vessel's lumen rather than the vessel wall. The extraction tool tends to remain more coaxial at the SVC–right atrial junction than left-sided leads.

The patient also has an indwelling Silastic (Port-a-Cath) catheter as another possible nidus for infection. However, since lead-related masses had been identified by TEE, it was elected to proceed with ICD lead extraction first. Since this extraction had higher risk characteristics such as dual-coil ICD leads implanted 11 and 5 years ago and no prior cardiac surgery, the procedure was done in the operating room environment.

PROCEDURE

The surgical incision site was marked in the preprocedure area. Consent and appropriate preoperative testing and evaluation were confirmed. The patient was intubated and an arterial line placed for continuous blood pressure monitoring during the procedure.

A large operating field extending from the base of the neck to the upper thigh was prepared. The patient first underwent placement of an 8.5-Fr sheath from the femoral vein and an intracardiac ultrasound placed. A smaller additional 6-Fr sheath was also placed. With the 2 femoral venous sheath technique, the 8.5-Fr sheath with the ultrasound can be used to easily place a guidewire into the most superior venous system to allow for placement of an SVC balloon if required, and the additional venous access can be used for fluid resuscitation or used to place a larger sheath as required. The ultrasound is used to identify and localize the adherent masses on the leads and monitor for the development or increase in pericardial fluid.

The patient's shoulder area had 2 incisions from the prior procedures. An elliptical incision was made encompassing the superior incision. The pocket was opened and the device removed. The leads were carefully dissected free, taking care to minimize lead injury. For any extraction procedure, careful dissection to avoid lead injury is critical. Technologies such as electrocautery (more correctly called electrosurgery) using an insulated blade or using electrical plasma as an energy source have been shown to be associated with reduced lead injury in clinical or bench studies.[17,18] When dissecting using any electrosurgery tools, the operator should use minimal power, avoid direct contact with the lead, keep the blade tip parallel to the lead, avoid a perpendicular blade orientation, and minimize overall use. With electrosurgery, different waveforms can be used. With a pure cut, a constant waveform with a relatively low voltage is delivered. In contrast, with coagulation, higher voltages are applied intermittently (current is delivered less than 10% of the time). Blended uses intermediate voltages and will deliver current intermittently but more than 10% of the time. When the blade is held closely to the tissue, with cutting, the underlying heat will vaporize the tissue, while with coagulation the higher voltages lead to the development of heating in a larger area with coagulum formation. Practically, the operator can cause coagulation formation with a cutting waveform and "cut" with the coagulation waveform. However, since the goal is to minimize voltages near the lead, only the cut waveform should be used when using electrosurgery adjacent to or near any lead. Dissection is performed close to the venous entry point, and since these leads were implanted using a subclavian approach, the leads were freed from all adjacent structures, particularly the clavicle.

Doing as much extravascular dissection as possible is beneficial since it minimizes any lead injury during the initial part of the extraction process. Attempts were made to retract the helices for both leads; unfortunately, they remained extended. The lead ends were prepared in the usual manner, and a locking stylet was advanced to the tip of both leads. This is an important step—if the locking stylet can be advanced to the tip, then the likelihood of leaving any lead remnants decreases, and the difficulty of the extraction decreases. The cables for both of these leads were then attached to a lead extender (Bulldog, Cook Medical). The lead extender is critical to allow additional tension on the lead along with the locking stylet and provides more control of all portions of the lead. This is particularly helpful when a redundant cable is present, e.g., in a lead with "inside-out" abrasion damage.

The extraction process was begun using a rotating mechanical extraction tool on both leads. A mechanical tool rather than a laser was chosen because of the laser-powered device's relative stiffness and the acute angles sometimes encountered with a right-sided extraction, although this preference is operator dependent with no published literature to support one technique over another. In this case, an Evolution sheath (Cook Medical) was chosen. Although the TightRail (Philips) has more flexibility in the body of the device, which could theoretically be beneficial for the acute angles encountered, the author has found the cutting mechanism with the current generation of the Evolution sheath is more effective. During the extraction process, continued evaluation of lead integrity is essential. A critical site is the proximal portion of the SVC coil. Care must be taken to maintain lead integrity, and often at this point, a larger-bore sheath (whether mechanical rotational or laser) is required. This is particularly important for right-sided leads where the distal end of the extraction sheath may impinge on the proximal portion of the SVC coil. If this region becomes problematic, it is important to change to a larger sheath if available. For right-sided leads that are associated with an acute angle, in my experience, using a mechanical rotational extraction tool without the outer sheath can sometimes provide even more flexibility. As the extraction proceeds to the inferior vena cava, it is important to stop and assess whether additional femoral venous access sites are required to allow for snaring the inferior portion of the lead from below, to allow for extra tension, and to decide whether a sheath should be placed superior to the leads to facilitate immediate placement of a tamponade balloon. Extraction was continued, and both leads were removed entirely. When removing multiple leads (regardless of lead entry point), it is critical to have all leads that are to be extracted to be prepared with locking stylets and to alternate among the leads to be removed using whatever tool is chosen. In addition, it is important to pay careful attention as the extraction tool is engaging the proximal portion of any ICD coil using fluoroscopy. If resistance is encountered, if possible, using an extraction tool with a larger internal diameter is extremely important and taking care to remain coaxial. The postprocedural intracardiac echocardiogram revealed no pericardial effusion (**Video 4.3**). **Figure 4.2** shows one of the extracted ICD leads and adherent tissue.

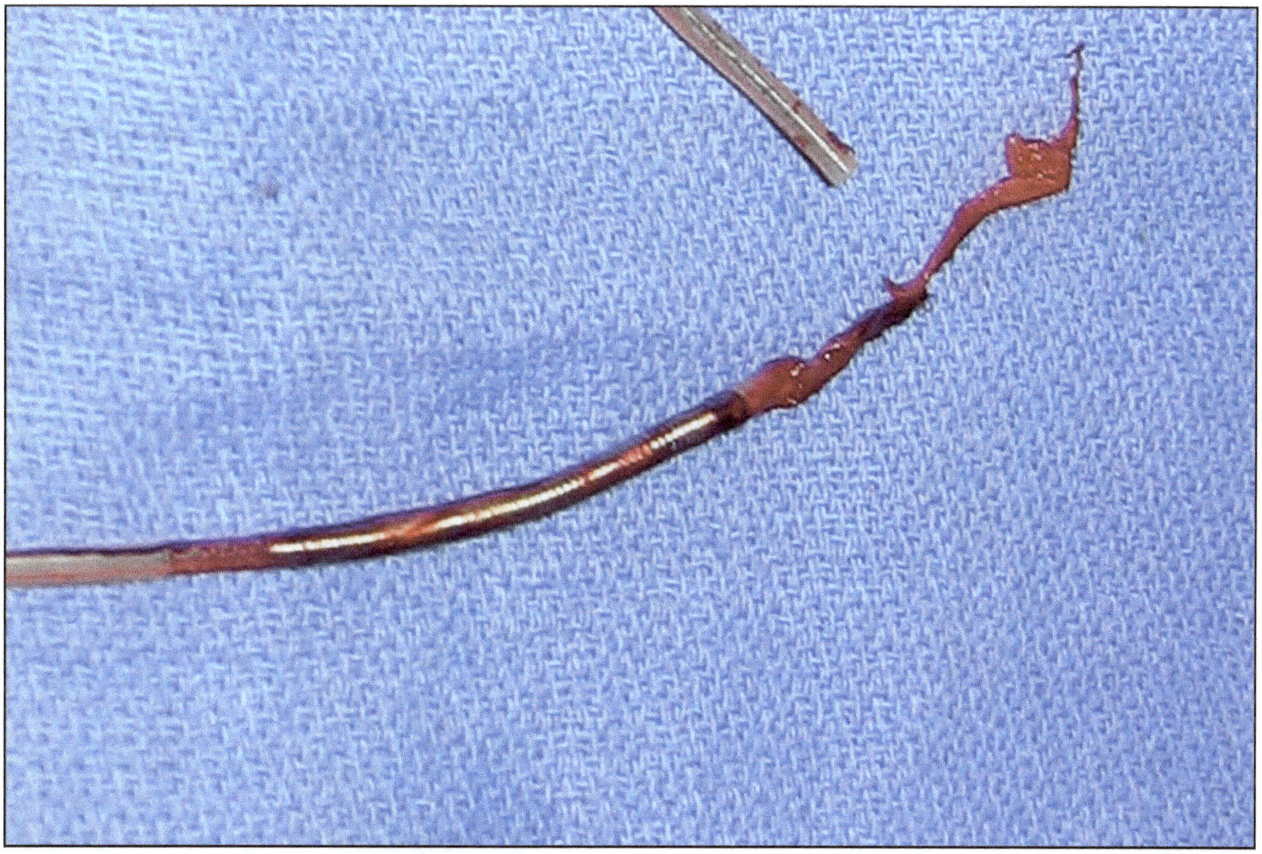

Figure 4.2 Gross specimen of the extracted Medtronic 6949 lead.

PROCEDURAL FOLLOW-UP

Postprocedural CXR identified no abnormalities (**Figure 4.3**) and TTE on postoperative day 1 showed no development of pericardial effusion and mild TR. All cultures from the leads and pocket were negative for growth. The patient continued to have fevers, and 7 days after lead extraction, after a failed attempt using interventional radiology techniques, she underwent removal of the indwelling Silastic catheter via sternotomy (**Figure 4.4**) with resolution of her signs of systemic infection. The patient was discharged with an external defibrillator vest and received a 4-week course of intravenous ampicillin.

The patient was seen as an outpatient 1 month after discharge. No arrhythmias were detected by the wearable external defibrillator, and subsequent 1-month ambulatory ECG monitoring revealed no ventricular arrhythmias. A cardiac MRI was performed, which demonstrated normal LVEF (**Video 4.4** and **Video 4.5**) and no late gadolinium enhancement. Our understanding of the sudden death risk of patients with recovered LVEF is less well established. In an analysis of the NCDR database of 26,197 Medicare-eligible patients who underwent ICD generator replacement, 7.3% of patients (average age, 77 years, and 34% with nonischemic cardiomyopathy) had recovery of LVEF by more than 50%.[19] At 3-year follow-up, LVEF greater than 50% was associated with significantly decreased readmission rates (12.2%) and reduced mortality 18.2% compared to patients with a persistent decrease in LVEF of less than 35% or those patients with partial recovery (LVEF 35%–50%). For comparison, the 3-year readmission and mortality rates for patients with persistent LVEF less than 35% were 27.5% and 32.7%, respectively. A single-center study found that patients with nonischemic cardiomyopathy and recovered LVEF (> 35%), absolute arrhythmia risk was low after a 4-year follow-up, and no arrhythmia events occurred in

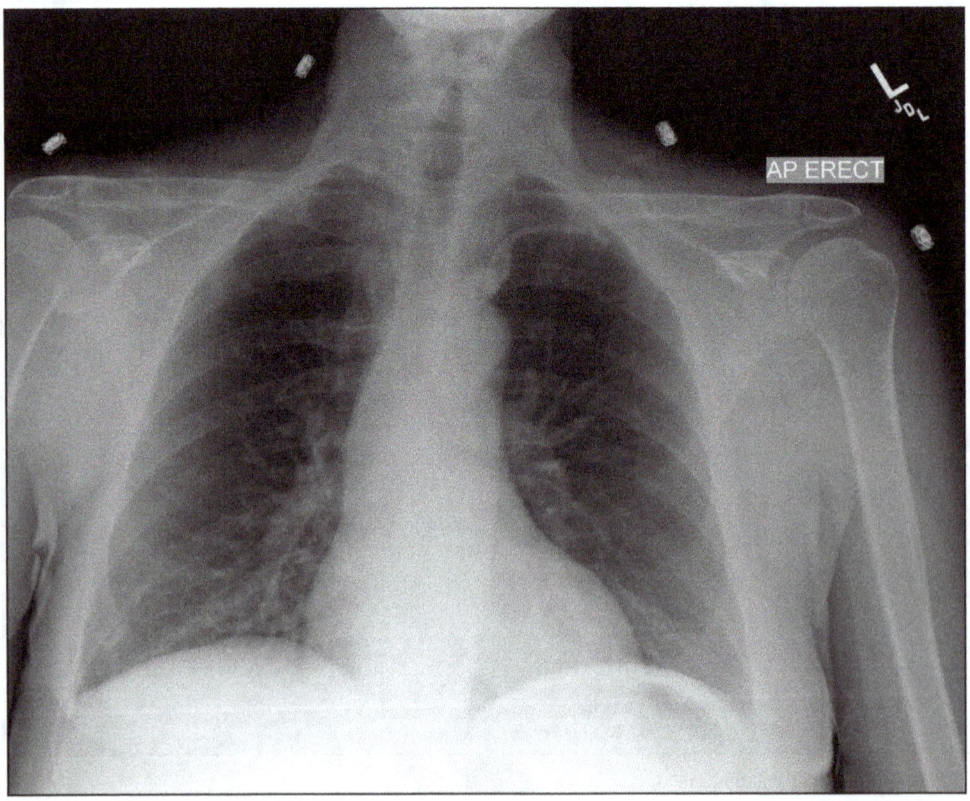

Figure 4.3 Postextraction, postero-anterior CXR shows no abnormalities. The indwelling Silastic catheter from the left can be seen.

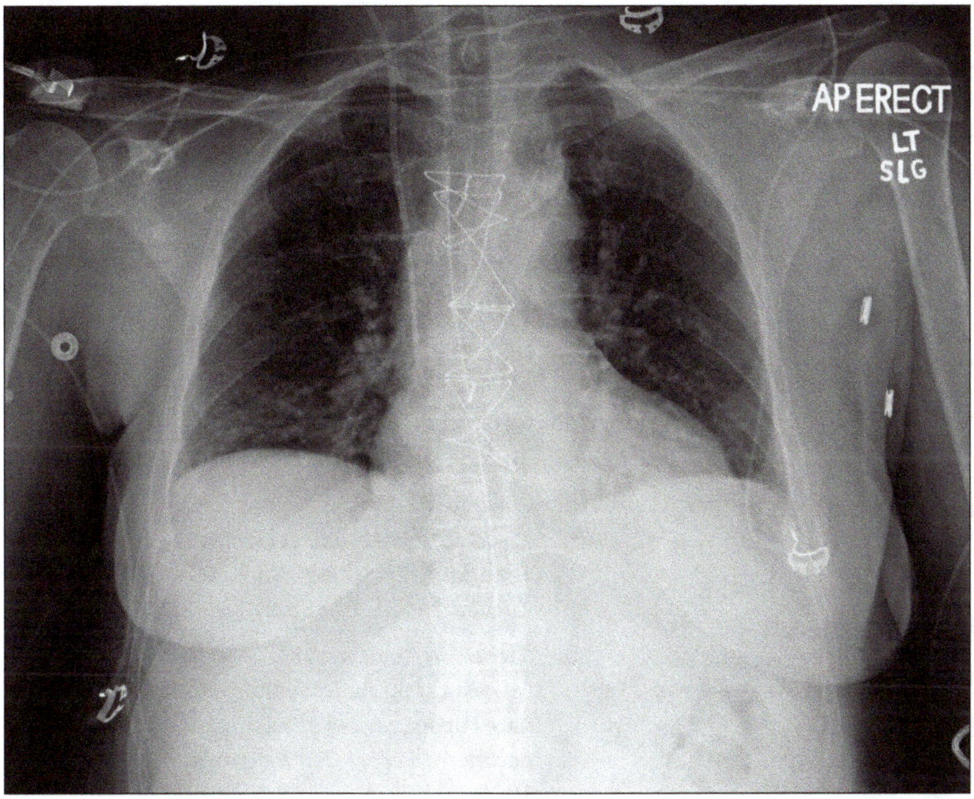

Figure 4.4 Removal of the Silastic catheter required a median sternotomy.

those patients with an LVEF of more than 50%.[20] After a shared decision-making process that included a discussion about the incomplete information available about appropriate therapies in the past, a decision not to implant an ICD was made. Continued follow-up is critical in patients even after long periods of apparent recovery of left ventricular function. This patient continues to do well and receives follow-up with the cardio-oncology service.[20]

SUMMARY POINTS

- Lead related masses are identified in 10%–15% of cases and their importance must be considered in clinical context, since at this time there are no specific imaging features that can consistently differentiate between infectious and noninfectious masses.
- The decision to not extract previously made this procedure more difficult. It is important to understand the implications of any decisions made over a patient's lifetime.
- During lead extraction, careful and continuous evaluation of lead integrity is critical.
- Important to identify all indwelling material in patients with bacteremia with a plan for management with continued infection.
- The decision on reimplantation of any device must be comprehensively addressed with the patient and a final decision made using a shared decision-making process.
- The evidence base for understanding the risk of recurrent arrhythmias in the setting of recovered left ventricular function is incomplete.

REFERENCES

1. Kusumoto FM, Schoenfeld MH, Wilkoff BL, et al. 2017 HRS expert consensus statement on cardiovascular implantable electronic device lead management and extraction. *Heart Rhythm.* 2017;14(12):e503–e551.
2. DeSimone DC, Sohail MR. Management of bacteremia in patients living with cardiovascular implantable electronic devices. *Heart Rhythm.* 2016;13(11):2247–2252.
3. Lo R, D'Anca M, Cohen T, Kerwin T. Incidence and prognosis of pacemaker lead-associated masses: A study of 1,569 transesophageal echocardiograms. *J Invasive Cardiol.* 2006;18(12): 599–601.
4. Downey BC, Juselius WE, Pandian NG, Estes MA 3rd, Link MS. Incidence and significance of pacemaker and implantable cardioverter-defibrillator lead masses discovered during transesophageal echocardiography. *Pacing Clin Electrophysiol.* 2011;34(6):679–683.
5. Robinson J, Wang WYS, Kaye G. Mobile echodensities on intracardiac device leads: Is it always a cause for concern? *Pacing Clin Electrophysiol.* 2020;43(4):388–393.
6. Cooper JM, Stephenson EA, Berul CI, Walsh EP, Epstein LM. Implantable cardioverter defibrillator lead complications and laser extraction in children and young adults with congenital heart disease: Implications for implantation and management. *J Cardiovasc Electrophysiol.* 2003;14(4): 344–349.
7. Pokorney SD, Parzynski CS, Daubert JP, et al. Temporal trends in and factors associated with use of single- versus dual-coil implantable cardioverter-defibrillator leads: Data from the NCDR ICD registry. *JACC Clin Electrophysiol.* 2017;3(6):612–619.
8. Boyle TA, Uslan DZ, Prutkin JM, et al. Impact of abandoned leads on cardiovascular implantable electronic device infections: A propensity matched analysis of MEDIC (Multicenter Electrophysiologic Device Infection Cohort). *JACC Clin Electrophysiol.* 2018;4(2):201–208.
9. Segreti L, Giannotti Santoro M, Di Cori A, et al. Safety and efficacy of transvenous mechanical lead extraction in patients with abandoned leads. *Europace.* 2020:euaa134.
10. Brunner MP, Cronin EM, Duarte VE, et al. Clinical predictors of adverse patient outcomes in an experience of more than 5000 chronic endovascular pacemaker and defibrillator lead extractions. *Heart Rhythm.* 2014;11(5):799–805.
11. Bongiorni MG, Kennergren C, Butter C, et al. The European Lead Extraction ConTRolled (ELECTRa) study: A European Heart Rhythm Association (EHRA) registry of transvenous lead extraction outcomes. *Eur Heart J.* 2017;38(40):2995–3005.
12. Pokorney SD, Mi X, Lewis RK, et al. Outcomes associated with extraction versus capping and abandoning pacing and defibrillator leads. *Circulation.* 2017;136(15):1387–1395.
13. Jacheć W, Polewczyk A, Segreti L, Bongiorni MG, Kutarski A. To abandon or not to abandon: Late consequences of pacing and ICD lead abandonment. *Pacing Clin Electrophysiol.* 2019;42(7): 1006–1017.
14. Elgaard AF, Johansen JB, Nielsen JC. Long-term follow-up of abandoned transvenous defibrillator leads: A nationwide cohort study. *Europace.* 2020;22(7):1097–1102.
15. Alqarawi W, Coppens J, Aldawood W, et al. A strategy of lead abandonment in a large cohort of patients with sprint fidelis leads. *JACC Clin Electrophysiol.* 2019;5(9):1059–1067.
16. Lewis RK, Ehieli WL, Hegland DD, et al. Hands on: How to approach patients undergoing lead extraction. *J Cardiovasc Electrophysiol.* 2020; 31(7):1801–1808.
17. Kypta A, Blessberger H, Saleh K, Hönig S, Kammler J, Neeser K, Steinwender C. An electrical plasma surgery tool for device replacement—Retrospective evaluation of complications and economic evaluation of costs and resource use. *Pacing Clin Electrophysiol.* 2015; 38(1):28–34.
18. Wasserlauf J, Esheim T, Jarett NM, Chan EKY, Schaller RD, Garcia FC, Knight BP. Avoiding damage to transvenous leads: A comparison of electrocautery techniques and two insulated electrocautery blades. *Pacing Clin Electrophysiol.* 2018;41(12):1593–1599.

19. Thomas IC, Wang Y, See VY, Minges KE, Curtis JP, Hsu JC. Outcomes following implantable cardioverter-defibrillator generator replacement in patients with recovered left ventricular systolic function: The national cardiovascular data registry. *Heart Rhythm*. 2019;16(5):733–740.

20. Berthelot-Richer M, Bonenfant F, Clavel MA, et al. Arrhythmic risk following recovery of left ventricular ejection fraction in patients with primary prevention ICD. *Pacing Clin Electrophysiol*. 2016;39(7):680–689.

21. Wilcox JE, Fang JC, Margulies KB, Mann DL. Heart failure with recovered left ventricular ejection fraction: JACC scientific expert panel. *J Am Coll Cardiol*. 2020;76(6):719–734.

VIDEO LEGENDS

Video 4.1 TEE showing a mobile mass attached to the lead in the right atrium (both 2D and 3D). [00:03]

Video 4.2 Another view with TEE showing a mobile mass attached to the lead in the right atrium (both 2D and 3D). [00:05]

Video 4.3 Postextraction intracardiac echocardiography shows no accumulation of pericardial fluid. [00:06]

Videos 4.4 and 4.5 Cardiac MRI after hospital discharge shows normal left ventricular function. [00:02] [00:02]

5 | Lead Management (Pocket Pain)

Fred M. Kusumoto, MD

CASE 5

CLINICAL VIGNETTE

A 66-year-old female with a long-standing history of atrial fibrillation underwent a dual-chamber pacemaker implant (Medtronic Advisa generator and 5076 atrial and ventricular leads) for bradycardia associated with sotalol 4 years ago. Pulmonary vein isolation because of continued atrial fibrillation was performed 3 years ago. She was referred to the Mayo Clinic for continued symptomatic atrial fibrillation and underwent a second ablation. Since then, she has not had recurrent atrial fibrillation identified by intracardiac electrograms. However, she has had continued pain at her pocket site since the implant. She denies any pain in her left arm. She describes the pain as intermittent, sharp, and more prominent with arm movement. A trial of low-dose NSAIDs (ibuprofen 200 mg daily) was tried for 2 months without a change in her symptoms. Her device was programmed to the DDI pacing mode, low rate of 30 bpm, 4 months ago to assess the need for rate support.

Her past medical history is significant for hypertension and diabetes mellitus, and her current medications are rivaroxaban, valsartan, and metformin.

Her pocket site shows no erythema or signs of infection or dermatitis. No swelling or prominent vessels are noted at the shoulder region, and the generator appears to be located in the correct tissue plane and in the usual location.

Her chest X-ray (CXR) is shown in **Figure 5.1**.

DECISION MAKING FOR LEAD EXTRACTION

Possible options were discussed and included continued observation, medications, generator relocation, removal of the generator, or removal of the generator and leads. The literature on pocket pain associated with CIEDs is sparse. Chronic pain is the reason for lead extraction in 1% to 3% of patients from several large single-center registries.[1–3] Chronic pain can have several different etiologies such as occult infection, upper extremity deep venous thrombosis, complex regional pain syndrome, placement of the device in the subcuticular space or in the axillary region, or component allergy. Still, a specific diagnosis often cannot be identified.[1–7] Case reports have discussed using lidocaine patches, generator relocation, and lead extraction.[3,6–9] In the largest study to date, investigators from several centers identified 27 patients who underwent lead extraction for pocket pain.[3] After extraction, 66% of patients had resolution of pain. There was no significant difference in the resolution of pain between those who had reimplantation of a device versus those who did not. In this and other case report studies, in patients with subcuticular device implant or superficial devices, repositioning of the device to the correct tissue plane or to a subpectoral position alleviated pain.[3,6,9]

Interrogation of the device on repeated evaluation demonstrated no continued requirement for rate support. Late (> 1 year after implant) device-related infection is rare and usually due to a recent generator replacement.[7] Lead extraction is associated with risk, and that risk will depend on multiple factors, including patient characteristics such as comorbidities or prior surgeries, device-related issues, such as device and lead type, time of initial lead implant, or the number of leads, and hospital site issues, such as total volume or experience.[7,10]

 ISBN: 978-1-942909-54-5

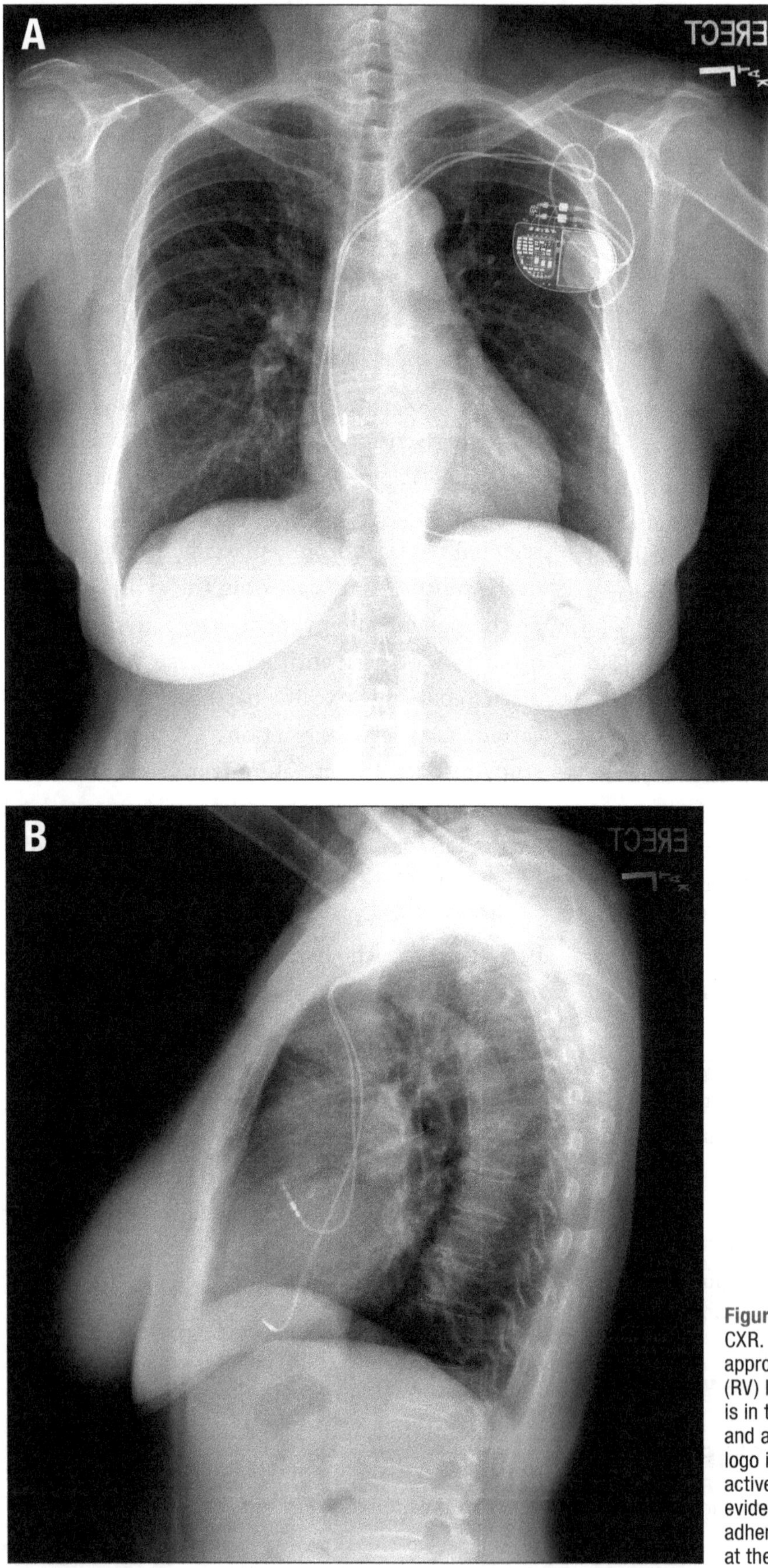

Figure 5.1 **Panel A:** Postero-anterior projection CXR. **Panel B:** Lateral projection. Confirmation of appropriate right atrial (RA) and right ventricular (RV) locations for the pacing leads. The RA lead is in the RA appendage, and the RV lead is apical and appears to be relatively septal. The Medtronic logo is seen on the generator, and the leads are active fixation and do not appear to have any evidence of loss of integrity. The leads may be adherent to each other or twisted on each other at the superior vena cava (SVC)–RA junction.

Chronic pain associated with a CIED that has been refractory to other strategies is a IIa indication for lead extraction.[7] No published data is available that evaluates the natural history of patients with abandoned leads only and no generator. From the physical examination, the generator appeared to be in a normally expected position. Since the device was implanted relatively recently, although lead extraction is associated with some risk, now would be the time to decide on a long-term strategy for the leads. After the discussion about the different options, the patient agreed on lead extraction and generator removal without reimplantation, understanding that pain may not resolve after the procedure since there was no preprocedure evidence for a specific cause for her symptoms.[3]

Since the leads are 4 years old and do not include an implantable cardioverter-defibrillator (ICD) or left ventricular (LV) leads, even though she has not had prior cardiac surgery, extraction in the electrophysiology laboratory was chosen.

PROCEDURAL PREPARATION

Before the procedure, the rivaroxaban was stopped. While lead extraction can be performed safely in the setting of anticoagulation, in this case, since the patient was not having atrial fibrillation, it was elected to hold her rivaroxaban for 48 hours before the procedure.[11] In addition, her angiotensin-receptor blocking (ARB) agent was also stopped. A randomized study from the anesthesia literature found that withholding ARBs and angiotensin-converting enzyme inhibitors before major noncardiac surgery were associated with a lower risk of death and postoperative vascular events.[12] A meta-analysis of 5 studies found that withholding immediate preoperative renin-angiotensin, aldosterone antagonist medications were associated with decreased incidence of intraoperative hypotension.[13] In addition to the routine preoperative blood testing, the patient was typed and crossed for 2 units of packed red blood cells.[7]

PROCEDURAL DETAILS

The surgical incision site was marked in the preprocedure area, and consent and appropriate preoperative testing and evaluation were confirmed. The patient was intubated and an arterial line placed for continuous blood pressure monitoring during the procedure.

In the electrophysiology laboratory, the entire chest and abdomen were prepared from the neck to the upper thigh area. The patient first underwent placement of an 8.5-Fr sheath from the femoral vein and an intracardiac ultrasound placed (**Video 5.1**). The ultrasound is used to identify any adherent masses on the leads and monitor for the development or increase in pericardial fluid during the procedure. The author prefers intracardiac echocardiography over transesophageal echocardiography (TEE) if only one intraoperative imaging modality is going to be used during the procedure, since having preextraction femoral venous access with a long sheath is beneficial if catastrophic large vessel tear occurs during the extraction and also can be used if lead snaring from an inferior approach is required.

An elliptical incision that encompassed the existing keloid scar from the initial implant was made. For patients with preexisting generators, multiple strategies for skin incision can be used. In this situation, the author generally uses an incision to remove the preexisting scar from the prior implant. The subcutaneous tissue was dissected in the usual manner, and the pocket was opened, and tissue cultures were obtained. On evaluation of the pocket, there was no overt evidence for infection, and the generator location was appropriate at the plane between the pectoralis major muscle and subcutaneous tissue. The patient was not pacemaker dependent, so the device was detached, and the leads were individually dissected to near the venous entry point, just under the clavicle. Since the adhesion of the lead to the posterior portion of the clavicle for those patients who had lead implant using subclavian vein puncture is often a site where lead damage can occur during the extraction process, the lead was freed completely from the clavicle. Since the leads have retractable helices, attempts were made to retract the helices. The RV lead helix retracted completely, but the RA helix would not retract.

The lead was prepared in the usual manner with the lead end cut to remove the connector and after using a standard stylet, a locking stylet advanced as far as possible. Twenty-five years ago, the development of locking stylets with an "active" fixation mechanism at the lead tip or along the entire body of the lead was a significant advance in technology that significantly improved the safety of the lead extraction procedure. Before the development of these stylets, "locking" was achieved by determining the lumen size of the lead and then choosing a stylet with a diameter that closely matched this lumen. These stylets were often difficult to advance to the tip of the lead, and when tension was applied during the extraction process would sometimes "slip." Using the modern generation of locking stylets, the stylet will often advance to the tip unless the lead lumen is obstructed by blood. It is critical to avoid any injury to the lead during this process of stylet exchanges. This is particularly important if a breach in lead integrity is suspected or known since these leads may be particularly fragile. Careful observation via fluoroscopy is critical when advancing or removing the stylet to ensure smooth transit through the lumen. Also, any locations where the locking stylet is difficult to advance or to remove should be noted. Once the locking stylet is in place, and the locking mechanism activated, it is important to assess how far the stylet has advanced through the lead's interior lumen. This provides the operator some sense of how much tension can be applied to the proximal portion of the lead, and conversely, how much forward pressure on the extraction tool can be used. Any distal portions of the lead where the locking stylet is not present will be more fragile and more likely to lose lead integrity. When the locking stylet has not advanced to the tip, it becomes far more likely that a combined approach from the femoral vein will be required to provide tension on the distal portion of the lead during the extraction process. In this case, the locking stylets were able to be advanced to both lead tips. Next, to help maintain lead integrity throughout the extraction process, it is critical to use sutures (2-0 silk in this case) or specialized compression coils to crimp the insulation to the conductor portion of the lead while trying to minimize any increase in the lead diameter. In addition to helping maintain lead integrity, using techniques to crimp the insulation to the conductor coil reduces the likelihood that the locking stylet will be pulled back during the extraction procedure.

At this point in the extraction procedure, gentle tension can be placed on each lead. By carefully observing the lead's behavior on fluoroscopy, this maneuver provides the operator some idea of where the potential adhesions may exist on each lead and whether the leads appear to be adherent to each other, and if the leads are twisted on each other. Since the helix on the RV lead had retracted, gentle tension alone was able to remove the lead (**Video 5.2**). In a recent study from a multicenter lead extraction registry, 27% of leads could be removed with simple traction. In a report from one center, more than 85% of leads were removed with traction and the use of a locking stylet even though these leads had a median implant time of 46 months.[14,15] Since even gentle traction could potentially cause loss of lead integrity, the author's practice is to place a locking stylet first before simple traction unless the lead has been implanted for less than 3 to 4 months.

To extract the atrial lead, mechanical rotational extraction tools were used. No randomized comparison of mechanical rotational extraction versus laser extraction has been done. A retrospective study from a single center that used both approaches suggest generally similar efficacy.[16]

First, the lead was freed at the vascular entry point and within the innominate vein using a shorter mechanical rotational extractor (9-Fr Shortie RL, Cook Medical). This sheath is relatively short (13.6 cm) and provides easier control of the tip. Fluoroscopy is used to ensure that the tool is being directed on the appropriate axis and to monitor for any lead damage. Although the Medtronic 5076 lead is 6-Fr in diameter, larger extraction sheaths are often required to accommodate any sutures or tools used to compress the insulation and any additional adherent fibrotic tissue. When evaluating what diameter extraction tool is required, it is best not to use a sheath with a "tight fit" as this may make removal of the tool from the lead to use another extraction tool difficult. After removing the rotational tool, the lead was examined, and adherent tissue exposed on the lead was removed to prevent reintroduction into the body.

A full-length mechanical rotational extractor (9-Fr Evolution RL, Cook Medical) was then used. As the distal portion of the extractor reaches the innominate vein–SVC junction, we pause to determine whether additional traction from below would be beneficial and whether an additional sheath should be placed in the SVC just superior to the innominate venous entry point if the placement of a SVC balloon could be required. For this patient, it was felt that neither of these additional techniques would be required, and the extraction process was continued. In cases where 2 (or more) leads need extraction using specialized sheaths (whether laser or mechanical rotational), it often is useful to alternate between leads, particularly if a region of binding between leads is encountered. With the removal of the extraction tools during the procedure, the leads should be examined for any debris. During extraction, forward pressure with the extraction tool and tension on the locking stylet is generally kept "equal," and throughout the process, fluoroscopy is used to evaluate for any degradation in lead integrity and to ensure that the extraction tool is coaxial to the lead.

When the distal portion of the extraction tool reached the distal electrode of the lead, the helix began to elongate (▶ **Video 5.3**) since it was still deployed and attached to the atrial myocardium. The extraction was paused, and the situation was reassessed. After discussion among all team members, it was elected to continue the procedure and not to employ any additional techniques. A sheath is present from below, and while it is often useful to be able to apply traction simultaneously from above and below a region where lead integrity is in question, in this case, since the helix extension was within the atrial tissue, it was felt that switching to an inferior approach or a simultaneous superior and inferior approach would not provide additional benefit. The extraction tool was kept coaxial to the lead body, and in addition to traction, counterclockwise pressure was exerted on the proximal portion of the lead, and the lead was freed from the atrial wall (▶ **Video 5.4**). Notice that the locking stylet has been pulled back even with the compression measures taken before extraction.

Once the lead was been freed, the patient was monitored and remained hemodynamically stable and no pericardial effusion developed as assessed by intracardiac echocardiography (▶ **Video 5.5**)

FOLLOW-UP

After the extraction, her CXR demonstrated no abnormalities (**Figure 5.2**) and transthoracic echocardiography (TTE) showed no pericardial effusion. Her ARB and rivaroxaban were restarted on postoperative day 2. Patient had complete resolution of her pain after the procedure. Over the last 2 years, she has not had recurrent symptomatic atrial fibrillation or symptomatic bradycardia but remains on rivaroxaban given her comorbidities.

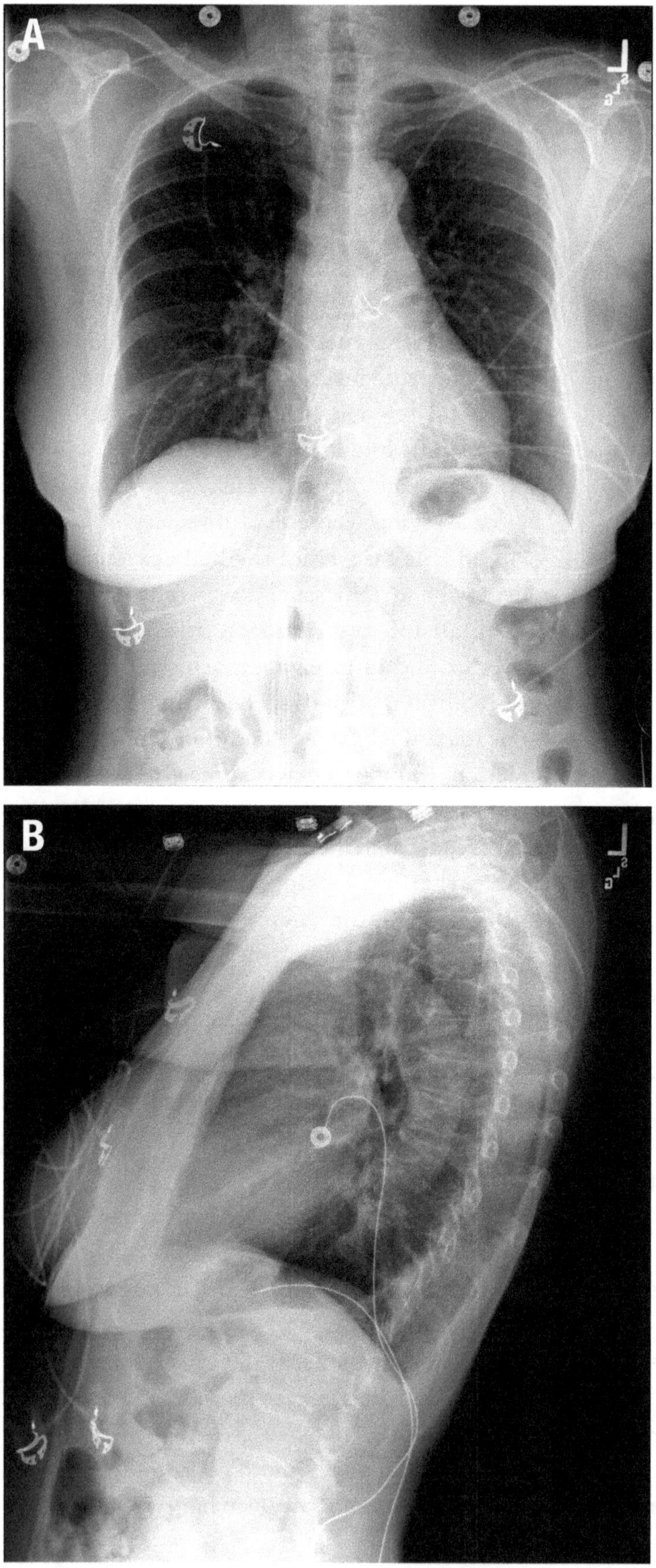

Figure 5.2 **Panel A:** Antero-posterior and **Panel B:** Lateral projection for the postoperative CXR that demonstrate no abnormalities and complete removal of all hardware.

SUMMARY POINTS

- The decision to extract and a discussion of all of the different choices along with risks and benefits in patients with chronic pain at the generator site and possible causes must be carefully considered.
- The possibility that the pain will not resolve after whatever is done must be discussed with the patient.
- Individualized decision making and preparation for issues such as anticoagulation status, perioperative drug strategies, and extraction site and techniques is critical.
- Careful dissection to the venous entry point and freeing the lead completely from any adjacent structures and removal of any adherent debris is important.
- During the extraction procedure, use specific "stop-points" just prior to any critical moments to assess current status of the patient and lead integrity, and whether or not any additional techniques or tools may be required. These "stop points" include after extravascular dissection has been completed, after all leads have been prepared and locking stylets have been deployed, at the innominate–SVC junction, at the point of freeing the lead from myocardial tissue, and immediately after removal of a lead.

REFERENCES

1. Gomes S, Cranney G, Bennett M, Li A, Giles R. Twenty-year experience of transvenous lead extraction at a single centre. *Europace.* 2014;16: 1350–1355.
2. Jones SO, Eckart RE, Albert CM, Epstein LM. Large, single-center, single-operator experience with transvenous lead extraction: Outcomes and changing indications. *Heart Rhythm.* 2008; 5:520–525
3. Lewis K, Dai M, Patton KK, et al. Lead extraction for reduction of chronic pain related to cardiovascular implantable electronic device. *Europace.* 2019;21(5):781–786.
4. Hayes DL, Loesl K. Pacemaker component allergy: case report and review of the literature. *J Interv Card Electrophysiol.* 2002;6(3): 277–278.
5. Mandal S, Pande A, Mandal D, Kumar A, Sarkar A, Kahali D, Mazumdar B, Panja M. Permanent pacemaker-related upper extremity deep vein thrombosis: A series of 20 cases. *Pacing Clin Electrophysiol.* 2012;35(10): 1194–1198.
6. Furman S, Curtis AB, Conti JB. Recognition and correction of subcuticular malposition of pacemaker pulse generators. *Pacing Clin Electrophysiol.* 2001;24(8 Pt 1):1224–1227.
7. Kusumoto FM, Schoenfeld MH, Wilkoff BL, et al. 2017 HRS expert consensus statement on cardiovascular implantable electronic device lead management and extraction. *Heart Rhythm.* 2017;14(12):e503–e551.
8. Hesselson AB. A simple technique for relocating chronic CIED leads to a subpectoral position for relief of erosion and pain. *Pacing Clin Electrophysiol.* 2018;41(7):834–838.
9. Espinosa J, Rueda JD, Rosselli D. Pacemaker implantation site neuralgia treated with lidocaine patches: Case report. *Universitas Médica.* 2012;53(2):208–211.
10. Lee JZ, Ling J, Diehl NN, et al. Mortality and cerebrovascular events after heart rhythm disorder management procedures. *Circulation.* 2018;137(1):24–33.
11. Zheng Q, Maytin M, John RM, Killu AM, Epstein LM. Transvenous lead extraction during uninterrupted warfarin therapy: Feasibility and outcomes. *Heart Rhythm.* 2018;15:1777–1781.

12. Roshanov PS, Rochwerg B, Patel A, et al. Withholding versus continuing angiotensin-converting enzyme inhibitors or angiotensin II receptor blockers before noncardiac surgery: An analysis of the vascular events in noncardiac surgery patients cohort evaluation prospective cohort. *Anesthesiology.* 2017;126(1):16–27.
13. Rosenman DJ, McDonald FS, Ebbert JO, Erwin PJ, LaBella M, Montori VM. Clinical consequences of withholding versus administering renin-angiotensin-aldosterone system antagonists in the preoperative period. *Hosp Med.* 2008;3(4):319–325.
14. Bongiorni MG, Kennergren C, Butter C, et al. The European Lead Extraction ConTRolled (ELECTRa) study: A European Heart Rhythm Association (EHRA) registry of transvenous lead extraction outcomes. *Eur Heart J.* 2017;38(40):2995–3005.
15. Lima NA, Cunha GS, Menezes NS, Silva ELD Junior, Lima CCV, Sampaio SMV. Lead removal without extraction tools: A single-center experience. *Braz J Cardiovasc Surg.* 2019;34(4):458–463.
16. Starck CT, Rodriguez H, Hürlimann D, et al. Transvenous lead extractions: Comparison of laser versus mechanical approach. *Europace.* 2013;15(11):1636–1641.

VIDEO LEGENDS

Video 5.1 Intracardiac ultrasound placed in the right atrium before the extraction (9 Mz mechanical, Boston Scientific Ultra Ice Plus). No pericardial effusion is present, and no echogenic masses are identified on the leads. [00:10]

Video 5.2 Gentle traction under fluoroscopy leads to removal of the right ventricular lead without requiring any sheaths. [00:03]

Video 5.3 When the extraction tool reached the distal electrode, traction-countertraction techniques lead to the elongation of the helix. The ultrasound catheter can be seen at the base of the right atrium. In this position, it does not interact with any of the extraction tools, and this location is extremely sensitive for identifying the presence of pericardial effusion. [00:03]

Video 5.4 Removal of the lead with traction and counterclockwise twisting of the lead. Notice that the locking stylet has retracted slightly during this final process (compare the location of the radiopaque tip of the locking stylet in Video 5.3 and Video 5.4). [00:06]

Video 5.5 Postextraction intracardiac echocardiography demonstrates no accumulation of pericardial fluid. [00:05]

6 | Superior Vena Cava Obstruction Due to Pacemaker Leads

Siva K. Mulpuru, MD, MPH

CASE 6

CLINICAL VIGNETTE

A 33-year-old male patient presented to the clinic with prominent neck veins, headaches, fatigue, and facial pain with minimal exertion. His past medical history included nephrolithiasis, multiple orthopedic surgeries, obstructive sleep apnea, and vasovagal syncope. He received a dual-chamber pacemaker for vasovagal syncope in 2003. Subsequently, he underwent lead replacement after an atrial lead fracture. The symptoms were more prominent over the previous 6 months. He endorses facial redness and fullness when he sleeps on 2 pillows (**Figure 6.1**). He also complained of shortness of breath with upper body exercise. The most recent device details are as follows:

Device Details

Device Component	Manufacturer/ Model	Date of Implant
Pulse generator	Guidant Insignia	03/2007
Right atrial lead	Medtronic 5076	03/2007
Right ventricular lead	Medtronic 5560	03/2003

His device was pacing less than 2% in both the right-sided chambers. Laboratory workup was unremarkable, and his echocardiogram revealed a structurally normal heart with an ejection fraction of 56%. As a part of the workup for his unexplained symptoms, he underwent a hemodynamic exercise study. His baseline superior vena cava (SVC) mean pressure was 18 mmHg (normal < 6 mmHg), and the pressure increased to 28 mmHg on arm exercise with the reproduction of symptoms. Venography confirmed complete occlusion of the SVC at the SVC–RA junction (**Video 6.1**).

PREPROCEDURAL PLANNING

The patient was evaluated by cardiac surgery and interventional radiology teams before the procedure. The device was turned to ODO mode 3 weeks before the procedure without any change in the patient's symptom burden. A preprocedural CT scan with contrast was also performed to understand venous anatomy for the procedure. The option of lead extraction and balloon venoplasty with or without a stent was discussed in detail with the patient.

PROCEDURAL DETAILS

A preprocedural huddle was performed with all teams in attendance. The patient was taken to the hybrid operating room and was prepped from the neck to the groin in a sterile manner. General anesthesia was administered, and a transthoracic echocardiography (TTE) probe was placed for monitoring during the procedure. Four units of blood cross-matched, packed red cells were available in the room for the procedure. Venous and arterial accesses were obtained using ultrasound guidance and modified Seldinger's technique. Dedicated arterial and venous sheaths were placed in the left femoral venous site for rapid initiation of peripheral cardiopulmonary bypass in the event of a complication. Multiple sheaths were also placed in the right common femoral vein. A 9-Fr sheath was placed in the right common femoral vein for high-volume crystalloid or blood product infusion. An 8-Fr SRO sheath (Fast Cath, Abbott) was placed in the right femoral vein for over a wire with the sheath's tip in the right atrium (RA). A 6-Fr sheath was also placed in the left common femoral vein for placement of a stiff

 ISBN: 978-1-942909-54-5

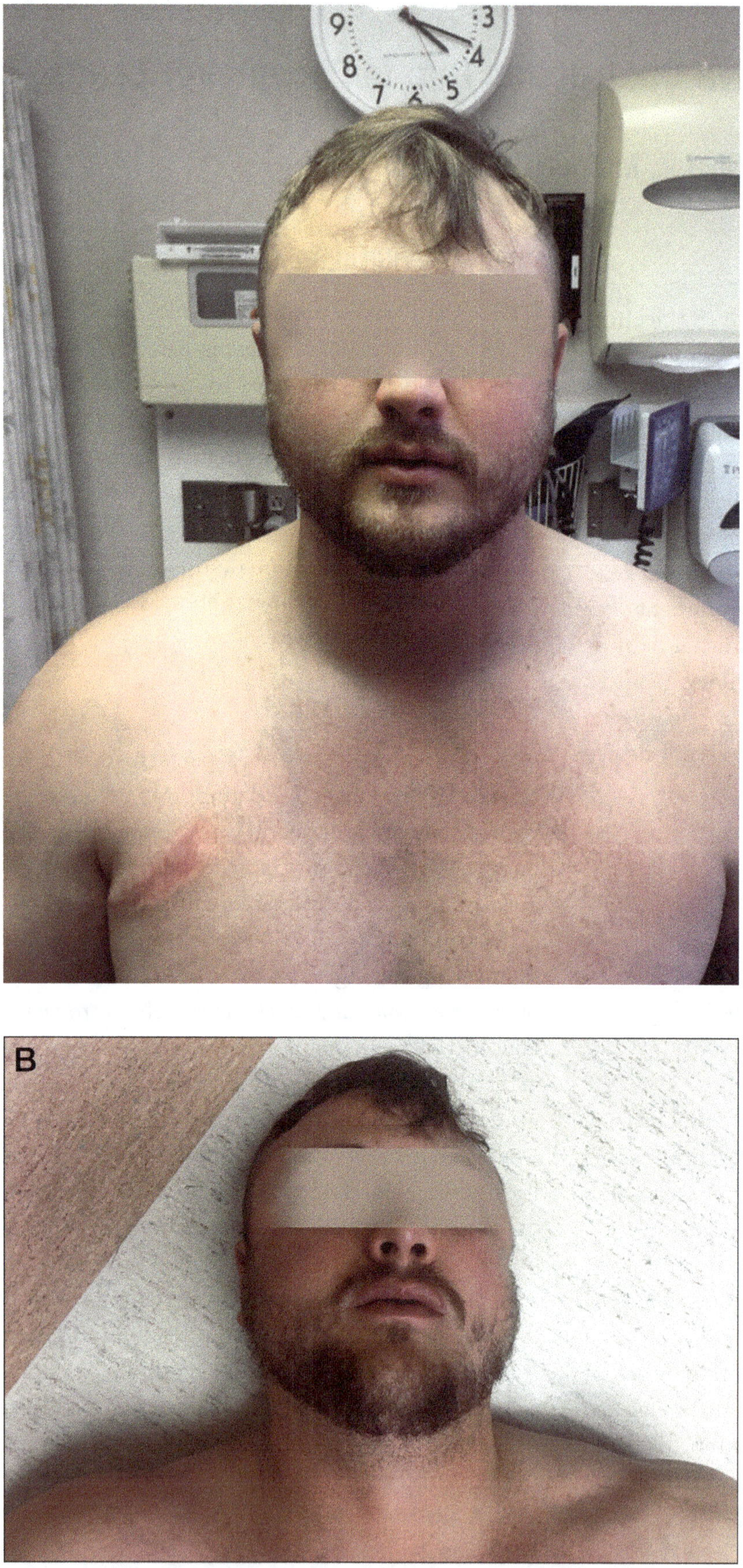

Figure 6.1 **Panel A:** A hypertrophic scar on the device site. Venous collaterals are noted on the chest wall suggesting the presence of central obstruction. The photograph was taken when the patient was standing up. **Panel B:** Facial plethora in a lying down position with the reproduction of his symptoms.

0.035-inch wire for the SVC occlusion balloon placement. The pocket was opened, and the leads were freed till the suture sleeves.

The sutures were cut, and the sleeves were pulled back. Stylets were placed in leads, and helices were retracted (**Video 6.2**). The leads were prepared using locking stylets (Lead Locking Device, EZ, Philips Medical). A 4-mm tip deflectable ablation catheter (Blazer, Boston Scientific) was used to engage the J portion of the atrial lead, and the lead tip was pulled towards the IVC to free the tip from the RA wall. (**Video 6.3**). A 15-mm Goose Neck snare (GN 1500, Medtronic) was used to go over the lead's tip and engage the body of the lead. The snare provided a way to apply downward traction on the lead and serve as a rail to advance sheaths from a superior access site (**Figure 6.2**).

A 14-Fr laser sheath (GlideLight, Philips) was placed on the ventricular lead. It was advanced using traction-countertraction technique, and the ventricular lead was eventually taken out of the vasculature (**Video 6.4**). Laser energy was used at the site of adhesions. The outer sheath was only advanced to the level of the tricuspid valve. The same 14-Fr laser sheath was then placed on the RA lead, and it was advanced to the level of the inferior vena cava. The Goose Neck snare was

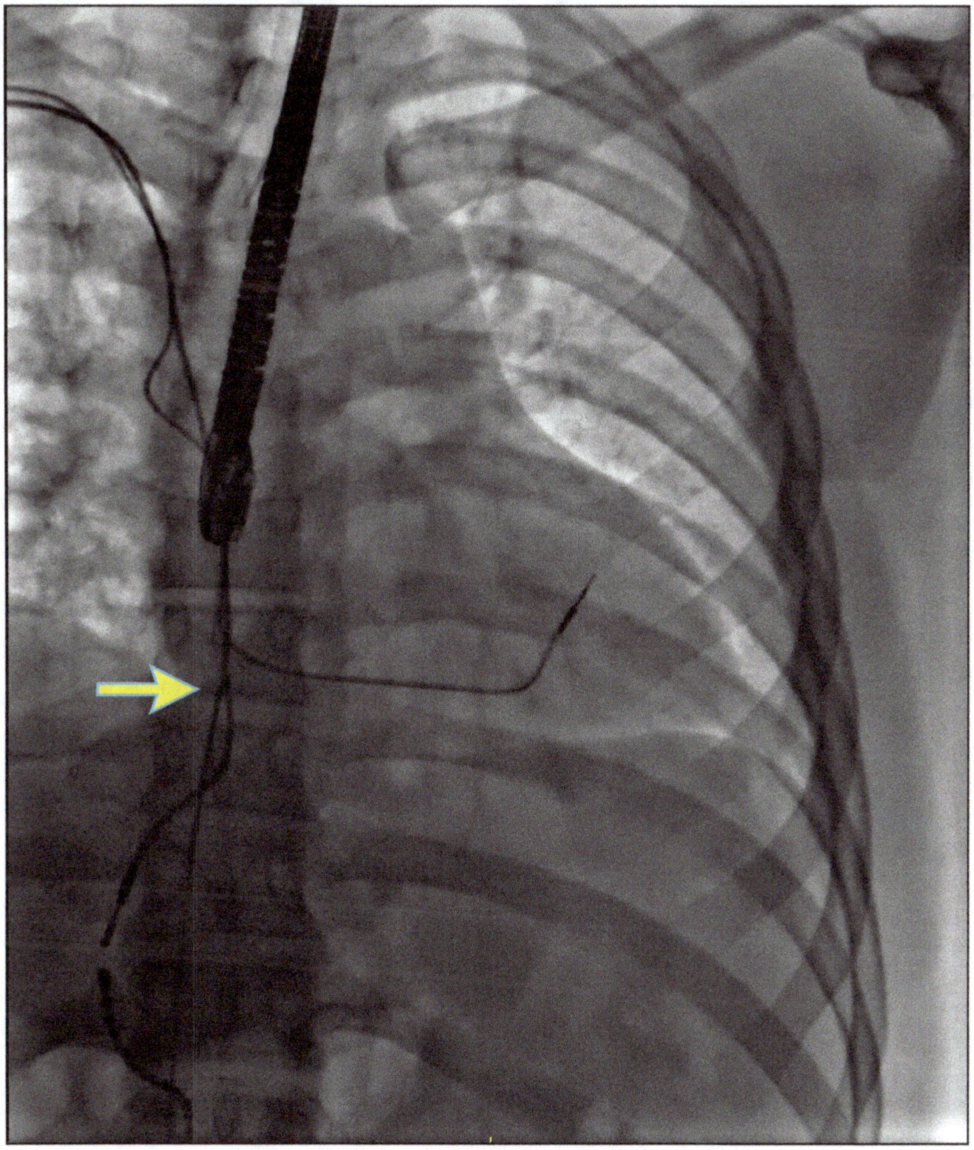

Figure 6.2 A 15-mm Goose Neck snare (GN 1500, Medtronic) was used to grab the body of the atrial lead to provide rail for extraction sheaths and to retrain vascular access.

then released, and the lead was pulled inside the outer sheath (**Video 6.5**). A long 7-Fr sheath was placed over the stiff wire, and a selective venogram was performed.

Venoplasty of the SVC-RA stenosis was performed using a 16-mm low-pressure balloon (PE-MT, Boston Scientific) (**Video 6.6**). After the inner laser sheath was taken, a stiff wire was placed into the IVC through the outer sheath for venoplasty. All sheaths were eventually removed, and hemostasis was achieved by manual compression. Transesophageal echocardiography (TEE) showed trivial pericardial effusion with mild tricuspid regurgitation (TR). As he did not have any symptoms when his device was set to ODO, a decision was made not to reimplant a pacemaker.

POSTPROCEDURAL COURSE

The patient was extubated in the recovery room and was transferred to the floor service. He was discharged from the hospital the next day. He felt a significant improvement in his symptoms after the procedure. However, 8 weeks after the procedure, he called back, saying symptoms were slowly returning. He was brought back for a repeat procedure. Venography showed redevelopment of the SVC RA stenosis. A covered stent (Viabhan VBX, Gore Medical) was placed in the SVC during a subsequent procedure (**Figure 6.3**). He was prescribed clopidogrel 75 mg a day and apixaban 5 mg twice daily for 6 months after the procedure. He remained symptom-free during his subsequent follow-up.

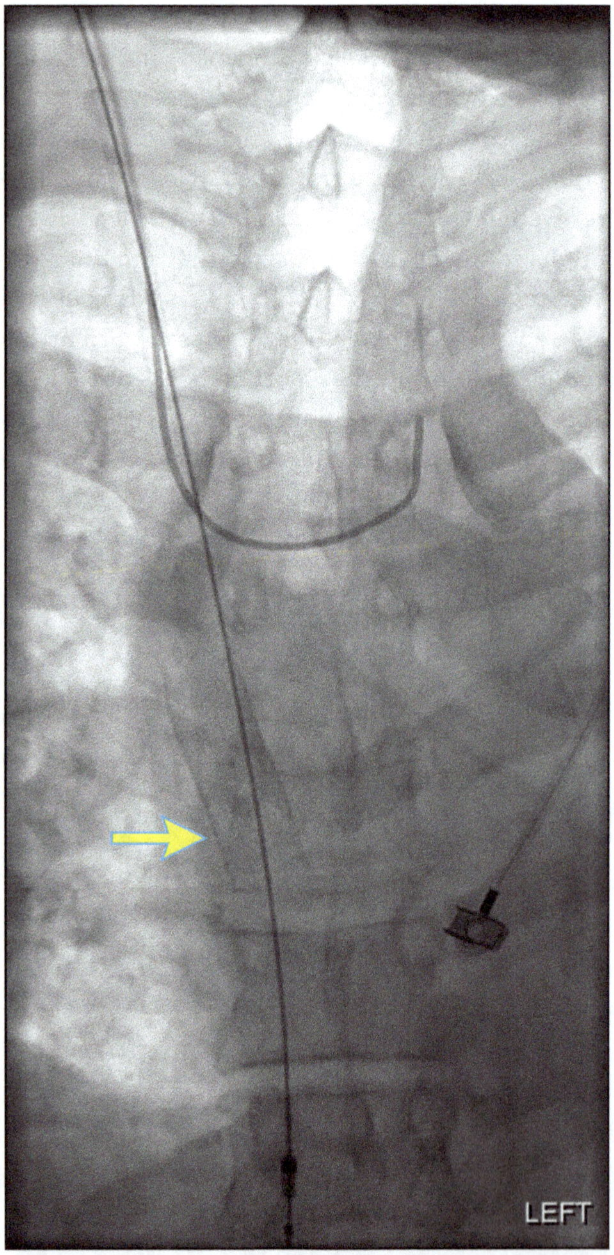

Figure 6.3 As there was a recurrence of restenosis, a 13 mm × 5 cm covered stent (Viabhan VBX, Gore Medical) was placed and postdilated during the subsequent procedure.

SUMMARY POINTS

- SVC syndrome can occur due to venous obstruction after pacemaker implantation. Symptoms include headaches, positional redness of the upper body, and facial swelling.
- Downward traction on the pacemaker leads provides rail to advance sheaths from superior sites without losing venous access.
- Venoplasty and stent placement are effective means of treating SVC stenosis.
- A trial period of turning the device "off – ODO mode" can provide information to make reimplantation decisions.
- Antiplatelet and anticoagulant therapy decision should be individualized based on shared decision making.

VIDEO LEGENDS

Video 6.1 Contrast venogram of the SVC was performed through a balloon-tipped catheter in the left anterior oblique (LAO 40) view shows complete occlusion of the SVC with the prominent azygous vein (arrow). [00:06]

Video 6.2 The lead helices were retracted, and the leads were prepared with locking stylets. [00:01]

Video 6.3 A deflectable catheter was used to hook the J portion of the atrial lead and pull the lead down to the IVC (RAO 30). [00:01]

Video 6.4 A 14-Fr laser sheath (GlideLight, Philips Medical) was used to break adhesions around the right ventricular lead. Notice that the other sheath is positioned in the RA, as it may be difficult to navigate additional curves across the tricuspid valve with the outer sheath. [00:05]

Video 6.5 After the 14-Fr laser sheath was advanced over the RA lead to the IVC level, the Amplatz Goose Neck snare (GN 1500, Medtronic) was released from the RA lead. The lead was pulled back into the inner sheath. The inner sheath was then pulled into the outer sheath, which was then used to retain access. [00:30]

Video 6.6 A 16-mm PE-MT low-pressure balloon (Boston Scientific) was used to dilate the region of stenosis. [00:05]

7 | Lead Extraction for Superior Vena Cava Occlusion

Charles J. Love, MD

CASE 7

CLINICAL VIGNETTE

The patient is a 61-year-old African-American female at the time of her presentation to our hospital at the end of July 2019. Her first pacemaker was a single-chamber device placed on her right chest in 1978 (41 years earlier) after an atrial septal and ventricular septal defect closure and development of a complete atrioventricular (AV) block. Then, on April 2, 1993, she had a Pacesetter Synchrony 2028L placed with new right atrial (RA) and right ventricular (RV) leads placed on the right side (Medtronic 5524 and 5024, respectively, both passive fixation), with a reported capping of her old RV lead. She subsequently had device replacements in 1998, 2005, and 2012. However, the leads apparently failed, and on May 27, 2014, she had the right-sided device removed and leads abandoned. A new dual-chamber pacemaker with St. Jude 2088 leads was implanted on the left side.

She has developed persistent atrial fibrillation/flutter (anticoagulated with apixaban) with AV block and has a slow escape rhythm at 35 bpm. She presented with intermittent presyncope, fatigue, and symptoms of congestive heart failure. She was found to have a markedly elevated capture threshold on the RV lead. She is now referred due to high threshold on the RV lead.

Device Details

Lead Performance Data	RA	RV
Lead Impedance (ohms)	280	250
Sensing (mV)	0.9	1.9
Capture (V@ms)	N/A	7.5V @ 1.0 ms (intermittent)
% Pacing	0%	99%

Additional Preprocedural Data

After the initial evaluation, it was found that she had undergone an assessment at another institution. A CT scan showed a 90% occlusion of her superior vena cava (SVC) and that she has intermittent symptoms of SVC syndrome (edema of the upper body, head, and neck, and pulsating headaches). The plan there was to have a patch repair of her SVC with open heart removal of her pacing leads and placement of an epicardial pacing system.

We considered and presented to her another option: a staged procedure. First, to get a reasonable heart rate and stabilize her hemodynamically, we would place a leadless pacemaker. Once she was recovered from that, we proposed to remove as much of the old lead systems as possible while leaving a guidewire through the SVC. We would then have interventional radiology (IR) place a stent into the SVC to help unload her venous system. After discussion with all parties (patient, IR, cardiac surgery, and electrophysiology), a decision was made to proceed with the less invasive option.

PREPROCEDURAL PLANNING (OVERALL)

Careful coordination with cardiac anesthesia, cardiac surgery (for backup), and IR was needed. We anticipated a long procedure time for the extraction and would need IR to be available immediately at the end of our part of the extraction. We also considered the patient's poor overall condition and her wishes with regard to the operation. We decided to start the staged procedure by doing the leadless pacemaker implant and then discharge her for several weeks to strengthen. We would then bring her back for the

 ISBN: 978-1-942909-54-5

more complicated extraction and stenting of the venous system. We also performed a CT scan to evaluate the intravascular structures and leads (**Figure 7.1**).

Leadless Pacemaker Implant (August 2019)

A leadless pacemaker (Micra, Medtronic) was placed without event during the first week of August of 2019. **Video 7.1** shows the position and condition of the 5 leads. **Videos 7.2–7.4** show the delivery of the leadless pacemaker. Note the difficulty in getting the catheter past the adhesions in the right atrium (Video 7.2). Postprocedure, the effective pacing provided immediate improvement regarding her lightheadedness, presyncope, shortness of breath, dyspnea on exertion, and heart failure symptoms. She was discharged the following day in a much-improved condition. After she was fully recovered and we were sure the new device was working well, she was brought back in October of 2019 for the next procedure.

PREPROCEDURAL PLANNING (EXTRACTION)

As is typical in our electrophysiology lab, the patient was prepped according to our protocol per the Heart Rhythm Society guidelines.[1] The patient was placed under general anesthesia (endotracheal

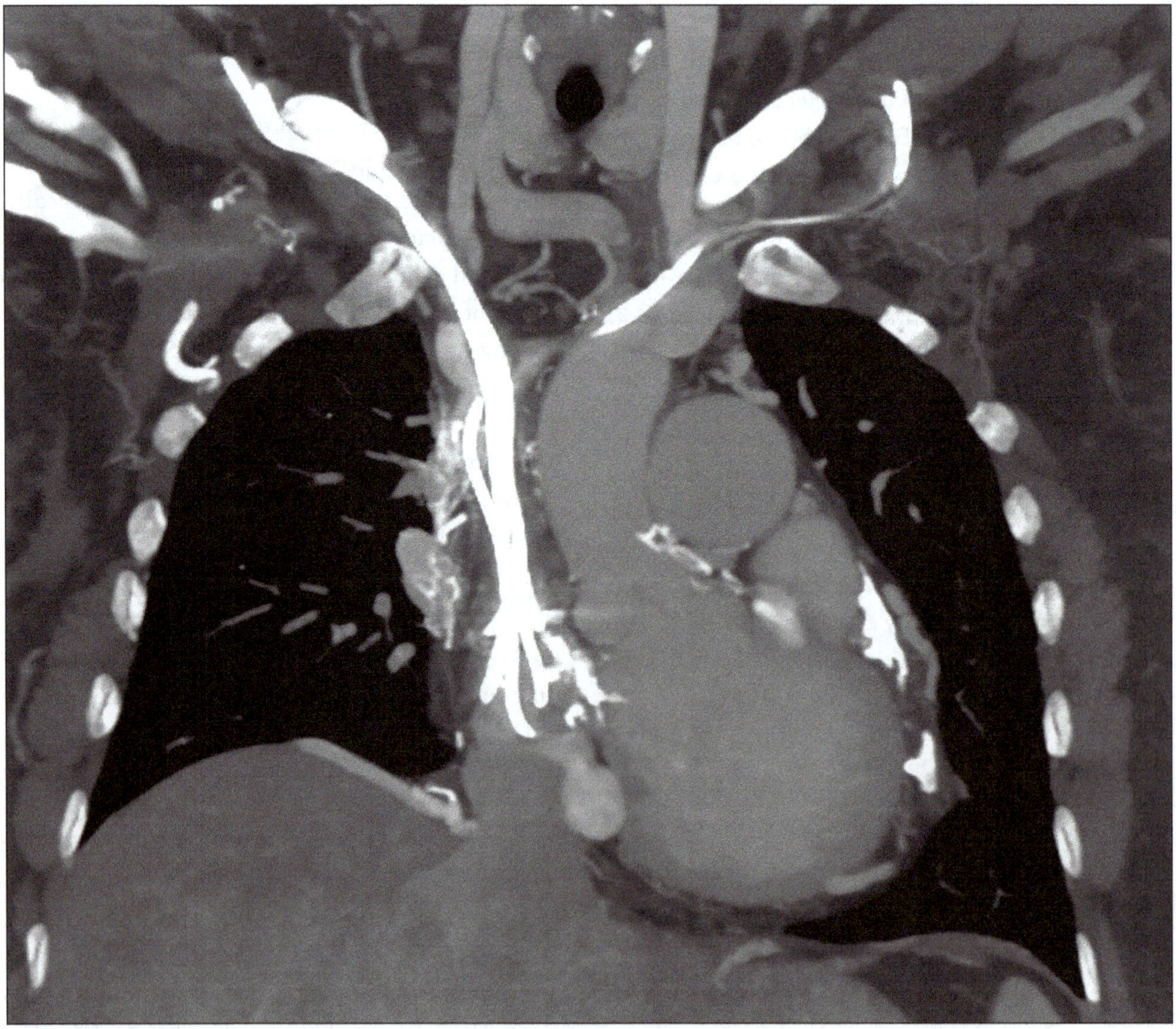

Figure 7.1 CT scan prior to our interventions showing 5 leads, 3 from the right and 2 from the left.

intubation) by our cardiac anesthesiology team. Intra-arterial pressure monitoring was established via the left femoral artery, given the history of prior sternotomy, so that a fem-fem bypass could be initiated quickly should the need for rescue by a cardiac surgeon become necessary. Getting on cardiopulmonary bypass via re-do sternotomy could take too much time. Sterile preparation and draping from the neck to the mid-thigh level were performed. Our cardiac surgeon was fully informed of the procedure and patient history and was immediately available, as was the perfusion team. Four units of packed red blood cells were in the room. We had planned to place a stiff guidewire via the femoral vein but found that the SVC was completely occluded, and we could not get any wire to pass from the femoral approach.

PROCEDURAL DETAILS

The extraction procedure took place in October 2019. In the description that follows, note that laser sheaths are sized by the outer diameter; all other sheaths are sized by the inner diameter.

System Removal, Left Prepectoral Region

Before the start of the procedure, cephazolin and vancomycin were given intravenously. A 4-Fr left femoral arterial line was placed. A 9-Fr high-volume central venous catheter was placed into the right femoral vein, followed by a 12-Fr sheath via a second right femoral venous access. However, a Bridge Occlusion Balloon was not placed, because neither the stiff wire nor a Terumo wire could be advanced into the SVC due to the occlusion. **Video 7.5** shows the appearance of the leads and devices before the start of the extraction.

Using sharp dissection, cautery, and blunt dissection, an incision was extended to the device pocket, which was opened sharply. The device was removed from the pocket, and the lead system was carefully dissected free from the fibrotic tissues to the venous entry site. The suturing sleeves were identified and removed, as was all suture material.

Both left-sided leads were cut, the suturing sleeves removed, and the inner conductor coils were exposed. The leads were prepared using a Liberator locking stylet and suture tie on each lead.

Lead #1, Right Atrium, St. Jude Medical/ Abbott Model 2088 Implanted on 5/27/2014

A Philips 14-Fr Laser was used initially but could not get past the clavicle; therefore, we switched to a Philips 11-Fr TightRail Sub-C to get past the obstruction under the clavicle. Going back to the 14-Fr Laser with an outer VisiSheath, we were able to advance along the lead and completely remove it (**Videos 7.6–7.9**). A long guidewire was then placed through the sheath and advanced to the inferior vena cava (IVC) for later use (**Video 7.10**).

Lead #2, Right Ventricle, St. Jude Medical/ Abbott Model 2088 Implanted on 5/27/2014

The 14-Fr Laser with an outer VisiSheath was advanced into the innominate vein and the SVC. However, the lead dislodged prior to getting the sheath down into the RA (**Video 7.11**). We could not get a second guidewire past the heart to have an extra wire in place due to the complexity of this patient's anatomy (**Video 7.12**).

At this point, the pocket was inspected for foreign bodies, then irrigated copiously with normal saline solution, and closed in multiple layers of an absorbable suture. The left subclavian to right femoral vein 0.35-inch J wire was retained and exited the pocket from the incision's lateral edge. Steri-strips were applied, and a sterile dressing was placed to cover the site and the retained 0.35-inch J wire for use by interventional radiology following this procedure.

Right-Sided Leads: Two in Right Ventricle, One in Right Atrium

At this point, we moved to the right side of the patient, where there were 3 retained leads. The skin was incised, and the leads were dissected free from the dense, calcified tissue surrounding it. Another incision was made over the right jugular vein to allow for a "straight-on access" to the oldest lead. The right-sided leads are described below.

Device Details

Device Component	Manufacturer/ Model	Date of Implant
Lead #3, right ventricle	Medtronic model 5024	1993
Lead #4, right atrium	Medtronic model 5524	1993
Lead #5, right ventricle	Unknown make/ model	1978

All the leads were cut, suturing sleeves removed, and inner conductors were exposed. Two of the leads were then prepared with locking stylets and suture ties. Lead #4 was damaged to the point that we could not advance a locking stylet.

We wanted to start with the "easiest" lead first, as this tends to free up the other leads. Since we could not get a locking stylet onto Lead #4, and Lead #5 was old, we started with the RV Lead #3. We first started with the 14-Fr Laser sheath on Lead #3 from the right prepectoral pocket. This got us around the bend near the junction of the innominate veins to the SVC. We were not able to pass the sheath beyond that point. We then switched to a 13-Fr TightRail without progress (**Video 7.13**). We subsequently used the Cook 13-Fr Evolution RL and freed the lead from the subclavian vein to the junction with the SVC (**Video 7.14**). However, at this point, none of the sheath technologies could pass the area of occlusion. We then switched to the RV lead placed from the right internal jugular vein, thinking that the "straight down" angle might allow us to advance through this area. Starting with a laser sheath, we could advance to the same area but could not pass through it. Using the 13-Fr Evolution RL, we were able to dissect the lead free down to the same innominate–SVC junction, where we reached the same obstruction when coming from the right subclavian. We could not overcome this obstruction with laser (**Video 7.15**), TightRail, or Evolution.

We then placed a Cook 16-Fr Byrd Femoral workstation using the access obtained for the 12-Fr sheath. We also left a second, shorter guidewire to retain access. We then used a Needle's Eye Snare to attempt to grasp one of the leads from below, but we could not snare any of the leads as they adhered to the venous and cardiac tissues. We then used a bioptome and were able to get hold of the RA lead (Lead #4). The lead was pulled into the femoral sheath and removed with traction along with the sheath. Once this lead was removed, Cine 16 shows the extensive calcification at the electrode tips of the 2 remaining RV leads, Leads #3 and #5, with the heaviest calcification around Lead #5, the oldest (upper) of the 2 leads (**Video 7.16**).

We then went back to the right subclavian ventricular lead (Lead #3). We were able to engage the lead with the bioptome. Using this technique, we could pull a portion of the lead into the IVC but could not fully extract it (**Video 7.17**). The lead was then snared using a Goose Neck snare, but the lead would not come free with traction alone. Finally, using the Goose Neck snare through a 13-Fr TightRail from the right femoral vein, we could free most of the lead. Still, it finally severed, leaving the distal end of the lead embedded in the fibrotic tissue of the ventricle (**Video 7.18**).

We now focused our attention on the oldest RV lead from 1978 (Lead #5). Using the bioptome through a large-curve Agilis sheath, we were able to engage the lead, but it would not come free from the myocardium, as it was heavily encased in fibrous tissue (**Video 7.19**). Given the length of the procedure, long fluoroscopy time, the encasement of the RV lead from 1978, and the high risk of proceeding further, we decided to abandon this lead in place. The right-sided pocket and internal jugular vein access sites were closed in the same fashion as the left side.

The patient was taken directly to IR. The "scout" look shows the lead fragments and the long guidewire from the left going down through the IVC (**Figure 7.2**). Using the previously placed 12-Fr

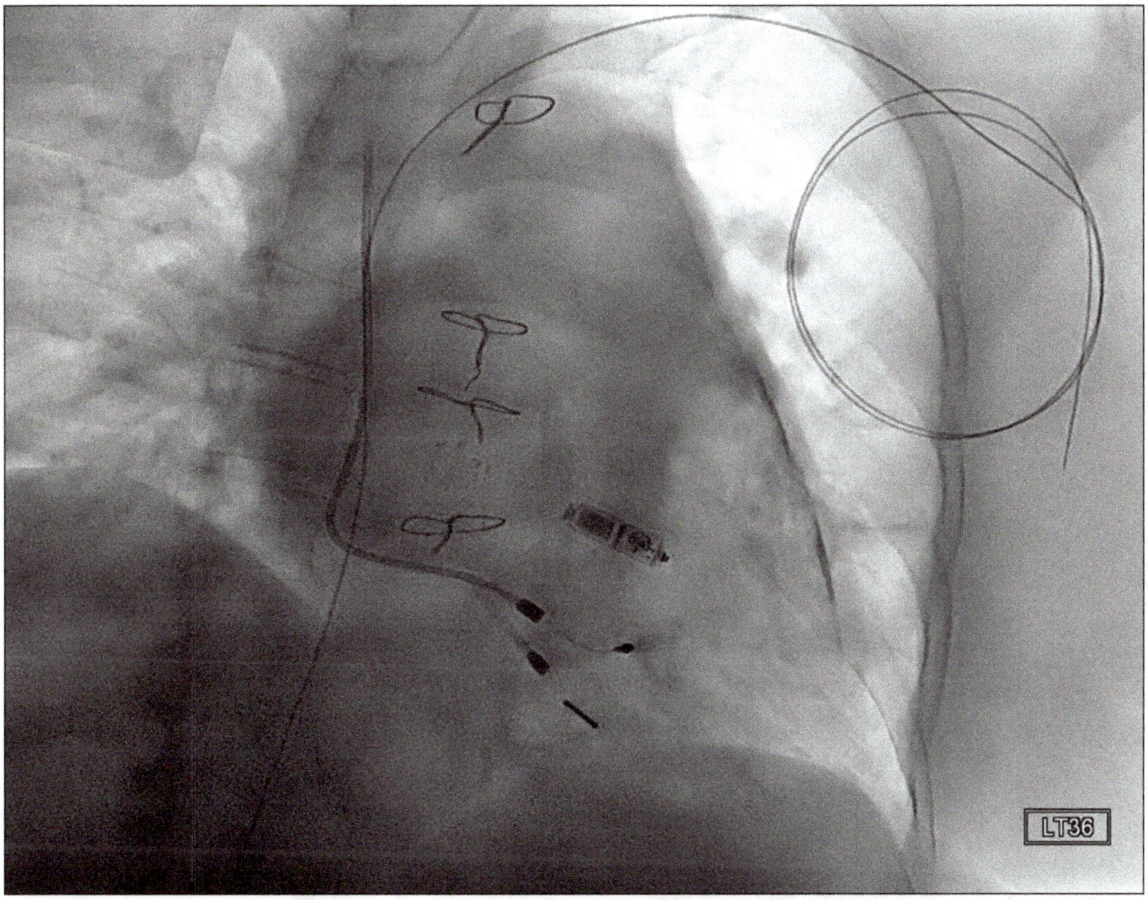

Figure 7.2 Postextraction/preintervention showing the 2 lead fragments and the guidewire placed through the occluded SVC.

right femoral venous sheath for access, a 15-mm Amplatz Goose Neck snare was placed and the end of the distal part of the guidewire was snared and pulled through the sheath (**Video 7.20** and **Video 7.21**). A 5-Fr catheter was advanced over the wire and into the mid brachiocephalic vein, and the guidewire was removed. Venography (**Video 7.22**) demonstrated that the right internal jugular was chronically occluded. There was flow-limiting severe stenosis of the proximal brachiocephalic and entire SVC. The hemiazygos and azygos veins were enlarged and provided the collateral flow.

The catheter was exchanged over a wire for a 16 × 80 mm Venovo stent was placed into the SVC and left innominate vein and expanded into place (**Video 7.23**). Then further expansion with a 10-mm × 8-cm conquest balloon and a 12-mm × 4-cm Atlas balloon was performed (**Figure 7.3**). A postvenoplasty venogram was performed, showing resolution of the hemiazygos and azygous collateral flow with the brisk flow into the RA via the SVC stent (**Video 7.24**). The 12-Fr sheath was removed, and a figure-eight suture was used for hemostasis.

POSTPROCEDURAL COURSE

The patient was taken to her room in stable condition after anesthesia recovery. The next morning, she noted being able to lie flat without symptoms of SVC syndrome for the first time in years. She was discharged home that morning. Her follow up in the device clinic showed that her leadless pacemaker was functioning well. Her exercise tolerance has improved significantly, and she no longer has any upper body swelling and her headaches resolved. Her heart failure symptoms have improved such that she has been able to resume her daily living activities again.

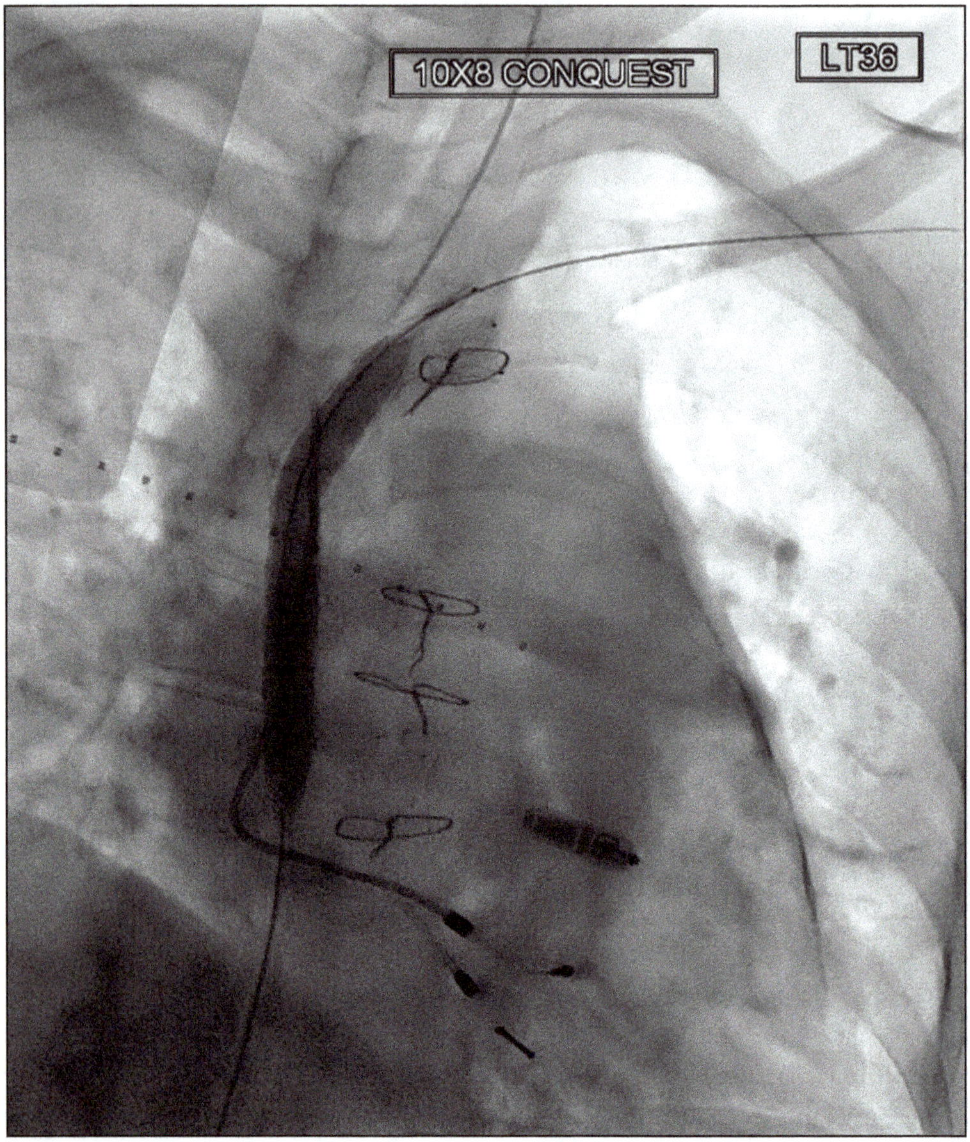

Figure 7.3 Balloon expansion of the stent.

SUMMARY POINTS

- It is important to get all the data available on previous studies and the anatomy before planning a complex procedure.
- Having as many options for sheaths, snares, and other tools will allow for the most success.
- Collaboration with other experts to come up with a good plan is always a great idea.
- Know when to stop! Sometimes it is OK to leave things behind. Don't "Win the battle and lose the war."
- Staging a procedure can make sense in some situations.

REFERENCE

1. Kusumoto FM, Schoenfeld MH, Wilkoff BL, et al. 2017 HRS expert consensus statement on cardiac implantable electronic device lead management and extraction. *Heart Rhythm.* 2017;14(12):e503–e551.

VIDEO LEGENDS

Video 7.1 Preleadless pacemaker implant. Note the 5 leads (2 from the left and 3 from the right), with the leads in the atrium moving together, suggesting that they are fibrosed to one another. [00:18]

Video 7.2 Leadless pacemaker deliver catheter being advanced to the right ventricle. Note that there was some difficulty crossing the tricuspid valve due to the leads and fibrosis in the right atrium. [00:56]

Video 7.3 Postdelivery of the leadless pacemaker showing that the tines are embedded into the myocardium. [00:04]

Video 7.4 The tether is removed from the pacemaker, and it rests securely in its final position. [00:31]

Video 7.5 Scout cine prior to lead extraction procedure showing the 5 leads once again. Note the superior track of the oldest lead that had been placed via the right internal jugular vein. Note also the leads moving in unison within the right atrium, suggesting they are bound together. [00:12]

Video 7.6 RA Lead part 1: The first lead attempted was the left atrial lead from 2013, using a laser sheath and VisiSheath together in a telescoping fashion. The subclavian vein is entered, remaining coaxial with the lead. [00:35]

Video 7.7 RA Lead part 2: Continuation of the laser/VisiSheath on the left-sided atrial lead, with advancement through the innominate vein. [00:45]

Video 7.8 RA Lead part 3: Further advancement of the laser/VisiSheath down the SVC to the RA. [00:30]

Video 7.9 RA Lead part 4: Final advancement of the sheath to the anode of the RA lead. Due to the acute angle and lack of room in the RA, countertraction could not be performed. However, by pushing the sheath inferiorly, the RA lead was able to be removed from the myocardium and then extracted. [00:55]

Video 7.10 Once the RA lead was removed while maintaining the extraction sheath through the occluded SVC, a guidewire was advanced (with some difficulty) into the IVC and was maintained for use later in the procedure. [00:56]

Video 7.11 The second lead attempted was the RV lead from 2013. The same sheath system was used. The RV lead pulled free from the myocardium before the sheath was entirely into the RA. [00:49]

Video 7.12 Once the left-sided RV lead was removed, an attempt was made to retain a second guidewire as a backup should we lose the first one. Despite multiple attempts, the wire was not able to be guided into the IVC. [00:56]

Video 7.13 From the right side, the first lead attempted was the RV lead from 1993. The TightRail was used due to its flexible nature and ability to cut through difficult and calcified binding sites. However, the sheath was stopped at the innominate vein and SVC junction, where the 3 remaining leads were bound together. [00:35]

Video 7.14 Working again on the RV lead from 1993, this time with a Cook Evolution RL, further progress through the binding of the 3 leads was not possible. [00:33]

Video 7.15 Using a laser/VisiSheath from the right internal jugular vein, the RV lead from 1978 was attempted next, again with the sheath being unable to pass the same binding site as noted for the RV lead from 1993. [00:53]

Video 7.16 This loop shows the heavy calcification around the electrodes of the RV leads. It also shows calcification in the right atrium just above the tricuspid valve. [00:01]

Video 7.17 Using a snare from the femoral vein, the RV lead from 1998 was captured, but it would not release from the myocardium due to the fibrous and calcified binding sites. [00:08]

Video 7.18 A 13-Fr TightRail was introduced over a snare, and the RV lead from 1998 was again captured. While attempting to bore through the binding site, the lead was severed. The proximal portion of the lead was pulled down from the SVC and removed, leaving the lead's distal end embedded in tissue. [00:56]

Video 7.19 Next, the RV lead from 1978 was captured using a bioptome (we were unable to grasp it with other snares). Though much traction was applied, the lead would not pull out of the RV, nor would it pull through the SVC. [00:27]

Video 7.20 The guidewire retained in the IVC from the left implant site is grasped using a Goose Neck-type snare. [00:06]

Video 7.21 The guidewire is pulled from the femoral vein through the introducer to allow for the introduction of interventional catheters, balloon, and stent. [00:09]

Video 7.22 Contrast injection via a catheter placed superior to the SVC obstruction showing the SVC occlusion extending up to the right internal jugular vein and major collateral flow through the azygous and hemizygous veins. [00:11]

Video 7.23 Deployment of a stent into the SVC. Note that a stent has already been placed in the left innominate vein. [00:10]

Video 7.24 Venogram superior to the SVC showing excellent blood flow down the SVC, with minimal flow via the collateral veins. [00:14]

8 | Management of a Patient with Lead Perforation

Klitos Konstantinidis, MD; Charles J. Love, MD

CASE 8

CLINICAL VIGNETTE

A 46-year-old female with a history of noncompaction cardiomyopathy had a single-chamber Medtronic implantable cardioverter-defibrillator (ICD) and single-coil active fixation defibrillator lead (Medtronic 6935M) implanted in December of 2015. The ICD implant was due to runs of nonsustained ventricular tachycardia detected on implantable loop recorder. She presented for system extraction due to symptomatic chronic perforation of the right ventricular (RV) lead. She started to develop symptoms of pericardial irritation and occasional discomfort shortly after the device was implanted. These symptoms were worse when the device was stimulating her heart. Subsequently, she developed a marked first-degree AV block of 400 ms with frequent and symptomatic periods of Mobitz 1 AV block. Her pericardial symptoms worsened over time, as did symptoms consistent with pacemaker syndrome. A transthoracic echocardiogram (TTE) in February 2020 showed that the lead had perforated through the RV free wall. The study also showed that her left ventricular (LV) function was normal but consistent with noncompaction cardiomyopathy. She was known to have a history of nonsustained ventricular tachycardia and thus remained at high risk for sudden arrhythmic death. Our plan was to extract the ICD lead, then place a new 3-chamber ICD system. The latter included a right atrial (RA) lead, RV ICD lead, and a His bundle pacing lead given her need for RV pacing.

PREPROCEDURAL PLANNING

A preprocedural CT was obtained to assess the lead position so the cardiac surgeon would have the best information about where the defect would be should he need to open the chest. The posteroanterior (PA) and lateral views (**Figure 8.1**, Panels A and B) show the lead to be high and anterior. The CT showed a lot of artifact, but there appeared to be a perforation of the lead through the anterior wall of the RV (**Figure 8.2**). Further evaluation by echocardiography provided additional evidence of perforation and a trace pericardial effusion (**Video 8.1** and **Video 8.2**). We discussed the option of prophylactic sternotomy or lateral thoracotomy; however, we decided that this would not be necessary. We also wanted to avoid the large scar (if possible) given her young age. Instead, to immediately address an acute pericardial tamponade and perform emergent rescue should cardiovascular complications occur during extraction, we planned to place a pericardial drain at the beginning of the procedure.

Due to the known issue of perforation and the high risk of tearing or causing a persistent leak of the RV, extra precautions were taken in addition to the typical preparations we perform in accordance with the HRS guidelines.[1] The patient was placed under general anesthesia (endotracheal intubation) by our cardiac anesthesiology team. Intra-arterial pressure monitoring was established. Sterile preparation and draping from the neck to the mid-thigh level were performed, with care being taken to allow good access to the left lateral thoracic area as well. Our cardiac surgeon was present in the EP hybrid procedure room, as was the perfusion team with the cardiopulmonary bypass pump primed. Before starting, blood products in the room included 6 units of packed red blood cells, 4 units of platelets, and 6 units of fresh frozen plasma.

Cardiotext Publishing. ISBN: 978-1-942909-54-5

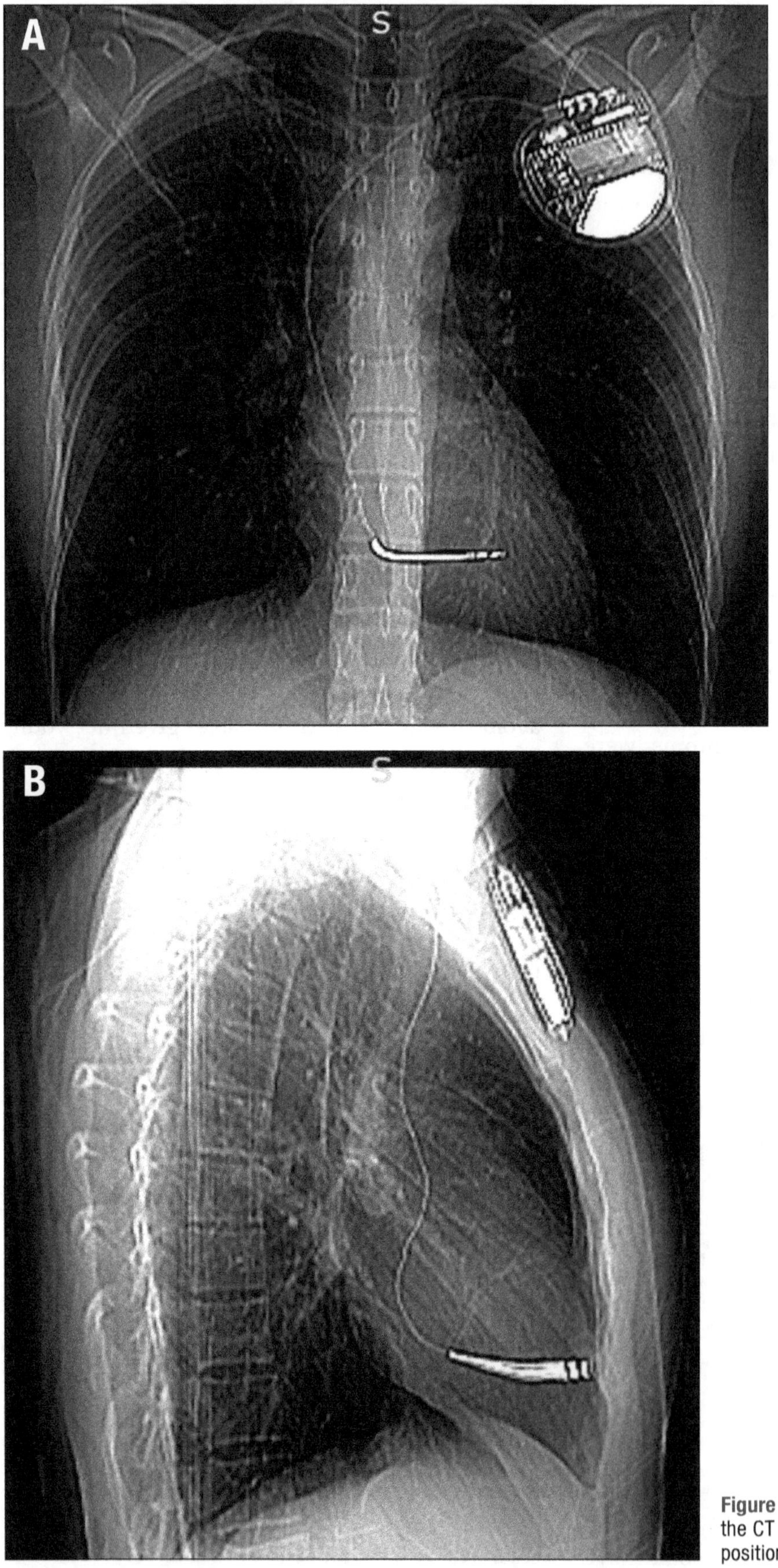

Figure 8.1 PA and lateral views of chest from the CT scan. These show a high and anterior position of the right ventricular lead.

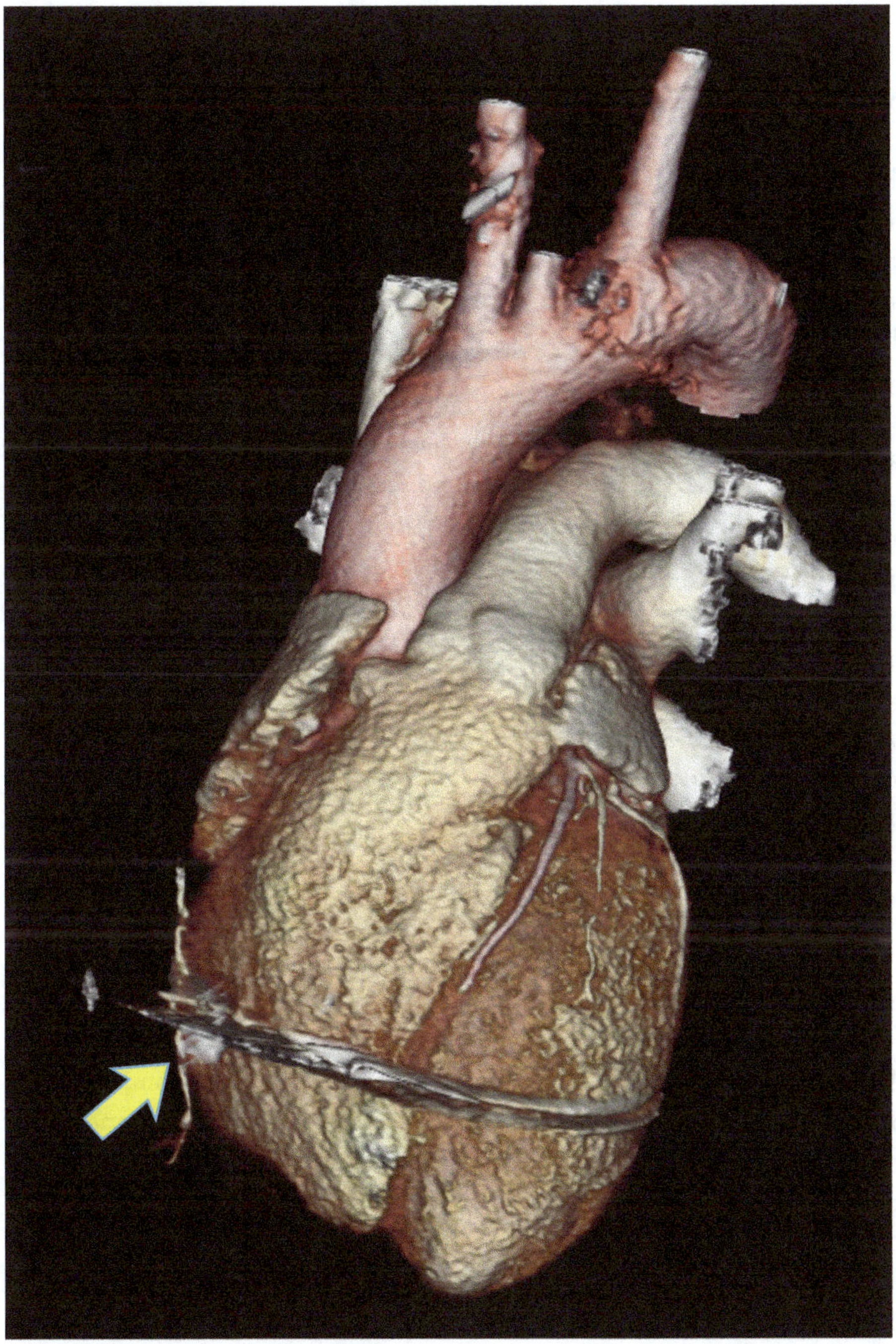

Figure 8.2 3D reconstruction of the patient's cardiac CT. The "band" around the lower part of the heart is the artifact. However, the **arrow** points to an area of probable perforation of the lead.

PROCEDURAL DETAILS

A transesophageal echocardiography (TEE) probe was advanced by the anesthesiology team to assist with hemodynamic monitoring throughout the procedure. At baseline, the TEE showed normal LV function with no pericardial effusion, normal tricuspid valve function, no evidence of atrial septal defect or patent foramen ovale, and no vegetations. The RV lead was attached to the anterior RV wall and appeared to be perforated through the wall about 2 cm above the RV apex. The initial PA and left anterior oblique (LAO) fluoroscopy showed that the lead was not pointing posteriorly in the LAO projection (**Video 8.3** and **Video 8.4**)

Pericardial Access

Pericardial access was then obtained for the elective pericardial tube placement as described previously.[2] Using an entry site 2 cm below the xiphoid process, with an epidural needle tip positioned just lateral to the pulmonic valve in the PA projection, the needle was inserted. The needle was advanced under fluoroscopy in lateral and PA views, ensuring that it would enter beneath the xiphoid process and stay away from the liver. Approximately 2 mL of contrast was injected, which outlined the pericardial space. The needle was further advanced until it traversed the pericardial space and confirmed with contrast injection (**Video 8.5**). A 0.014-inch wire was advanced into the pericardial space (**Video 8.6**). We confirmed circumferential looping of the wire to confirm its presence in the pericardial space. The wire was exchanged with a 0.035-inch floppy J wire through a 6-Fr dilator, and the position was confirmed (**Video 8.7**). A pericardial drain was inserted in the pericardial cavity, with positioning confirmed by fluoroscopy and the TEE (**Video 8.8**).

Device Removal

For prophylaxis, cephazolin and vancomycin were given intravenously before the incision. Using ultrasound guidance, a 9-Fr high-volume central venous catheter was placed into the right and left femoral veins for rapid infusion of fluid and blood product should it become necessary. Under ultrasound guidance, a second venous access was performed on the right femoral vein. An Amplatz Super Stiff guidewire was placed and advanced under fluoroscopic guidance to the right internal jugular vein serve as a rescue wire should a Bridge Occlusion Balloon be required.[3] A 12-Fr introducer was placed on the wire and positioned at the entry to the femoral vein, after which the wire was then clamped to the drape at the proximal end of the dilator. Following infiltration with 1% lidocaine/0.5% bupivacaine mixture, an incision was made to accommodate the left upper chest device. Using sharp dissection, cautery, and blunt dissection, the incision was extended to the device pocket, which was opened sharply. The device was removed from the pocket, and hemostasis was then obtained using cautery. The lead system was carefully dissected free from the fibrotic tissues down to the venous entry site. The suturing sleeve was identified and removed, as was all suture material.

Lead Extraction

The cathodal pin was rotated to retract the fixation helix, then the lead was cut, the suturing sleeve removed, and the inner conductor coil was exposed. A purse-string suture was placed around the lead insertion site for hemostasis and placed through a piece of rubber tubing, then clamped to the drape. The lead was prepared for extraction using a Liberator locking stylet (Cook Medical), a Bulldog lead extender (Cook Medical) snaring the high-voltage cables for additional traction, and then a suture around the lead, which was tied to the locking stylet and the Bulldog. We did not expect a great deal of fibrosis based on the initial fluoroscopic evaluation of the lead, which showed good movement of the lead in the superior vena cava (SVC). Therefore, we started with a 10-Fr Cook Byrd polypropylene sheath, which advanced easily along the lead to the SVC–innominate junction. Traction was placed on the lead to maneuver around into the SVC, but this resulted in the RV becoming inverted, and the patient's blood pressure dropped significantly. The tension was released, and blood pressure recovered quickly (**Video 8.9**). TEE did not show any effusion, and the ventricles were filling well. We were then able to advance to the RV but could not easily get past the mid-portion of the RV coil. At this point, we switched to a rotating mechanical sheath, a Philips 13-Fr TightRail (**Video 8.10**). This was slowly advanced over the shock coil through the binding site until it reached what appeared to be the RV wall. Using constant, careful traction, the lead was completely removed with countertraction (**Video 8.11**). Note the fixation helix could not be retracted but elongated as the lead was pulled into the sheath. The sheath was pulled back into the right atrium, and the lead was removed from the sheath. A guidewire was then placed through the sheath and advanced to the inferior vena cava. Then, the sheath was withdrawn (**Video 8.12**). Hemostasis was then obtained using the previously placed purse-string suture.

The TEE continued to show an absence of pericardial effusion, and the pericardial drain remained dry. Once the patient was deemed to be stable, the cardiothoracic surgeon was able to leave the room. The new implant proceeded without event, with the placement of the 3 leads (RA, RV, and His bundle) and the new device as planned (**Video 8.13**). A TYRX antibiotic envelope (Medtronic) was used to decrease infection risk.[4] The pericardial drain was removed at the end of the procedure. There was no evidence of pericardial effusion on TEE at the end of the case. The patient went to the recovery room, then our telemetry unit in stable condition.

POSTPROCEDURE FOLLOW-UP

Though no immediate complications were noted, the postprocedure chest X-ray (CXR) the following morning revealed a 5-cm left-sided pneumothorax (**Figure 8.3**). The patient was asymptomatic, hemodynamically stable with normal oxygen saturation on room air. A repeat CXR 6 hours later showed it slightly worsened, thus a pigtail catheter was used to re-expand the lung. The air leak resolved by postoperative day 3. The pigtail catheter was removed with the CXR showing a minimal residual left pneumothorax. The patient was discharged to home stable on a postoperative day 4. The etiology of the pneumothorax was not clear, as there was no new venous access performed on this case, noting that the extraction sheath followed the lead into the central circulation. We speculate that the perforated RV lead had been attached to the pleura of the left lung, and when this was pulled back into the heart, a small avulsion of the pleura/lung tissue might have occurred.

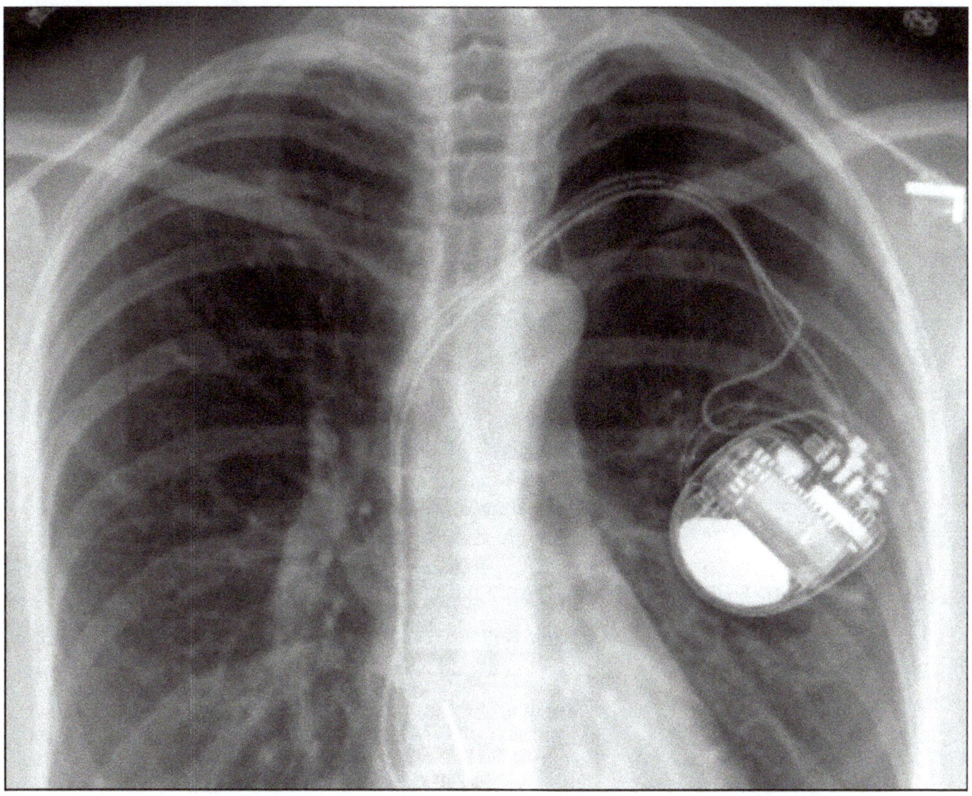

Figure 8.3 PA CXR showing a left-sided pneumothorax.

SUMMARY POINTS

- System extraction due to chronic perforation of transvenous leads is a high-risk procedure, but often can be performed without extravasation of blood into the pericardium.
- Preprocedural planning to immediately address any complications should they occur during the procedure is a critical part of the procedure.
- Pericardial drain insertion at the beginning of the procedure to drain any hemodynamically significant pericardial effusion should be considered when a perforation is present.
- Cardiothoracic surgery team, including the surgeon and the perfusion team with a primed pump, should ideally be present in the operating room during the extraction part of the procedure.

REFERENCES

1. Kusumoto FM, Schoenfeld MH, Wilkoff BL, et al. 2017 HRS expert consensus statement on cardiac implantable electronic device lead management and extraction. *Heart Rhythm*. 2017;14(12):e503–e551.
2. Keramati AR, DeMazumder D, Misra S, et al. Anterior pericardial access to facilitate electrophysiology study and catheter ablation of ventricular arrhythmias: A single tertiary center experience. *J Cardiovasc Electrophysiol*. 2017;28(10):1189–1195.
3. Azarrafiy R, Tsang DC, Boyle TA, Wilkoff BL, Carrillo RG. Compliant endovascular balloon reduces the lethality of superior vena cava tears during transvenous lead extractions. *Heart Rhythm*. 2017;14(9):1400–1404.
4. Tarakji KG, Mittal S, Kennergren C, et al. Antibacterial envelope to prevent cardiac implantable device infection. *N Engl J Med*. 2019;380(20):1895–1905.

VIDEO LEGENDS

Video 8.1 2D echo showing perforation of the lead through the RV wall. [00:19]

Video 8.2 3D echo showing perforation of the lead through the RV wall. [00:11]

Video 8.3 The lead in a high position; however, one cannot tell if it is anterior or septal in this projection. [00:02]

Video 8.4 The lead pointing towards the image intensifier and not to the right (i.e., not posterior), suggesting that it is in the RV free wall. [00:05]

Video 8.5 Preextraction access to the pericardium. The access needle is advanced slowly, using a small amount of contrast. The needle is seen at the end of the cine as it enters the pericardial space. [00:56]

Video 8.6 After the pericardial access needle is in the pericardial space, an 0.014-inch guidewire is advanced into the pericardial space. [00:06]

Video 8.7 The 0.014-inch guidewire is then exchanged for a long 0.035-inch guidewire, which is advanced to show that it is not in the right ventricle. [00:08]

Video 8.8 The pericardial drain tube is advanced over the 0.035-inch guidewire. This has been placed prophylactically to be able to both immediately detect a hemopericardium and drain it should it occur. [00:08]

Video 8.9 Initial use of a Cook Byrd telescoping polypropylene extraction sheath. The sheath was easily advanced to the SVC, but a binding site prevented further advancement. [00:52]

Video 8.10 Use of a Philips TightRail extraction sheath. This passed through the biding site and was advanced to an area near where the lead was perforated through the RV free wall. [00:23]

Video 8.11 Further advancement of the TightRail to slowly advance to the myocardium, then use countertraction to extract the lead. The patient remained completely stable at this point, without evidence of pericardial effusion on TEE or blood from the pericardial drain. [00:22]

Video 8.12 Access to the central circulation was retained by placing a guidewire through the TightRail. [00:09]

Video 8.13 Final view of the new leads in the right atrium, right ventricle, and Bundle of His positions. [00:02]

9 The Use of Shockwaves to Facilitate Lead Management (Intravascular Lithotripsy)

Walid M. Barake, FRCPC; Paul A. Friedman, MD

CASE 9

CLINICAL VIGNETTE

A 68-year-old man with past medical history of dilated cardiomyopathy, atrial fibrillation, and status post atrioventricular node ablation and cardiac resynchronization therapy (CRT), presents with progressive heart failure despite excellent CRT response for several years. Cardiac investigations, including device check and imaging, confirm left ventricular (LV) lead dislodgement. After discussion with the patient, the decision was to perform LV lead revision especially in the context of undisputed LV ejection fraction (LVEF) decline from 55% to 40% on transthoracic echocardiogram (TTE).

The left axillary vein was occluded (**Video 9.1**) and venous access was attempted with no success. The existing LV lead was removed over the wire, which was then exchanged to an Amplatz Extra-Stiff wire (Cook Medical) for better support. Attempts to serially dilate the vein were met with resistance. Venoplasty was attempted using a 6-mm non-compliant balloon (OPTA Pro, Cordis) (**Video 9.2**) followed by Flextome cutting-balloon (Boston Scientific) with minimal lumen expansion. The LV lead delivery sheath could not be advanced due to the multiple calcified stenotic lesions.

ALTERNATIVE OPTIONS

The following alternate options were considered:

- Right-sided pacing system with lead tunneling to left device pocket
- Leadless LV endocardial pacing
- Ultrasound-based therapy (shockwave lithotripsy) for venoplasty
- Conservative (noninvasive) approach, including maximizing medical therapy and close follow-up without further procedural interventions

We felt that calcifications would remain a barrier for right-sided system given the unsuccessful venoplasty of the SVC stenosis as shown previously (**Video 9.3**; **Figure 9.1**, Panel A). In addition, the patient had a strong preference to keep the device system on the left side. He did not qualify for LV endocardial pacing. The patient preferred an invasive approach over medical therapy alone since he has responded well in the past with CRT.

After vigilant consideration and discussion with the patient and his family, knowing that shockwave balloon is not FDA-approved for this indication, we decided to use intravascular lithotripsy (Shockwave balloon, Shockwave Medical).[1]

PREPROCEDURAL PLANNING

New baseline echocardiogram, defibrillator interrogation, and chest imaging were performed. Blood type and cross-match was completed. Informed consent was obtained, and the patient was brought to the pacing lab. Two large-bore peripheral intravenous (IV) accesses were established. A wide chest preparation was performed. Close monitoring of the heart rhythm and lead parameters was planned and implemented. A standard preprocedural time-out was performed. IV antibiotics were administered. General anesthesia was provided and a radial arterial line was established for invasive blood pressure monitoring.

 ISBN: 978-1-942909-54-5

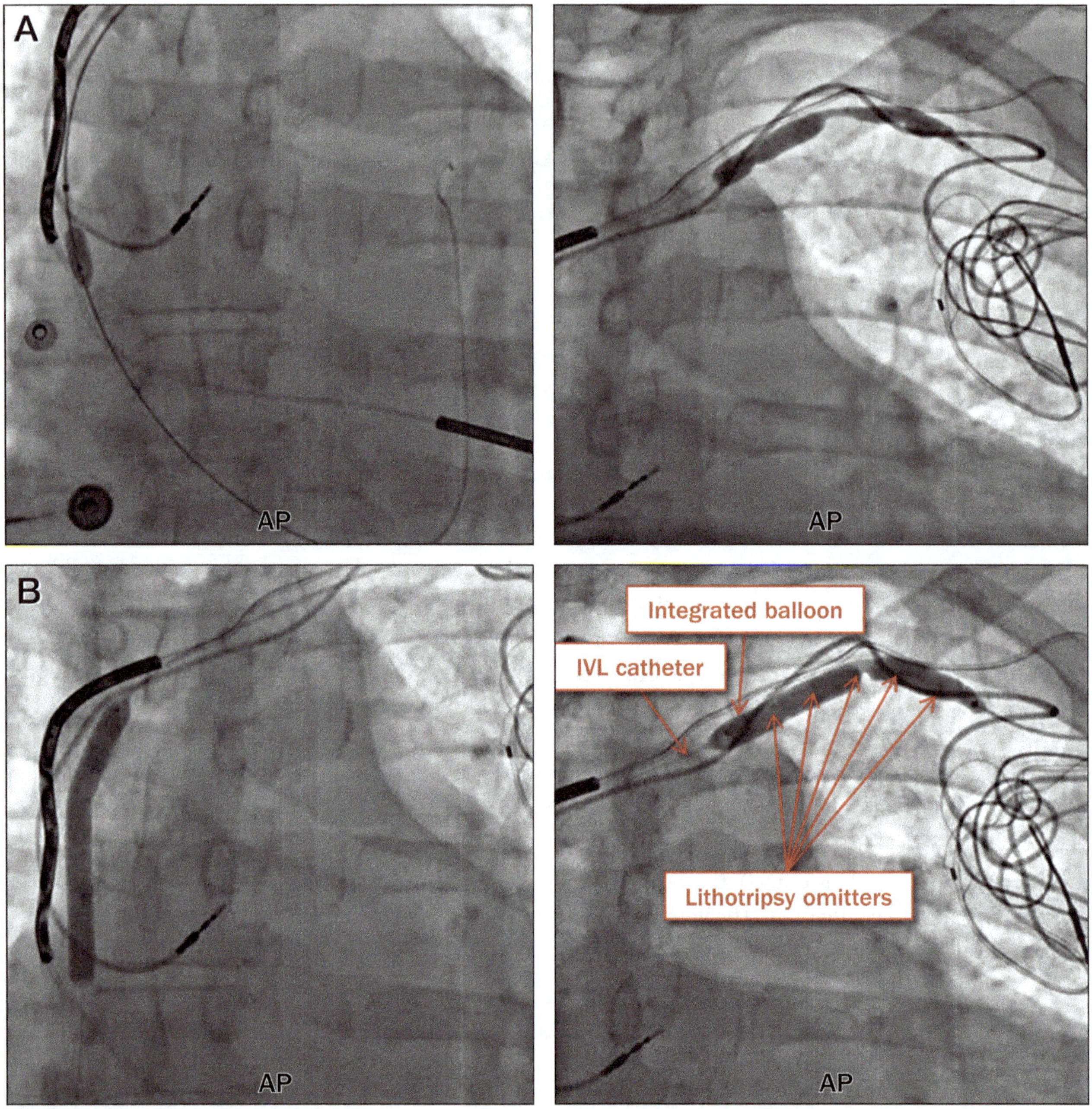

Figure 9.1 **Panel A:** Severely stenotic lesions despite the multiple venoplasty attempts described (prior to sound-wave delivery). **Panel B:** The excellent venoplasty results with shockwave therapy except for a residual 50% stenosis at the clavicular level. *Abbreviations:* AP, anteroposterior; IVL, intravascular lithotripsy.

PROCEDURAL DETAILS

A 0.014-inch wire was used to guide the Shockwave balloon (5 mm × 60 mm). The balloon was used to predilate each lesion by expansion to near-burst pressure. The balloon was then expanded to 4 atmospheres (recommended pressure for therapy delivery) and shockwaves were delivered for a total treatment of 300 seconds (proximal-to-distal). Sound waves cracked most calcifications with desirable angioplasty results except for the lesion at the clavicle level, which remained moderately stenotic (see Figure 9.1, Panel B). The delivery sheath was then easily advanced and His-bundle lead was fixated with paced QRS duration of 100 ms.

POSTPROCEDURAL CARE

The patient has tolerated the procedure well and remained hemodynamically stable throughout. In follow-up, the patient did very well with stable lead parameters (perioperative and follow-up parameters) and no heart failure or complications.

DISCUSSION

Calcification leading to vein stenosis frequently involves significant challenges to lead revision/extraction. Sound waves have been widely used for urinary tract stone disruption since 1980 with a longstanding safety record.[2] More recently, ultrasound-enhanced therapy was FDA-cleared to treat peripheral arterial lesions.[3] Sound-wave treatment is currently not FDA-cleared for venoplasty. Sound waves create a localized field effect that preferentially affects vessel wall calcium. The current mechanical extraction tools disturb those calcifications but at the expense of vascular/lead trauma. The rhythm should be carefully monitored during shockwave delivery. Although rare, shockwaves have been reported to cause depolarization affecting the cardiac rhythm.[4] This unique lead management technology warrants future study.

SUMMARY POINTS

- Calcifications remain a major impediment for device operators when faced with challenging vascular stenoses.
- Sound-wave-based therapy has a longstanding safety record, yet is often not utilized.
- Ultrasound-based therapy assisting in lead management is a novel and promising approach. This unique lead management technology warrants future study.

REFERENCES

1. Barake W, Madhavan M, Kowlgi GN, Cha YM, Asirvatham SJ, Friedman PA. Sound wave balloon-assisted device implantation: A novel approach that merits consideration. *Europace* 2021 Feb 13;euaa281. Online ahead of print. doi:10.1093/europace/euaa281.
2. Chaussy C, Brendel W, Schmiedt E. Extracorporeally induced destruction of kidney stones by shock waves. *Lancet.* 1980;2: 1265–1268.
3. Shockwave Medical, Inc. Shockwave Medical Intravascular Lithotripsy (IVL) system; U.S. Food and Drug Administration; [cited 07/26/2018]. https://www.accessdata.fda.gov/cdrh_docs/pdf18/K180958.pdf
4. McQuillan C, Alkhalil M, Johnston PW. A paced heart without a pacemaker. *Eur Heart J.* 2019;40(10):819.

VIDEO LEGENDS

Video 9.1 Left axillary venogram cine is depicted. The contrast injection (venogram) suggests severe narrowing and possible occlusion in the left axillary vein as it crosses below the clavicle and becomes subclavian vein. A prominent collateral venous circulation can be also noted. [00:03]

Videos 9.2 and 9.3 Cine clips obtained at maximum inflation (near burst pressure) at the different stenotic lesions. Over-the-wire balloon venoplasty was attempted with a 6-mm non-compliant OPTA Pro, Cordis. Note the inadequate venoplasty results limited by the hard calcification lesions. [00:01] [00:01]

10 | Lead Extraction in a Patient with Patent Foramen Ovale and Paradoxical Embolism

Adetola Ladejobi, MD, MPH; Siva K. Mulpuru, MD, MPH

CLINICAL VIGNETTE

A 52-year-old female with a history of childhood seizures and multiple syncopal events was evaluated for fever, incision site tenderness, erythema, and drainage despite completing a 1-week course of oral cephalexin. She had undergone a subpectoral dual-chamber implantable cardioverter-defibrillator (ICD) generator change 2 weeks earlier. Cephalexin had been initiated given the onset of incision site drainage 3 days after the generator change. All her blood cultures were negative. Her ICD was initially inserted 17 years ago after an electrophysiologic study demonstrated inducible ventricular tachycardia/fibrillation in the setting of mitral valve prolapse and numerous spontaneous PVCs. She had multiple appropriate shocks after device implantation. She also had multiple generator changes with a *Staphylococcus aureus* device infection necessitating device extraction 14 years ago. Her RV lead had been revised multiple times, most recently in 2009. Her other medical history included asplenia secondary to a motor vehicle accident, chronic atypical chest discomfort, congestive heart failure, patent foramen ovale (PFO) with a left-to-right shunting (▶ **Video 10.1A** and **B**), multiple idiopathic cerebrovascular accidents, chronic idiopathic leukocytosis and thrombocytosis, and a diagnosis of lupus with negative anti-nuclear antibodies. Components of her infected device are listed in the device details. **Figure 10.1** shows a baseline chest X-ray (CXR) with the device in situ.

Device Details

Device Component	Manufacturer/Model	Date of Implant
Pulse generator	Medtronic Evera XT DR	06/2017
Right atrial lead	Medtronic 5076	01/2003
Right ventricular lead	St. Jude 6947	06/2009

PROCEDURAL DETAILS

The infectious disease and surgical teams were consulted by the heart rhythm service to aid in planning for the device extraction, which proceeded as anticipated. The right subpectoral generator was removed from the pocket, and suture sleeves were dissected free of extensive adhesions. The leads were then amputated, and with the aid of universal locking stylets and laser sheaths, removed from the right atrium and ventricle (**Figure 10.2**). The surgical team helped with pocket closure. Apart from a brief period of hypotension during traction on the right ventricular lead, no complications were noted during the procedure. After the device extraction, the patient was noted to have new-onset right-sided weakness and aphasia when she woke up. A diagnosis of left middle cerebral artery territory stroke was made and was thought to be related to her recent device extraction in the setting of a PFO. Given the unclear timing of her stroke onset, the patient was not felt to be a candidate for intravenous thrombolysis or thrombectomy. A transesophageal echocardiogram (TEE) showed a new, highly mobile, multilobulated 4.3 × 0.5-cm long mass in close proximity to the PFO (▶ **Video 10.2**).

 Cardiotext Publishing. ISBN: 978-1-942909-54-5

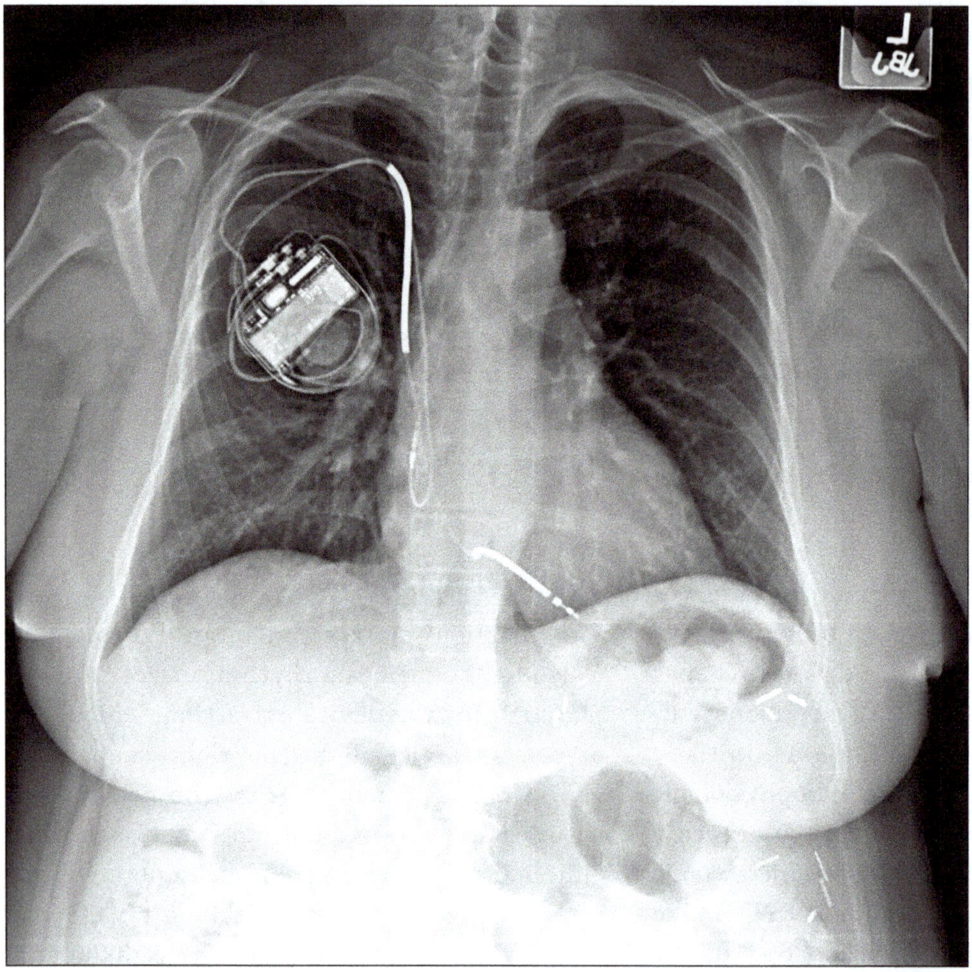

Figure 10.1 CXR showing infected device dual-chamber ICD in situ. The right ventricular has a dual-coil ICD.

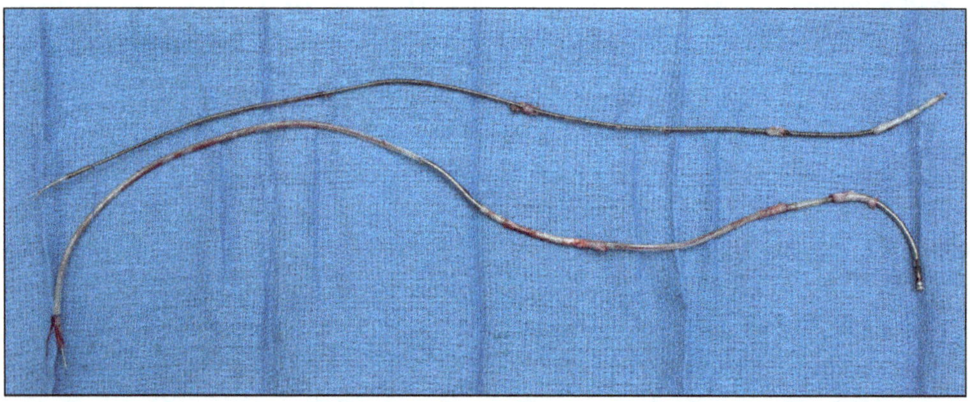

Figure 10.2 Infected device leads after transvenous removal.

This was thought to represent a fibrin sleeve developed after endocardial surface denudation secondary to laser-assisted lead extraction. Intraoperative pocket cultures grew methicillin-resistant *Staphylococcus epidermidis*, methicillin-sensitive *Staphylococcus aureus*, and oxacillin-resistant *Staphylococcus haemolyticus*. All were sensitive to vancomycin.

PATENT FORAMEN OVALE CLOSURE

After obtaining clearance from Infectious Diseases, a team discussion, and shared decision making with the patient, a decision was made to proceed with percutaneous PFO closure to prevent a subsequent stroke from mobile mass debris. However, the initial PFO closure plan was postponed, given the observed thrombus was so close to the superior limbus on intracardiac echocardiography (ICE) (**Video 10.3**). The patient was continued on heparin anticoagulation, and her vancomycin course was extended. The PFO closure attempt was made a week later. At procedure onset, ICE imaging showed reduced but persistent right atrial thrombus. Carotid filters in both common carotid arteries were placed first to prevent cerebral emboli. A 7.0 SpiderFX filter was advanced from the femoral artery into the common carotid arteries bilaterally (**Video 10.4**, red arrows). Following this, a straight wire and a balloon wedge were used to transverse the PFO, after which the balloon wedge was placed in the pulmonary vein. After switching out for an Amplatz Super Stiff wire, a Gore Cardioform 30-mm device was successfully deployed across the PFO (**Video 10.5**). After device deployment, there was no shunting across the PFO and no evidence of left atrial thrombus. The carotid filters were then successfully retrieved. No adverse postprocedural neurologic sequelae were noted.

POSTPROCEDURAL COURSE

The patient did well in the postoperative period. She also continued to have physical and speech therapy and regained some of her neurologic function. She then had a subcutaneous ICD placed a month after being initially discharged with a LifeVest.

DISCUSSION

Estimates suggest that approximately 1 in 4 persons in the general population have a PFO. These have been postulated to be a mechanism for cryptogenic stroke.[1,2] The presence of a PFO is associated with a greater than 3-fold increase in the risk of embolic cardiovascular events in patients with endocardial device leads.[3] This is thought to be secondary to the ability of endovascular leads to serving as a nidus for thrombus formation. Transvenous lead removal (TLR) is associated with mobilization of endocardial debris attached to the leads, which may transverse a PFO and result in paradoxical embolization (**Figure 10.3**). Debris may represent adherent material (e.g., fibrous sheaths, thrombus, or vegetation) sheared off by the telescoping motion of lead removal devices. Endocardial damage during the lead removal process may also serve as a nidus for new thrombus formation. Embolization may also occur from in situ left-sided vegetations. A few case reports indicated that lead fragments trapped in PFOs, paradoxical lead fragment embolization, and air embolism across the PFO.[4–7] Existing registry data of stroke rates after lead extraction range from 0.07%–0.11%.[8,9] However, in a more focused study by Lee et al., an overall stroke rate of 1.0% was seen in patients with infected CIEDs after TLR.[10] Ideally, one would close the PFO before TLR. In cases of lead extraction due to device infection, permanently implanting another intracardiac device into the infectious milieu is ill-advised. From our experience, three options can be considered for addressing this conundrum: temporary percutaneous PFO closure with a PFO closure device, extraction following an embolic protection device (EPD), or balloon occlusion of the PFO during lead extraction.

Temporary Percutaneous PFO Closure with a PFO Closure Device

A PFO closure device can be used to plug the PFO prior to lead extraction in the same procedure. If blood cultures are negative, a permanent device can simply be left in situ. However, when blood cultures are still positive, the septal occluder must be removed. A significant drawback of this approach is that atrial septal dilation, which may be required for device placement, often creates a bigger defect than the initial PFO. Therefore, after the closure device removal, the hole in the interatrial septum can be larger than the original defect. However, this may be an acceptable tradeoff as the larger defect may still be amenable to percutaneous closure after blood cultures turn negative. **Video 10.6**A shows the placement of a Gore-Tex septal occluder ahead of TLR. Video 10.6B shows the septal occluder being retrieved after extraction completion.

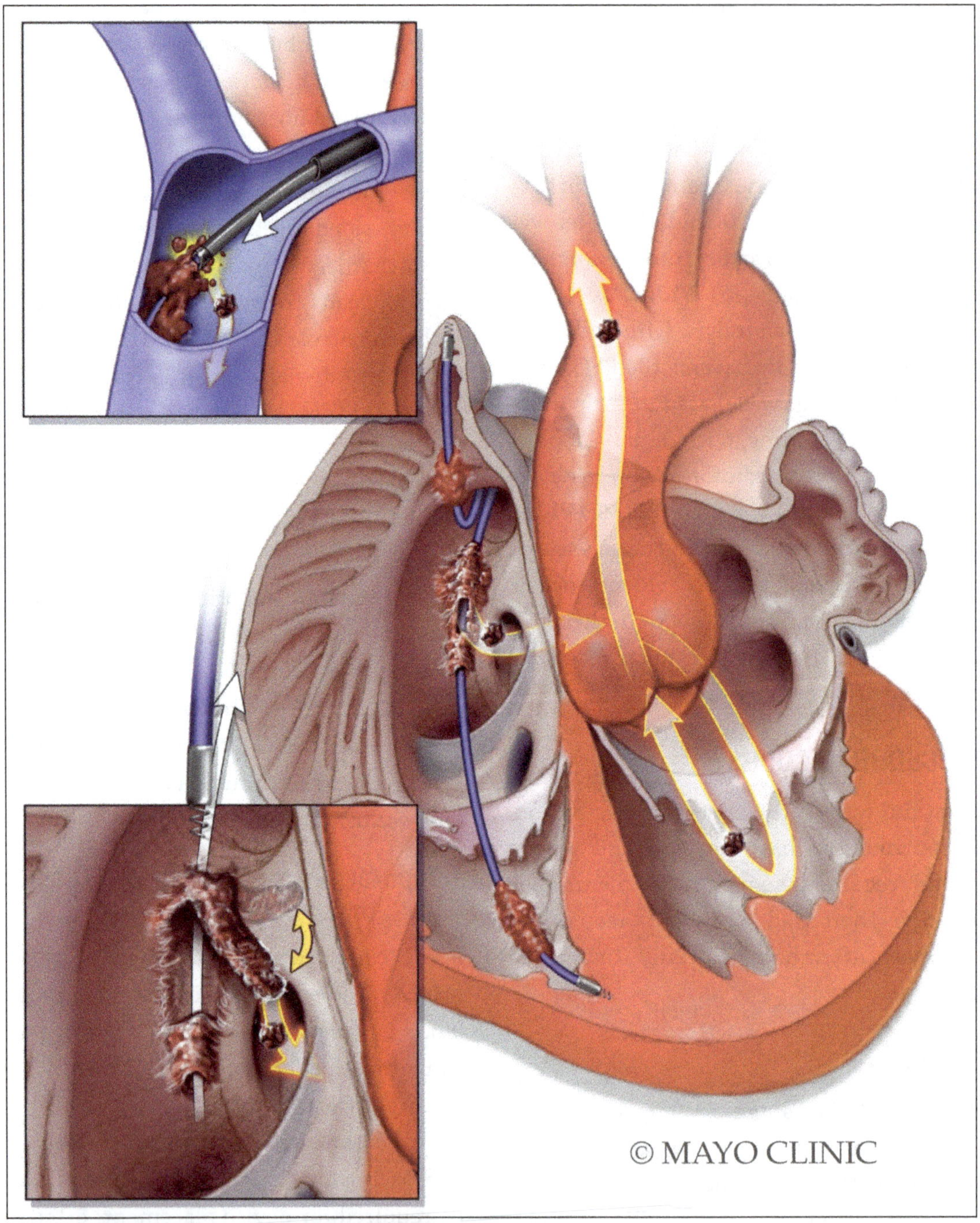

Figure 10.3 Illustration of the mechanism of paradoxical embolization during transvenous lead removal (TLR). **Panel A:** Debris is liberated when lead removal equipment (e.g., TightRail, Laser sheath) is telescoped over the device lead. **Panel B:** Debris is also liberated when the device is freed from its previous endocardial attachment. **Panel C:** The liberated debris can cross the PFO and get into the systemic circulation from where it may embolize to the cerebral or other systemic vascular bed.

Lead Extraction After Insertion of an Embolic Protection Device

Several EPDs exist for protecting the cerebral circulation during potential embolus-producing procedures.[11,12] Case reports exist of their successful use in TLR.[13,14] A major limitation of their use is that their use requires therapeutic anticoagulation with an activated clotting time of at least 250 seconds. This increases the risk of bleeding complications during lead extractions. A second major limitation is that they cannot be left in for prolonged periods of time. For example, the Sentinel Cerebral Protection System (Boston Scientific) is only approved for an indwell time of 90 minutes by the FDA. As such, they may have to be removed prior to completion of the lead extraction procedure. Another limitation is the conflicting data on their effectiveness when used for cerebral embolic protection—for example, in transcatheter aortic valve replacement.[15,16] Apart from the previously mentioned case reports, their effectiveness in TLR remains unknown. In our case, we employed the Sentinel EPD during the procedure to close the PFO to prevent a recurrent stroke from thromboembolism.

Balloon Occlusion of the PFO During Lead Extraction

Temporary PFO closure can be achieved with a balloon (**Video 10.7**). Rials et al. reported the successful use of an atrial septal occluder balloon in a patient with an atrial septal defect and device lead vegetation undergoing TLR.[17] However, in our experience, the use of balloon occlusion can result in thrombus formation around the balloon and the supporting wire, which can then increase the risk of embolization.

SUMMARY POINTS

- This clinical vignette demonstrates the real risk of cerebrovascular accidents arising from paradoxical emboli in patients with PFO undergoing TLR.
- As such, a serious consideration should be made to include routine PFO evaluation in the work up of patients undergoing TLR.
- If identified, shared decision making as well as a team approach can be employed to optimize a stroke risk reduction strategy.
- While several options exist for minimizing paradoxical emboli, they all have potential downsides that must be discussed with the patient and the team.
- PFO can be permanently closed before the TLR in noninfection cases, while a temporary PFO closure may be considered during the extraction in patients with bacteremia.

REFERENCES

1. Hagen PT, Scholz, DG, Edwards WD. Incidence and size of patent foramen ovale during the first 10 decades of life: An autopsy study of 965 normal hearts. *Mayo Clinic Proc.* 1984;59:17–20.
2. Lechat P, Mas JL, Lascault G, et al. Prevalence of patent foramen ovale in patients with stroke. *N Engl J Med.* 1988;318:1148–1152.
3. DeSimone CV, Friedman PA, Noheria A, et al. Stroke or transient ischemic attack in patients with transvenous pacemaker or defibrillator and echocardiographically detected patent foramen ovale. *Circulation.* 2013;128:1433–1441.
4. Arnott C, Kelly K, Wolfers D, Cranney, G, Giles R. Paradoxical cardiac and cerebral arterial gas embolus during percutaneous lead extraction in a patient with a patent foramen ovale. *Heart Lung Circ.* 2015;24:e14–e17.

5. Dieuzaide P, Savon N, Chalvidan T, LeTallec L, DeHaro JC, Djiane P. A complication of pacemaker lead extraction: Paradoxical embolism of a lead fragment in a leg artery. *Pacing Clin Electrophysiol.* 1998;21:2699–2700.

6. Larsen JM, Theuns DA, Thøgersen AM. Paradoxical thromboembolic stroke during extraction of a recalled St. Jude Medical Riata defibrillator lead with conductor externalization. *Europace.* 2014;16:240–240.

7. Le Dolley Y, Thuny F, Bastard E, et al. Images in cardiovasclar medicine: Pacemaker lead vegetation trapped in patent foramen ovale: A cause of hypoxemia after percutaneous extraction. *Circulation.* 2009;119, e223–e224.

8. Bongiorni MG, Kennergren C, Butter C, et al. The European Lead Extraction ConTRolled (ELECTRa) study: A European Heart Rhythm Association (EHRA) registry of transvenous lead extraction outcomes. *Eur Heart J.* 2017;38:2995–3005.

9. Wazni O, Epstein LM, Carrillo RG, et al. Lead extraction in the contemporary setting: The LExICon study: An observational retrospective study of consecutive laser lead extractions. *J Am Coll Cardiol.* 2010;55:579–586.

10. Lee JZ, Agasthi P, Pasha AK, et al. Stroke in patients with cardiovascular implantable electronic device infection undergoing transvenous lead removal. *Heart Rhythm.* 2018;15: 1593–1600.

11. Macdonald S. New embolic protection devices: A review. *J Cardiovasc Surg.* 2011;52:821–827.

12. Mousa AY, Campbell JE, Aburahma AF, Bates MC. Current update of cerebral embolic protection devices. *J Vasc Surg.* 2012;56:1429–1437.

13. Harrison JL, Patel R, Jogiya R, Redwood S, Rinaldi CA. Use of a cerebral protection device for the laser extraction of a pacemaker lead traversing a patent foramen ovale. *Heart Rhythm.* 2017;3:447–449.

14. Thosani A, Raina A, Liu E, Lasorda D, Chenarides J. Malpositioned endocardial left ventricular pacing lead extraction with transcatheter cerebral embolic protection in the setting of multiple prior embolic strokes. *Heart Rhythm.* 2019; 5:552–554.

15. Alkhouli M, Alqahtani F, Harris AH, Hohmann SF, Rihal CS. Early experience with cerebral embolic protection during transcatheter aortic valve replacement in the United States. *JAMA Intern Med.* 2020;180:783–784.

16. Testa L, Latib A, Casenghi M, Gorla R, Colombo A, Bedogni F. Cerebral protection during transcatheter aortic valve implantation: An updated systematic review and meta-analysis. *J Am Heart Assoc.* 2018;7(10):e008463.

17. Rials SJ, Good AP, Nicholson DJ. Temporary occlusion of an atrial septal defect to prevent paradoxical embolization during extraction of infected defibrillator leads. *J Innov Card Rhythm Manag.* 2014;5:1626–1629. doi:10.19102/icrm.2014.050506

VIDEO LEGENDS

Video 10.1 (A) Transesophageal echocardiographic (TEE) image showing the PFO. Note the device lead in the right atrium. [00:03] (B) PFO shown in Figure 10.1 with color flow Doppler imaging. Note left to right shunting as indicated by the blue color jet. [00:01]

Video 10.2 TEE image showing new mobile echodensities seen in the right atrium after transvenous lead extraction. The right panel is an orthogonal view of the left one at the level indicated by the white dotted line. [00:06]

Video 10.3 Intracardiac echocardiographic image showing debris attached to the right atrial side of the interatrial septum. The close proximity of the debris to the patent foramen ovale precluded initial PFO closure, given the high risk of systemic embolization. [00:06]

Video 10.4 Fluoroscopic image showing the SpiderFX embolic protection device in the right and left common carotid arteries. [00:01]

Video 10.5 Fluoroscopic image showing PFO closure with an Amplatzer device. [00:01]

Video 10.6 (A) Fluoroscopic image showing the deployment of an Amplatzer device across a patent foramen ovale [00:06] (B) Retrieval of the Amplatzer device after use to temporarily close a PFO during transvenous lead removal. [00:04]

Video 10.7 Fluoroscopic image showing temporary PFO closure with a balloon occluder (yellow arrow points to dog bone effect on the balloon as it passes through the PFO). [00:06]

11 | Large Lead Mass

Justin Z. Lee, MBBS; Siva K. Mulpuru, MD, MPH

CASE 11

CLINICAL VIGNETTE

A 72-year-old male with end-stage renal failure on dialysis, ischemic cardiomyopathy with prior stenting of the left anterior descending and right coronary arteries, paroxysmal atrial fibrillation, prior dual-chamber implantable cardioverter-defibrillator (ICD) 8 years ago followed by biventricular ICD upgrade procedure 2 years ago, presented with septic shock secondary to pacemaker lead endocarditis.

Eight years ago, he was diagnosed with ischemic cardiomyopathy with a left ventricular ejection fraction (LVEF) of less than 35%. As a result, he underwent primary prevention dual-chamber ICD implantation, which was implanted via a right-sided approach. His ejection fraction initially recovered, but he later developed left bundle branch block and worsening ejection fraction to 25%, prompting a biventricular ICD implantation via the left-sided approach 2 years ago. The pulse generator on the right side was removed, and the right atrial (RA) lead and dual-coil right ventricular (RV) ICD lead on the right side were abandoned.

Two years later, he presented with fever and chills and was found to be in septic shock. He underwent intubation and mechanical ventilation, and he required vasopressors for hemodynamic support. Blood cultures grew *Staphylococcus capitis*. Transthoracic echocardiogram (TTE) revealed a LVEF of 25%. Transesophageal echocardiogram (TEE) showed a sizeable mobile echo density measuring 3.2 × 1.9 cm with multiple lobulations attached to the RV and RA lead as it passes into the RV (**Figure 11.1**, **Video 11.1**). No tricuspid valve masses were visualized. No shunt was identified with color flow Doppler and agitated saline.

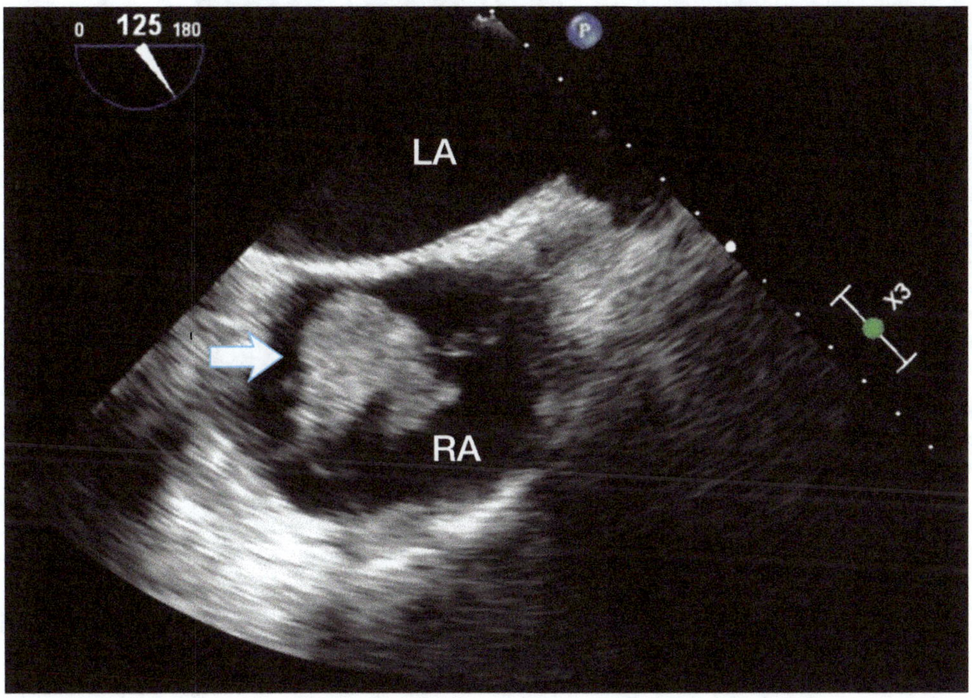

Figure 11.1 TEE showing a 3.2 × 1.9 cm mass attached to the device lead.

Cardiac Lead Extraction: A Case-Based Contemporary Approach.
 ISBN: 978-1-942909-54-5

The underlying rhythm was sinus rhythm. His chest X-ray (CXR) (**Figure 11.2**) showed that he had 5 leads. The details of his leads are noted below.

Device Details

Lead	Laterality	Manufacturer/Model	Date of Implant
Right atrial lead	Left	Medtronic 5076 CapSureFix Novus	3/20/2018
Right ventricular single-coil ICD lead	Left	Medtronic 6935M Sprint Quattro Secure S MRI SureScan	3/20/2018
Coronary sinus lead	Left	Medtronic 4598 Attain Performa S MRI SureScan	3/20/2018
Right ventricular dual-coil ICD lead	Right	Not available, abandoned	2012
Right atrial lead	Right	Not available, abandoned	2012

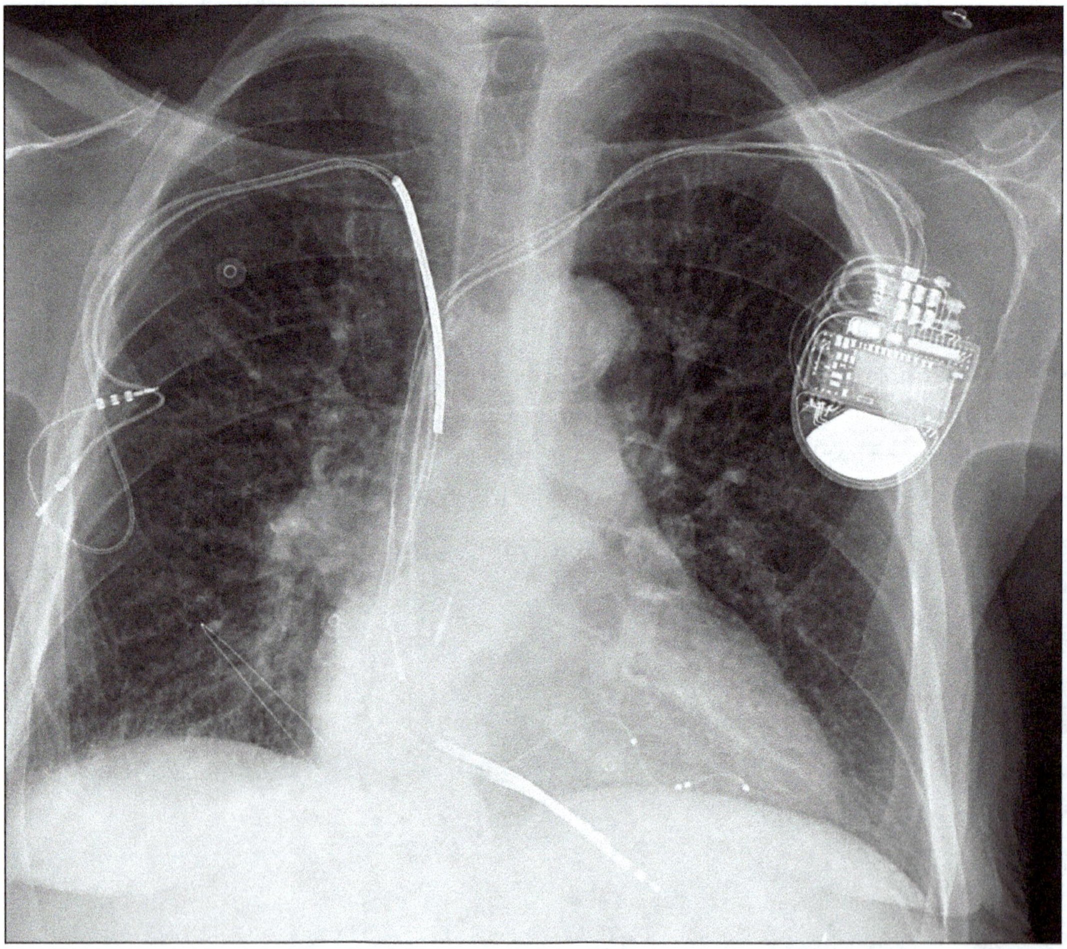

Figure 11.2 CXR showing 3 left-sided leads (RA, coronary sinus, and single-coil RV defibrillator lead) and 2 abandoned right-sided leads (RA and dual-coil RV lead).

PREPROCEDURAL PLANNING

A CT venogram was performed to guide device reimplantation. The bilateral subclavian and innominate veins were narrowed but patent. The SVC was also narrowed but patent. The plan is for the extraction of all 5 leads with debridement of both right and left pockets. Although he has a large 3.2 × 1.9 cm vegetation, following shared decision making with the patient on open surgical extraction and transvenous lead extraction (TLE), the decision was made to proceed with TLE with immediate extracorporeal circulation or extracorporeal membrane oxygenation (ECMO) if acute right heart failure or significant embolism with hemodynamic instability develops.

PROCEDURAL DETAILS

The procedure was performed under general anesthesia with a TEE probe placed for monitoring during the procedure. A 4-Fr sheath was placed in the left femoral artery, and a 5-Fr sheath was placed in the left femoral vein. These were in preparation for possible cardiopulmonary bypass or ECMO. In the right femoral vein, a 12-Fr sheath was placed for Bridge Occlusion Balloon (Philips Medical) deployment, a 9-Fr triple lumen catheter was placed for possible crystalloid resuscitation or blood transfusion, and a 5-Fr sheath was placed for possible upsize to a Cook workstation (Cook Vascular Inc.) if needed. Cardiac surgery was on stand-by, and 4 units of cross-matched, packed red blood cells were available in the room for the procedure. Through the 12-Fr sheath, a stiff 0.035-inch wire and a Bridge Occlusion Balloon was advanced. The balloon was positioned in the inferior vena cava (IVC) after test inflation.

Incision and dissection were made over the pulse generator; the pulse generator was freed from the pocket and disconnected from the leads. With simple traction, the RA lead and the coronary sinus lead was extracted. Both the GlideLight laser sheath and TightRail mechanical sheath (Philips Medical) was used to free the RV ICD lead.

Following extraction of the left-sided leads, an incision was then made over the right infraclavicular area to free the right-sided leads from the suture sleeves. With the laser sheath, the dual-coil ICD lead was successfully extracted. On TEE, the mobile mass was still attached to the RA lead. During the process of extracting the RA lead, the mobile mass was visualized to have embolized on

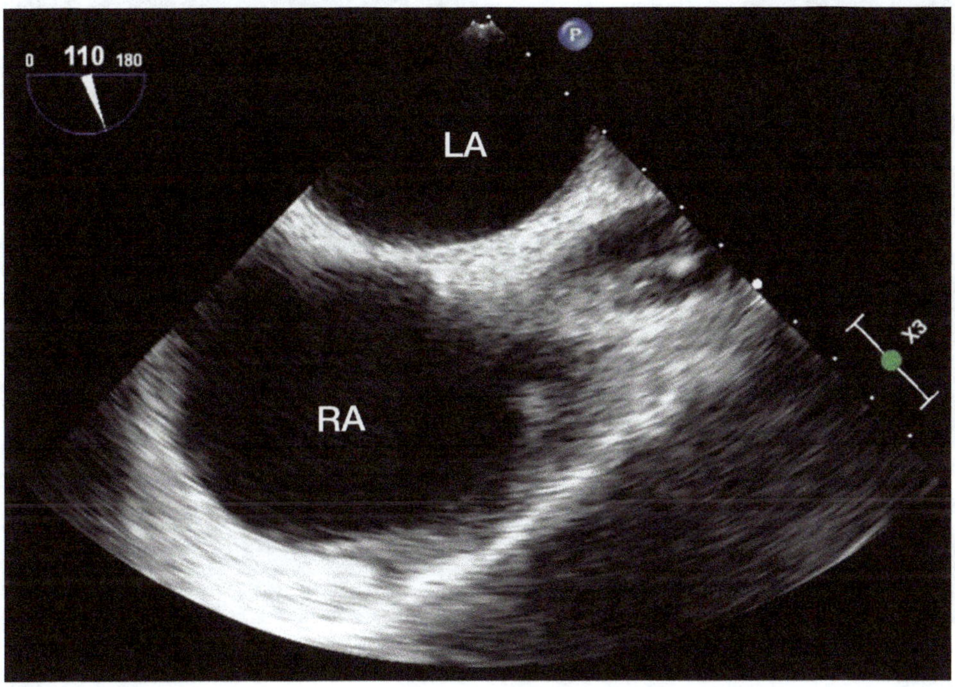

Figure 11.3 TEE showing that the mass had embolized.

TEE (**Figure 11.3**, **Video 11.2**, and **Video 11.3**). There were no desaturations or hemodynamic instability. The RA lead was then successfully extracted. The right- and left-sided pocket wounds were debrided and irrigated, and vacuum-assisted wound closure devices were applied bilaterally. Postprocedural TEE did show an increase in tricuspid regurgitation (TR) postextraction from mild-moderate to moderate in severity. There was no change in RV function.

POSTPROCEDURAL COURSE

With the embolization of the mobile mass, a preemptive chest CT-scan was performed, which showed a new, large, near-occlusive acute pulmonary embolism in the distal right main pulmonary artery with extension into the right upper lobar, interlobar, right middle lobar, and right lower lobar pulmonary arteries (**Figure 11.4**, **Video 11.4**). During the postprocedural course, his oxygen saturations remained normal at room air following extubation. He underwent additional wound debridement 2 days later. He was restarted on intravenous heparin and warfarin. He was subsequently discharged, and CRT-D was reimplanted following completion of intravenous antibiotic therapy.

DISCUSSION

Large vegetations greater than 2.5 cm offer a risk of obstructing the main stem of the pulmonary artery.[1] The options for approaches to lead extraction in the context of large vegetations can be summarized in **Table 11.1**. These include open surgical extraction, vacuum-assisted removal of the vegetation with the AngioVac device (AngioDynamics),[2] clot aspiration of the vegetation with the Penumbra Aspiration System

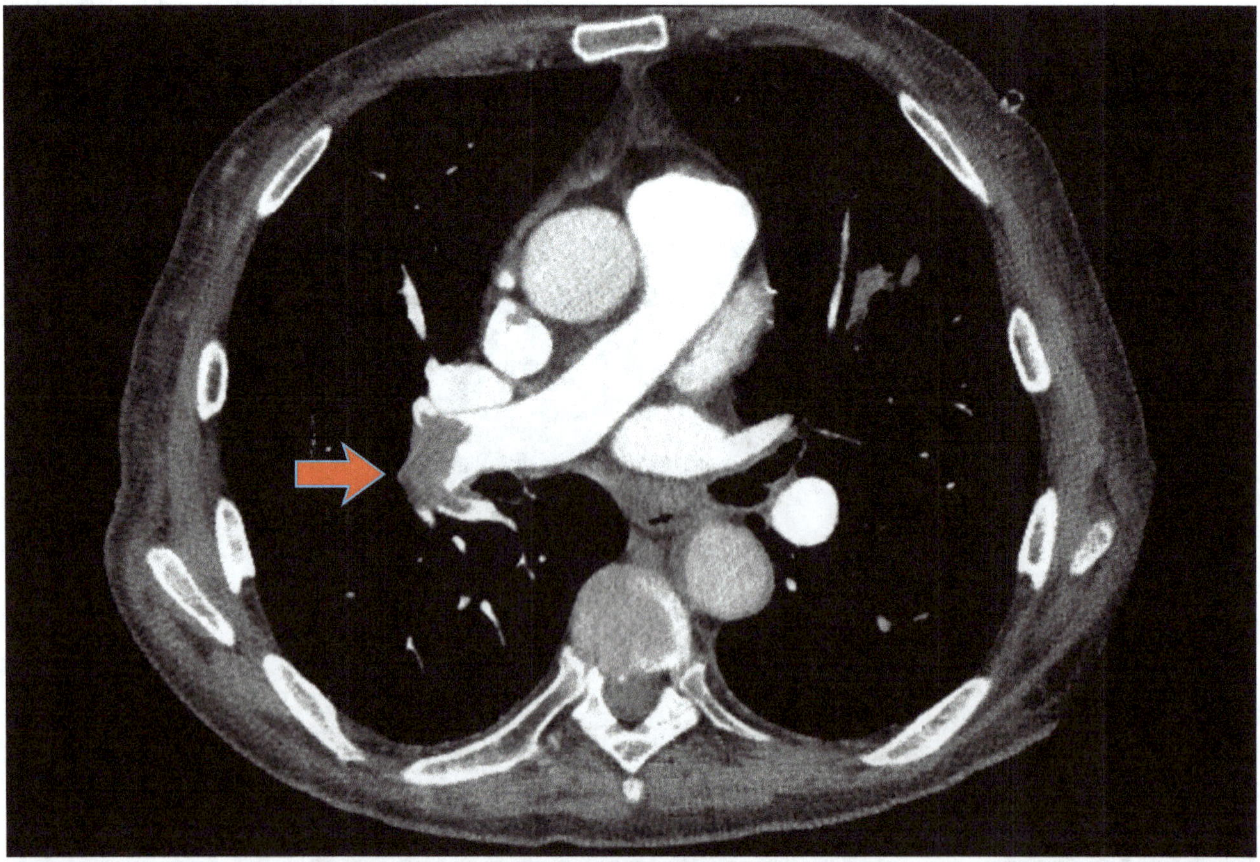

Figure 11.4 CT angiogram of the chest showing a large, near-occlusive acute pulmonary embolism in the distal right main pulmonary artery (**arrow**).

(Penumbra Inc.),[3] or fulguration of the vegetation—that is, use of a Needle's Eye Snare or other snares to break the vegetation. In a study of 24 patients with large lead vegetations who underwent surgical lead removal, perioperative mortality was 5.7%.[4] In a study where vacuum-assisted removal was used in 101 patients with large lead vegetations, complete removal of all vegetative material was achieved in 95% of patients.[5] There are also patients who may do reasonably well without using those approaches, such as in the described case, but the risk of hemodynamic instability from obstructive shock is high. Flow Triever mechanical thromboembolectomy device (Inari Medical) can be used to retrieve thrombi or large emboli from the pulmonary arteries in patients with persistent symptoms or hemodynamic instability with embolism.

Table 11.1 Options for extraction in large vegetations

Options
Open surgical extraction
AngioVac device (AngioDynamics)
Penumbra aspiration system (Penumbra Inc.)
Fulguration (use a Needle's Eye Snare or any other snare to try to break it up)

SUMMARY POINTS

- In patients with large vegetations, open-heart surgical extraction may be considered.
- In patients with large vegetations who are high risk for open-heart surgery, a transvenous approach may be considered.
- If the transvenous approach is adopted in patients with large vegetations, it should be performed only in an operating room with full equipment for immediate extracorporeal circulation if acute right heart failure or major embolism with hemodynamic instability develops.

REFERENCES

1. Kusumoto FM, Schoenfeld MH, Wilkoff BL, et al. 2017 HRS expert consensus statement on cardiovascular implantable electronic device lead management and extraction. *Heart Rhythm.* 2017;14:e503–e551.
2. Godara H, Jia KQ, Augostini RS, et al. Feasibility of concomitant vacuum-assisted removal of lead-related vegetations and cardiac implantable electronic device extraction. *J Cardiovasc Electrophysiol.* 2018;29:1460–1466.
3. Richardson TD, Lugo RM, Crossley GH, Ellis CR. Use of a clot aspiration system during transvenous lead extraction. *J Cardiovasc Electrophysiol.* 2020;31:718–722.
4. Ruttmann E, Hangler HB, Kilo J, et al. Transvenous pacemaker lead removal is safe and effective even in large vegetations: an analysis of 53 cases of pacemaker lead endocarditis. *Pacing Clin Electrophysiol.* 2006;29:231–236.
5. Starck CT, Schaerf RHM, Breitenstein A, et al. Transcatheter aspiration of large pacemaker and implantable cardioverter-defibrillator lead vegetations facilitating safe transvenous lead extraction. *Europace.* 2020;22:133–138.

VIDEO LEGENDS

Video 11.1 TEE showing a 3.2 × 1.9 cm mass attached to the right ventricular and right atrial lead. [00:04]

Video 11.2 TEE showing a free-floating mass in the right atrium. [00:05]

Video 11.3 TEE showing that the mass had embolized. [00:04]

Video 11.4 CT angiogram of the chest showing a large, near-occlusive acute pulmonary embolism in the distal right main pulmonary artery. [00:31]

12 | Using AngioVac for Lead Extraction

Yong-Mei Cha, MD

CLINICAL VIGNETTE

A 69-year-old female has morbid obesity, hypertension, nonischemic cardiomyopathy, and chronic kidney disease stage III. In 2017, she received a dual-chamber pacemaker for complete AV block and syncope. In 2018, she had an episode of *Proteus* sepsis and was treated with intravenous antibiotics. In 2019, she was readmitted for fatigue and hypotension. She was found to have candidemia. Subsequently, she developed respiratory failure and was intubated.

Labs

HB: 10.3 mg/dl; WBC: 7600 × 10^9/L;
Platelets: 173,000 × 10^9/L; Creatinine: 1.1 mg/dL
Blood culture: *Candida albicans*
Urine culture: *Candida albicans*

Imaging

Transthoracic echocardiogram (TTE) showed normal left ventricular (LV) function, ejection fraction 57%. There was no evidence of valvular heart disease, endocarditis, or vegetations.

A transesophageal echocardiogram (TEE) showed a large vegetation, measuring approximately 3 × 2 cm, attached on the atrial aspect of the right ventricular (RV) lead. It is mobile and prolapsing into the RV (**Video 12.1**). Moderate tricuspid valve regurgitation (TR) was present around the device lead and vegetation (**Video 12.2**). The atrial septum was intact.

Device Details

Device Component	Manufacturer/Model	Date Implanted
Generator	Medtronic A2DR01 Advisor DR MRI	2017
RA lead	Medtronic 5076 CapSure Fix Novus SureScan	
RV lead	Medtronic 5076 CapSure Fix Novus SureScan	
Underlying rhythm: Complete AV block and pacemaker dependency		

CASE 12

Clinical Diagnosis and Indication for Lead Extraction

- Pacemaker lead endocarditis with *Candida albicans*
- Fungemia with sepsis and hypotension
- Complete AV block; status post permanent pacemaker implantation and pacemaker dependency

The patient has persistent fungemia despite IV capsofungin, and also has hypotension associated with systemic fungal infection. There is a clear pacemaker lead infection. Although thrombus can have a similar appearance, given the patient's verified *Candida* infection, the TEE findings are most consistent with fungal vegetation. Lead extraction is indicated to eradicate systemic infection. A large fungal ball attached to the ventricular lead is a concern as it may dislodge and cause a large pulmonary artery embolization.

 ISBN: 978-1-942909-54-5

PREPROCEDURAL PLANNING

This complicated case requires multispecialty collaboration for the procedure, including anesthesiology, cardiovascular surgery standby for potential sternotomy, interventional radiologist for application of AngioVac (AngioDynamics), electrophysiologist, and general surgery for wound debridement and vacuum-assisted suction device placement in the hybrid operating room.

- Arterial line for BP monitoring
- Intraoperative TEE
- Extraction supplies: Excimer laser sheath and laser system, TightRail rotating dilator sheath, Evolution sheath, locking stylet
- Bridge Occlusion Balloon available
- Venous access: Left femoral vein, one for temporary pacing for pacemaker dependency, one for 19-Fr return cannula; 3 right femoral vein access, one for fluid/blood resuscitation, one for 26-Fr AngioVac suction cannula, and one extra for potential need of extraction workstation from below. Right internal jugular access for possible need of inserting AngioVac suction cannula

The AngioVac catheter is considered to break the vegetation away from the lead and suck it out of circulation. AngioVac is venous-to-venous extracorporeal circuit consisting of an outflow line, a central pump, a filter, and an inflow line. The AngioVac cannula has a shaped tip that opens like a tulip, creating a flow through the cannula into a filter (**Figure 12.1**).The thrombus or vegetation is trapped in the filter while blood is returned to the body through a second venous cannula. The AngioVac cannula and circuit are used with a standard centrifugal pump, bubble trap, and reinfusion cannula (**Figure 12.2**).

PROCEDURAL DETAILS

The patient was intubated under general anesthesia. Bilateral femoral vein access and right internal jugular access were obtained. The chest and abdomen were prepped and draped in a sterile fashion. A temporary pacing electrode was placed on maintaining pacing.

AngioVac Thrombectomy

Heparin was given to keep the activated clotting time at ~300 seconds after venous accesses were obtained. A 19-Fr return cannula was placed in the left femoral vein, and a 26-Fr, 65-cm DrySeal sheath (W. L. Gore & Associates, Inc.) in the right femoral vein. The patient was placed on an external bypass and the angiographic cannula passed up through the inferior vena cava up to the right atrium. A 2-0 silk suture was placed across one of the site leaves of the distal end of the AngioVac to ease directional control. With transesophageal ultrasound assistance, engaging in the vegetation was attempted, but it proved impossible because of the angulation toward the RV (**Video 12.3**). TEE shows that the AngioVac, inserted from

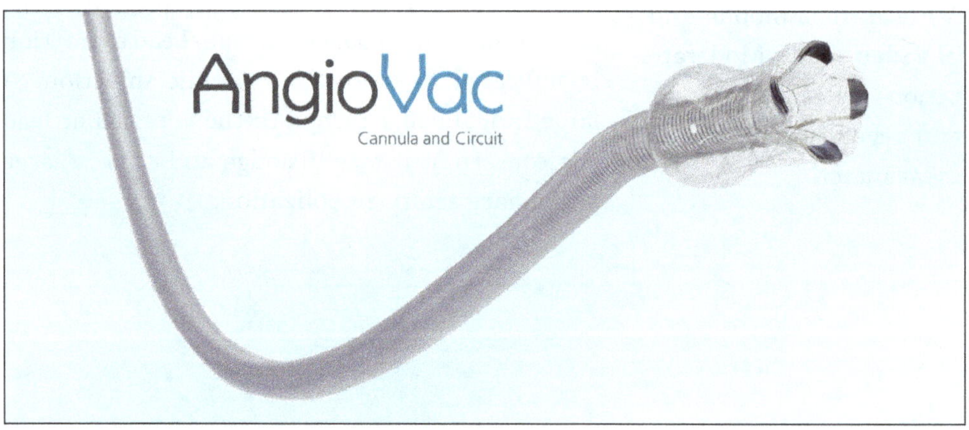

Figure 12.1 The AngioVac cannula has a shaped tip that opens like a tulip, creating a suction that pulls blood flow through the cannula into a filter.

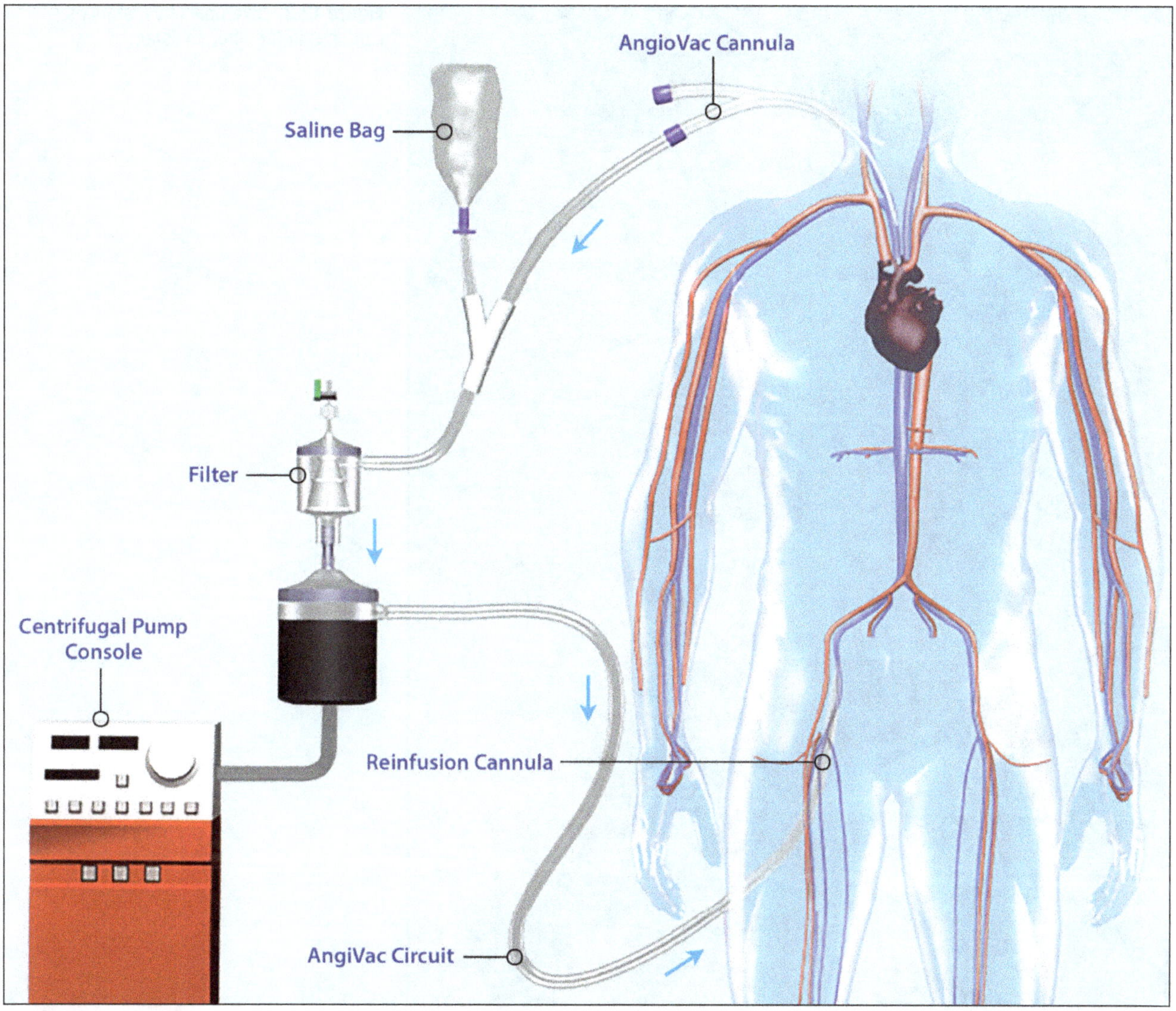

Figure 12.2 AngioVac cannula and circuit system. AngioVac is a venous-to-venous extracorporeal circuit consisting of an outflow line, a central pump, a filter, and an inflow line. The cannula has been inserted into the right internal jugular vein. Blood and thrombus are aspirated through the filter canister, allowing clot capture utilizing a centrifugal pump canister before returning blood to the patient via the reinfusion cannula placed into the femoral vein.

below, is not able to bend and reach the vegetation. Right internal jugular vein access was utilized. A 26-Fr, 35-cm DrySeal sheath was placed into the right internal jugular vein and advanced down to the right atrium. (**Video 12.4** shows the right internal jugular approach to place the AngioVac suction cannula). We were now able to engage the vegetation with the AngioVac (**Video 12.5** shows the AngioVac cannula in contact with vegetation). Large bits of the vegetation were aspirated, and on TEE, no remnant was noted on the leads (**Video 12.6**, TEE showing that the vegetation is no longer apparent after the suction). The vegetation fragments were noted in the bypass pump filter (**Figures 12.3** and **12.4**); culture of these fragments grew *Candida albicans.*

Subsequently, the AngioVac was removed. Both 26-Fr introducer sheaths were removed, and purse-string sutures were placed at the puncture site. The 19-Fr return cannula in the left common femoral vein was also removed, and a purse-string suture placed around it.

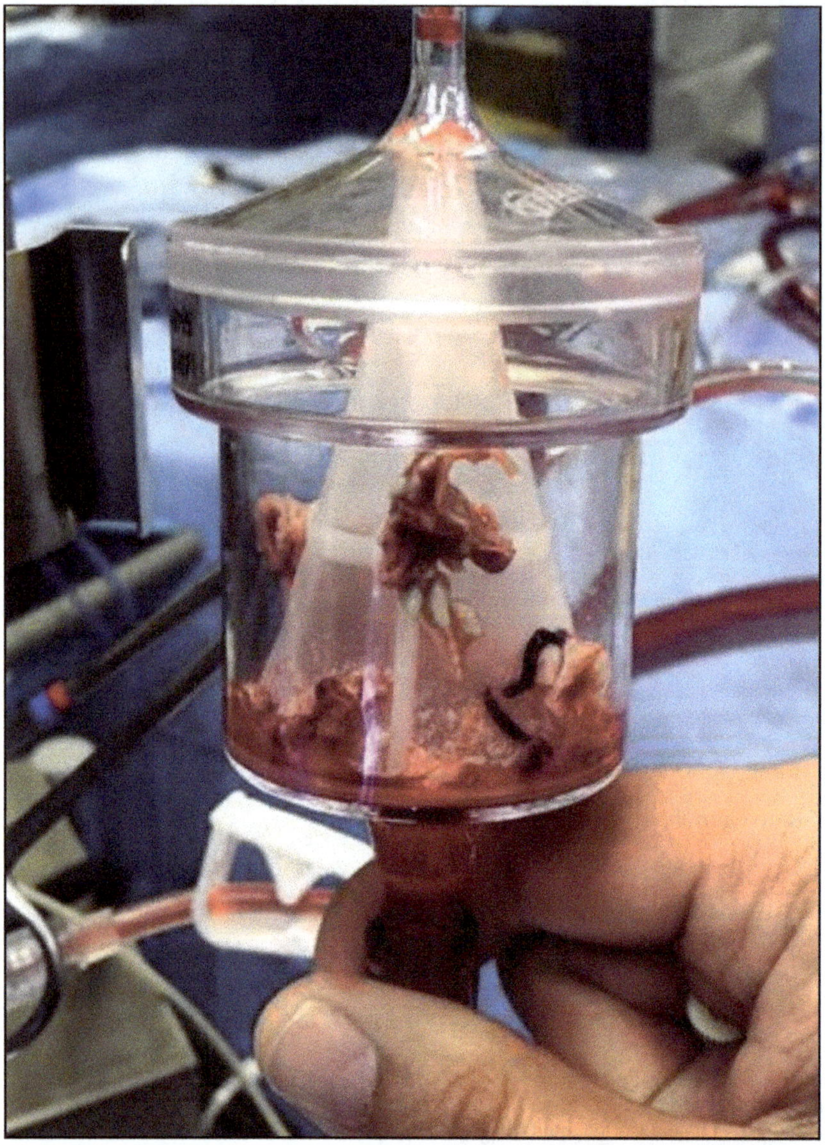

Figure 12.3 Example of vegetations captured in the filter canister.

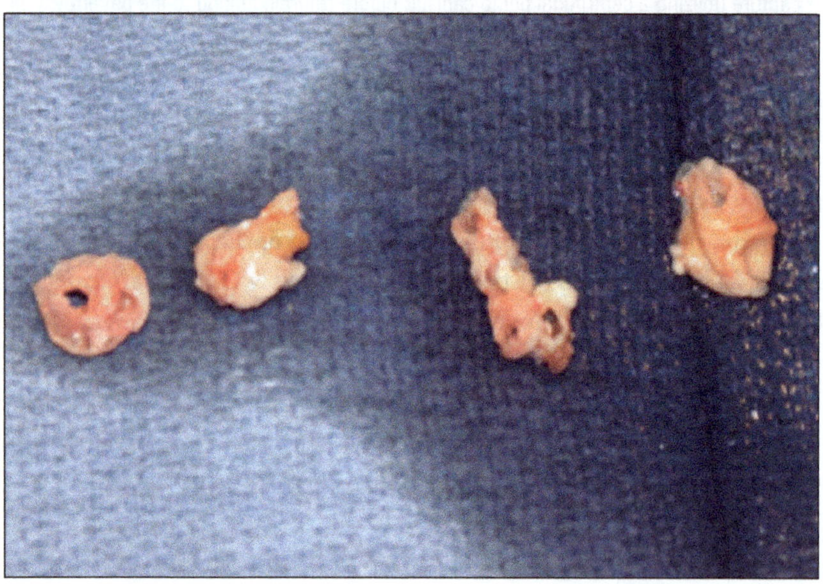

Figure 12.4 Photo shows vegetation pieces (broken by the cannula). The vegetation culture grew *Candida albicans*.

After removing the large vegetation, Heparin was reversed by protamine sulfate. The left-side device pocket was opened. Leads were freed from the pocket. Both atrial and ventricular lead active fixations were retracted. The atrial lead was able to be removed without difficulty by gentle pulling. The ventricular lead encountered fibrosis at the superior vena cava (SVC)–right atrial junction. A 12-Fr laser catheter was selected and tested in good function. The RV lead was amputated and locked in place using a universal locking stylet. The laser sheath was advanced over the lead. A few episodes of laser deployment were required to free and removed the lead. A permanent lead was placed via the right internal jugular vein and connected to an external pacemaker generator for temporary pacing.

The general surgeon took over the procedure and performed wound debridement and wound vac placement. At the end of the procedure, the final TEE showed no residual vegetation or mass in the cardiac chambers. There was no pericardial effusion.

POSTPROCEDURAL COURSE

The patient recovered well after the procedure. No symptoms were reported suggesting pulmonary emboli. One week later, the patient received a permanent dual-chamber pacemaker on the right side.

SUMMARY POINTS

- Fungemia is a serious systemic infection.
- Lead extraction is indicated in patients who have persistent fungemia and pacemaker lead infection (vegetation).
- An adequate planning of the procedure includes the selection of team members and supplies.
- AngioVac should be considered when extracting the lead that has one or more sizeable (> 2 cm) mobile vegetations or thrombi to avoid massive embolic complications.
- Cannula assignment to the vegetation is critical. Although a femoral vein approach is more often used, an internal jugular vein approach is a good alternative to facilitate aspiration of vegetation.

VIDEO LEGENDS

Video 12.1 TEE shows mobile vegetation attached to the RV lead moving between the right atrium and right ventricle (red arrow), 3 × 2 cm in size. [00:04]

Video 12.2 TEE illustrates TR was present around the device lead and vegetation. [00:01]

Video 12.3 TEE shows that the AngioVac inserted from the right femoral vein cannot reach the vegetation, instead directing into the atrial septum. [00:04]

Video 12.4 Right internal jugular approach to place the AngioVac suction cannula 35-cm DrySeal sheath, which is advanced down to the lower right atrium and tricuspid annulus. [00:01]

Video 12.5 TEE shows AngioVac cannula (red arrow) in contact with vegetation (blue arrow). [00:06]

Video 12.6 Following the AngioVac suction, TEE shows the large vegetation is removed, and no remnant was noted on the lead. [00:04]

13 | Extraction Case Complicated with Superior Vena Cava Tear Due to Intramural Pacemaker Lead

Freddy Del-Carpio Munoz, MD; Gregory A. Cogert, MD; Samuel J. Asirvatham, MD

CASE 13

CLINICAL VIGNETTE

A 25-year-old, left-handed male with a history of neonatal myocarditis and subsequent complete heart block had a pacemaker implanted when he was 17 days old. An initial abdominal generator and epicardial lead system was exchanged for a right infraclavicular dual-chamber transvenous system when he was 6 years old. By the age of 14, he underwent a pulse-generator change out due to battery depletion and the right ventricular (RV) lead was noted to be stretched with inadequate slack. Attempts to advance the lead failed, and due to concerns of dislodgement with further body growth, a new right subclavian active fixation RV lead was implanted, and the chronic lead was kept in place. Eleven years later, he underwent another pulse-generator replacement; at that time, both functioning leads had inadequate slack. The most recent RV lead could be easily advanced to provide more slack, but the right atrial (RA) lead would not advance. Three weeks later, the patient noted the right infraclavicular pacemaker incision was open and the leads were exposed with some clear fluid draining. He had no local signs of infection like erythema, pain, or fever. He was pacemaker dependent with no underlying intrinsic escape rhythm. On physical examination, the right infraclavicular scar was hypertrophic, there was a 4-mm open wound with mild purulent drainage, and the device header was visualized through the medial aspect of the incision. His blood work included normal blood cell counts. A 2-view chest X-ray (CXR) (**Figure 13.1**) showed a right infraclavicular implant with 3 active-fixation transvenous leads in addition to an abandoned epicardial abdominal lead. The lack of slack in all 3 leads was obvious, albeit more evident in the abandoned RV lead. There was no clear calcification around the leads throughout the extracardiac lead courses. Transthoracic echocardiogram (TTE) and transesophageal echocardiogram (TTE) revealed 2 small, mobile masses (1.5 × 0.9 cm and 1 × 0.7 cm) attached to the pacing leads in the right atrium, which could not be defined as being thrombus versus vegetation. The interatrial septum was intact. There was normal valvular function without valvular vegetation, global left ventricular dysfunction, and an estimated ejection fraction of 40%.

Device Details

Device Component	Manufacturer/Model	Date of Implant
Pacemaker generator	Medtronic 7941 Thera DR	3/27/1995
RA lead	Medtronic 6957 Spectraflex	8/13/1987
RV lead (active)	Medtronic 4057M Screw-In	3/27/1995
RV lead (abandoned)	Medtronic 6957 Spectraflex	8/13/1987
RV epicardial lead (abandoned)	Medtronic 5985 Spectrax SX (left lower abdominal)	10/16/1981

Clinical Decision

A decision was made to extract the system, implant a temporary permanent pacemaker, and once the infection was treated, to implant a new biventricular pacemaker device.

PREPROCEDURAL PLANNING

A temporary right internal jugular screw-in pacemaker lead was placed in high anterior RV. The incision was opened and the generator removed. At the time of this procedure, the Bridge Occlusion

 Cardiotext Publishing. ISBN: 978-1-942909-54-5

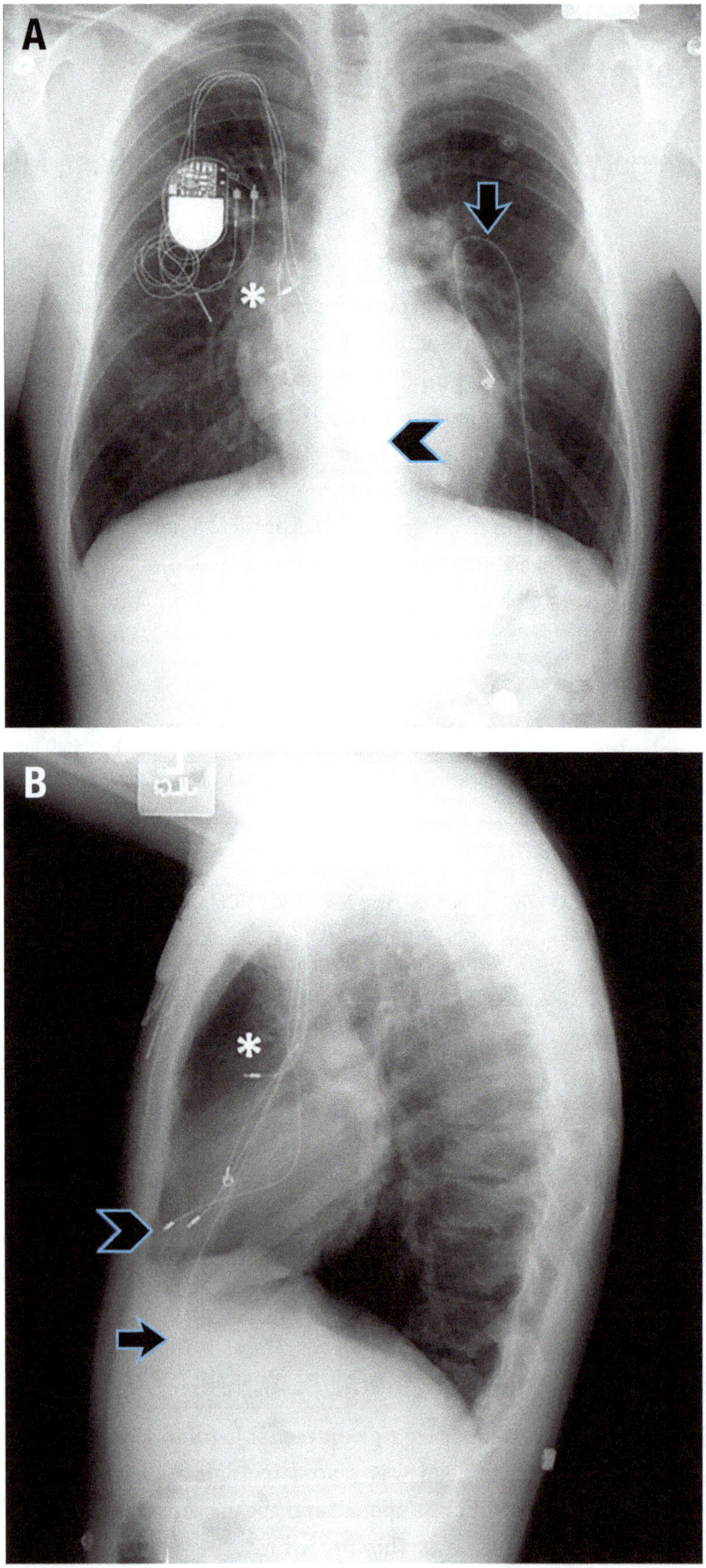

Figure 13.1 Two-view CXRs. Two pacemaker leads are observed in the RV (**black arrow heads**) and another in the RA appendage region (*). The disconnected epicardial lead is visible (**black arrows**). The CXR shows deep inspiration and hyperinflated lungs with a normal cardiac silhouette. No obvious calcification can be observed around the leads. The abandoned RV lead has prominent lack of slack.

Balloon was not available clinically. Femoral access was obtained to provide backup temporary pacing through a deflectable catheter.

EXTRACTION PROCEDURAL DETAILS

The procedure was performed in the electrophysiology laboratory, at the time this was a common practice. He was placed under general anesthesia. Extensive dissection of the leads was completed in order to separate them from marked fibrosis in the pocket. Stylets were advanced to the tips of the atrial and current RV lead; a stylet would not advance in the abandoned RV lead. Screws were retracted on all 3 leads without difficulty. First the abandoned RV lead pin was cut off and a locking stylet was advanced close to the tip. Gentle traction was applied but failed to retract the lead. A laser sheath (Philips Medical) was deployed and freely advanced from the subclavian vein to the superior vena cava (SVC). An area of linear calcification was noted in the SVC. It was difficult to position an outer sheath over the laser catheter. With gentle manipulation, the sheath was advanced 2 cm farther down the SVC. Cardiac pulsation was felt through the lead traction. On release of traction, the patient suddenly became hypotensive. He received fluids, transfusions, and epinephrine, and he required chest compressions. A cardiac surgeon performed an emergent median sternotomy, and there was no blood in the pericardium. An immediate right anterior thoracotomy revealed a right hemithorax and a 3-cm linear tear in the lateral wall of the SVC was the source of bleeding. The pacemaker lead was firmly adhered to a heavily calcified area in the SVC wall. Using 2 3-0 Prolene sutures, the massive hemorrhage was partially controlled. After a transfusion of total of 24 units of packed red blood, no cardiac output could be restored, and the patient expired.

Autopsy

Figure 13.2 shows macroscopic findings of the autopsy. In Panel A, the SVC is intact and contains the extraction sheath. In Panel B, the SVC and the innominate vein were incised. Dense fibrosis can be observed. On manual examination, there was palpable calcification around the leads. In **Figure 13.3**, Panel A shows a segment of the SVC and the junction of the right atrium with the leads running from cranial to caudal. In Panel B, microscopic transversal cuts at the specified levels are shown. The SVC had a perforation 1 cm from the innominate vein confluence at a site of intramural incorporation or "tunneling" of the chronic RV pacemaker lead into the vein wall, with heavy fibrosis and calcification. At least one lead had a proximal and distal intramural course in the SVC.

DISCUSSION

The pathophysiology of the interaction of an implanted transvenous lead and the cardiovascular system involves a process that starts with acute inflammation leading to thrombus formation at sites of endovascular and endocardial contact. The thrombus then organizes and becomes fibrotic tissue that typically is observed along the lead at the vascular entry site, the curve from the innominate vein into the SVC, anodal ring to tip and in cases of ICDs in-growth around the coils. Over time and usually in younger patients, old leads can undergo a process of calcification incorporated into the fibrosis. Transvenous lead extractions are feasible and safe when the fibrotic tissue is freed from the lead assuming that the tensile strength of the vessel exceeds that of the scar tissue. Thus, a friable vessel will not permit a transvenous extraction despite the skill of the operator. We also assume that the lead travels within the vein lumen into the heart, but in some instances when the lead erodes the vessel wall and it becomes excluded from the vein or becomes part of the transmural vein thickness, the result of the extraction procedure will carry a high risk of vascular tear and perforation. It is possible that this process of lead intramural vein incorporation happens at the time of lead placement after damage to the vein endocardium similar to a vein wall dissection with part of the lead

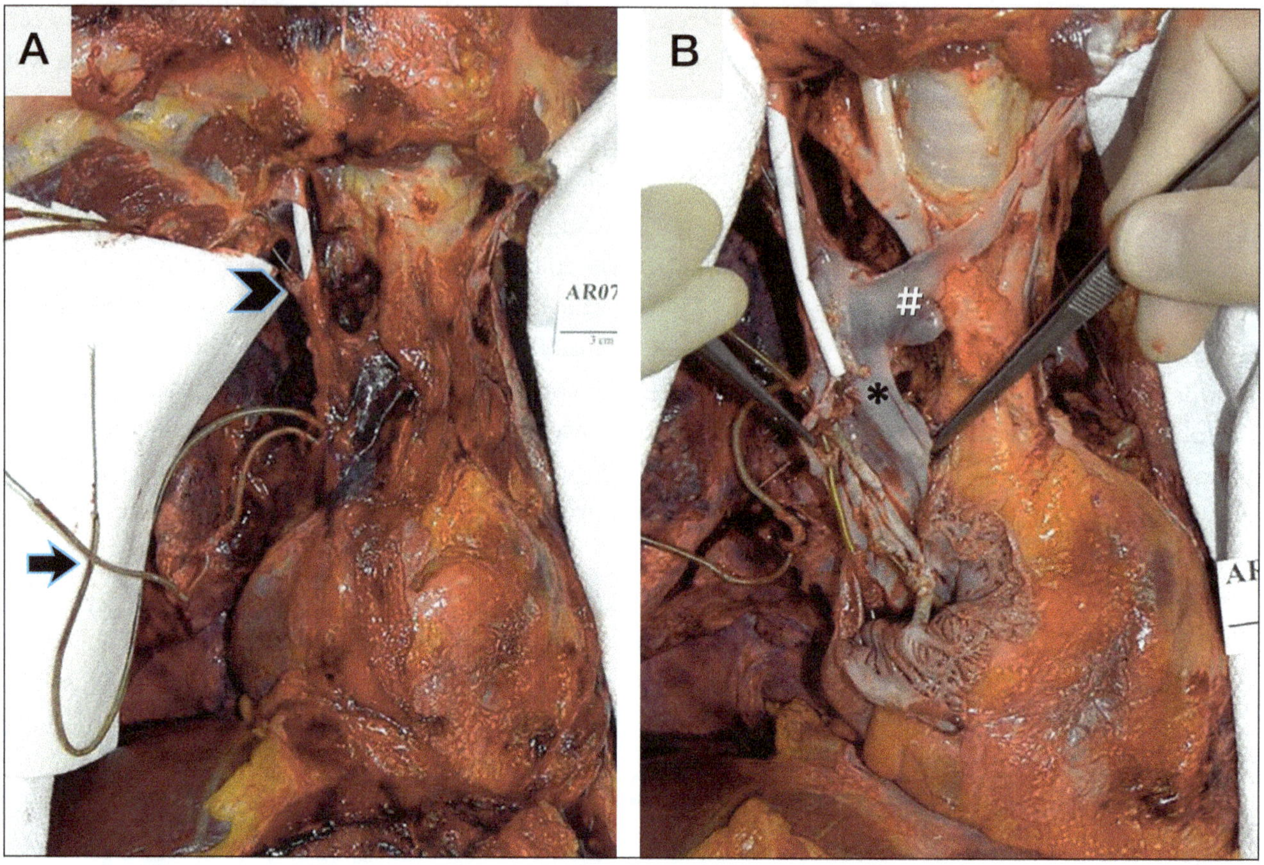

Figure 13.2 Autopsy findings. **Panel A:** Left panel shows the mediastinum with the heart in situ in an anterior view. An extraction sheath (**white color**) can be observed inside the SVC (**black arrow head**). Two of the leads are seen to the left of the picture (**black arrow**). **Panel B:** The SVC and the right atrium were incised open. The tip of the extraction sheath contains the chronic RV lead and its tip (**asterisk**) is located the level of the SVC tear approximately 1 cm from the confluence with the innominate vein (**#**). There is dense scar around all leads with heavy calcification reported after manual examination.

tunneled inside the vein wall thickness.[1] These circumstances can make it potentially impossible with current techniques and tools to separate the strongly adhered lead without provoking transmural vessel wall injury. As discussed in Chapter 3 about lead extraction imaging, preprocedural evaluation with CT angiogram can reveal the extravascular or intramural course of chronic leads and plan for a high risk procedure accordingly.

Lead extraction carries a 1%–2% risk of vascular damage to the SVC that can lead to tear and catastrophic vascular complications associated with high mortality rate. In spite of better tools for lead extraction, the risk of vascular tear has remained stable and has not been eliminated. In a study of more than 800 extraction leads, Tarakji and colleagues analyzed microscopically the vascular tissue adhered to extracted leads and found that in 9%–10%, there was histological evidence of full-thickness (endothelial, muscular, and adventitial layers) vascular tissue.[2] In spite of microscopically transmural vascular compromise, the extraction case was not always associated with a catastrophic or clinically evident vascular injury of the SVC.

In a large retrospective analysis of all extraction cases in a tertiary center over a 16-year period, the reported incidence of catastrophic vascular complications requiring emergent surgical or endovascular interventions was 0.8% that carried a mortality rate of 36%.[3] The most common site of vascular injury was the SVC, typically at the junction with the right atrium. The time to decompensation in the majority of patients was within minutes of the precipitating procedural event, and in 66% of cases, required immediate rescue surgical

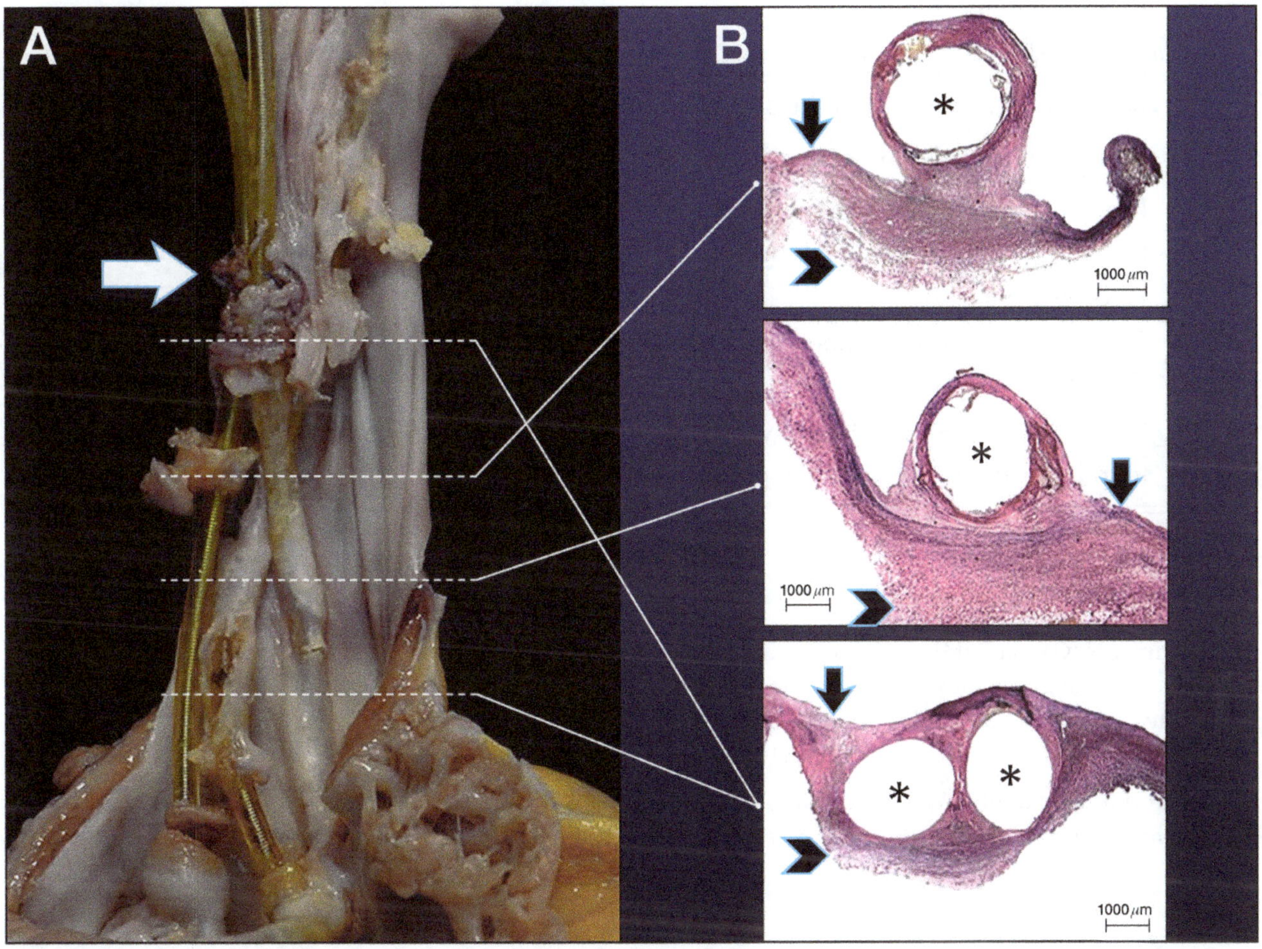

Figure 13.3 **Panel A:** Autopsy picture showing the junction of the SVC and right atrium. The anterior wall of the SVC and right atrium were cut open. There was palpable calcified fibrosis around the pacemaker leads. A residue of the Prolene suture placed at time of surgery to contain the vascular tear is still observed in the upper part (**white arrow**). **Panel B:** Histopathological specimens were obtained at different levels of the SVC, as shown by the transversal lines. The specimens were processed with Verhoeff-van Gieson stain. Collagen appears **red**, elastin is **black**, and everything else is tan-pink. Observe that in the superior (level of the SVC tear) and the inferior transversal cuts, the leads had an intramural or "tunneled" course; they were embedded into the SVC wall and there was minimal vascular tissue separating the lead from the adventitia of the vein (**lower panel**). In the other segments, it can be seen that the adhesions around the leads were attached to the wall SVC, but they were not engrained into the wall. The endothelium is marked by **black arrows** and the adventitia by **black arrowheads**. The **asterisks** mark the space occupied by the leads.

intervention. The main predictors of catastrophic vascular complications included longer lead implant duration, the use of powered sheaths, and the need for femoral approach, while the factors associated with mortality included older patient age, lead extraction for infection, and performing surgery or vascular intervention in the electrophysiology lab compared to the operating room.

This information has major implications for the proceduralist performing lead extractions. First, it is not uncommon to injure the entire vessel wall containing the leads. Second, not all transmural vascular compromise leads to vascular tear and complications, probably due to the supporting role of fibroadipose tissue and myocardial sleeves surrounding the SVC, which can contain major hemorrhage. Finally, the ingrowth of the lead in the wall of the SVC can lead to major vascular injury regardless of the technique used, and the extraction of high-risk patients should always be performed in a setting where a cardiothoracic surgeon is readily available to perform a rescue thoracotomy to repair the vascular damage. This case prompted a change in our clinical practice, and all these cases since then are carried out in the hybrid operating room.

SUMMARY POINTS

- Leads can get engrained or incorporated into the wall of the veins.
- Extraction of leads tunneled into the vein wall frequently compromise the entire vein wall.
- High-risk extraction cases should be carried out in a setting where a cardiac surgeon is readily available. It is our common practice to perform these high-risk cases in a hybrid surgical room.
- The Bridge Occlusion Balloon to temporarily occlude an SVC tear should be considered in these high-risk cases.
- Imaging (CT scan) can aid in revealing leads with heavy calcified fibrosis, intra- or extra-mural vascular course, and the procedure can be planned accordingly.

REFERENCES

1. Suraci N, Garcia P, Mihos C, Rosen G, Santana O. Right atrial, right ventricular, superior vena cava dissection caused by Swan-Ganz catheter placement. *J Invasive Cardiol.* 2019;31(5):E95.
2. Tarakji KG, Saliba W, Markabawi D, et al. Unrecognized venous injuries after cardiac implantable electronic device transvenous lead extraction. *Heart Rhythm.* 2018;15(3):318–325.
3. Brunner MP, Cronin EM, Wazni O, et al. Outcomes of patients requiring emergent surgical or endovascular intervention for catastrophic complications during transvenous lead extraction. *Heart Rhythm.* 2014;11(3):419–425.

14 | Early Detection of Superior Vena Cava Tear Using Video-Assisted Thoracoscopy During Lead Extraction

Yong-Mei Cha, MD; Fatima A. Al-Ahmed, MD; Arman Arghami, MD

CLINICAL VIGNETTE

The patient is a 61-year-old male with a significant medical history of diabetes mellitus, peripheral vascular disease, and osteomyelitis, which has led to bilateral below-the-knee amputation and ischemic cardiomyopathy, left ventricular ejection fraction (LVEF) 30%. A cardiac resynchronization defibrillator (CRT-D) was implanted in 2009 for heart failure and primary prevention. LVEF improved to 44% in 2010. His first system became infected shortly after insertion, requiring removal and replacement. He did well subsequently until he had an elective pulse generator replacement in 2016. He noted almost immediately after that that the site was swollen and became progressively red and more swollen. The incision then broke down with serosanguineous drainage. He was initially treated with doxycycline, which did not alter the progressive course, and the drainage cultures demonstrated coagulase-negative *Staphylococcus*. He was treated with vancomycin and transferred to Mayo Clinic. The pacemaker site was slightly erythematous, and there was an area of tissue breakdown in the lateral third of the incision. Blood culture was negative. Transesophageal echocardiography (TEE) showed no evidence for infective endocarditis and no vegetations identified. There was no mass or vegetation identified in the right atrial (RA) and right ventricular (RV) leads. The LVEF was 35% with an intact atrial septum. The patient was diagnosed with CRT-D pocket infection.

Device Details

Device Component	Manufacturer/Model	Date of Implant
Pulse generator	St. Jude Medical 3357-40 Unify Assura Device CRT-D	March 5, 2010
LV lead	St. Jude Medical 1056T QuickFlex GG145370	
RA lead	St. Jude Medical 1642T TN041119	
RV lead	St. Jude Medical 7120 Durata AHA47819	

PREPROCEDURAL PLANNING

The patient was evaluated by cardiac surgery, electrophysiology, and general surgery teams before the procedure. The patient was not pacemaker dependent. We planned TEE to monitor pericardial effusion and tricuspid valve regurgitation (TR) during extraction. Video-assisted thoracoscopy surgery (VATS) was considered to monitor superior vena cava (SVC) to monitor potential SVC tear.

EXTRACTION PROCEDURE

General

The patient was intubated and ventilated throughout the procedure. A TEE probe was placed. A double-lumen tube was used to facilitate video-assisted thoracoscopy (VAT) surveillance during the procedure (left lung intubation only, **Figure 14.1**). The patient was prepped and draped in the usual aseptic fashion. A time-out was performed. An antibiotic (cefazolin [Ancef], 2.0 g) was given intravenously.

Cardiac Lead Extraction: A Case-Based Contemporary Approach.
 Cardiotext Publishing. ISBN: 978-1-942909-54-5

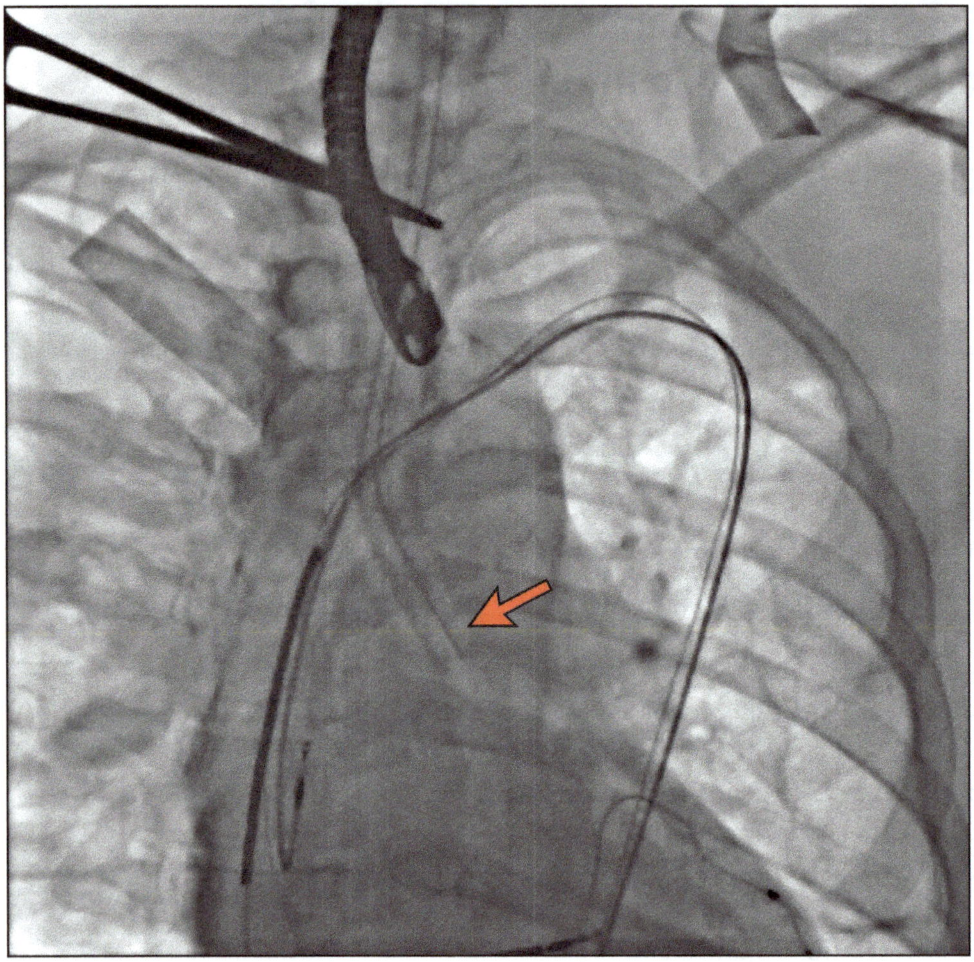

Figure 14.1 **Red arrow** points endotracheal tube insertion for left lung ventilation only.

Vascular Access

A 4-Fr radial arterial line was obtained to monitor blood pressure. A 9-Fr sheath was inserted into the left femoral vein for fluid resuscitation and potential blood transfusion. The femoral Cook workstation (Cook Medical) was placed in the right femoral vein.

VATS

The VATS port was placed in the right fourth intercostal space using a 5-mm port. Using videoscopic technique right chest cavity was entered safely and mediastinal structures were surveyed and observed throught the extraction process. **Figure 14.2** shows the setup of VATS in the right chest, and **Figure 14.3** shows that the operators can visualize the SVC lateral wall and pericardium on the screen throughout the extraction course. **Video 14.1** shows an example of video observation using VATS.

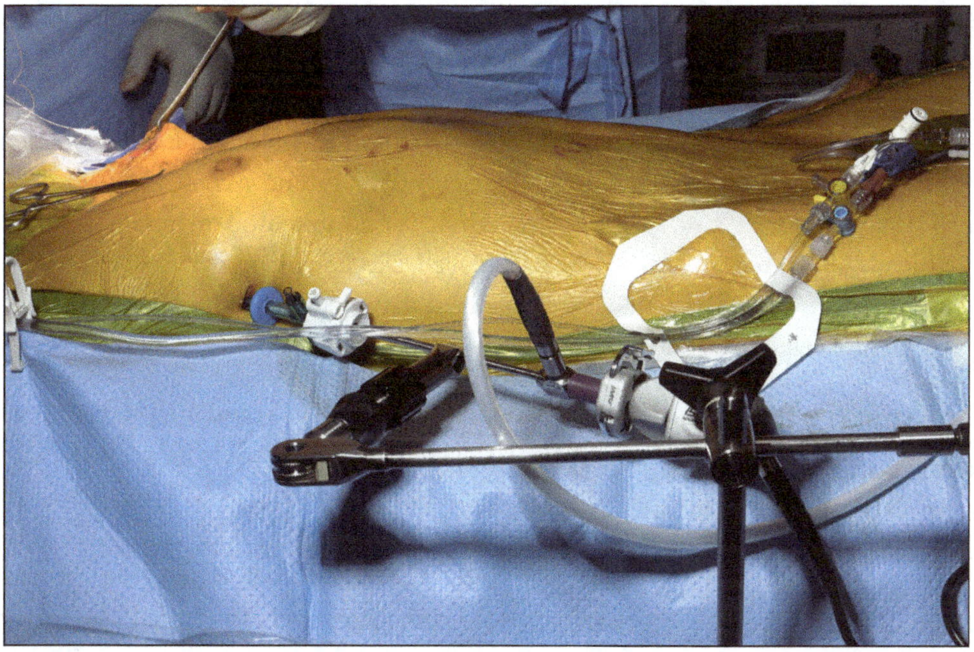

Figure 14.2 The setup of VATS in the right chest.

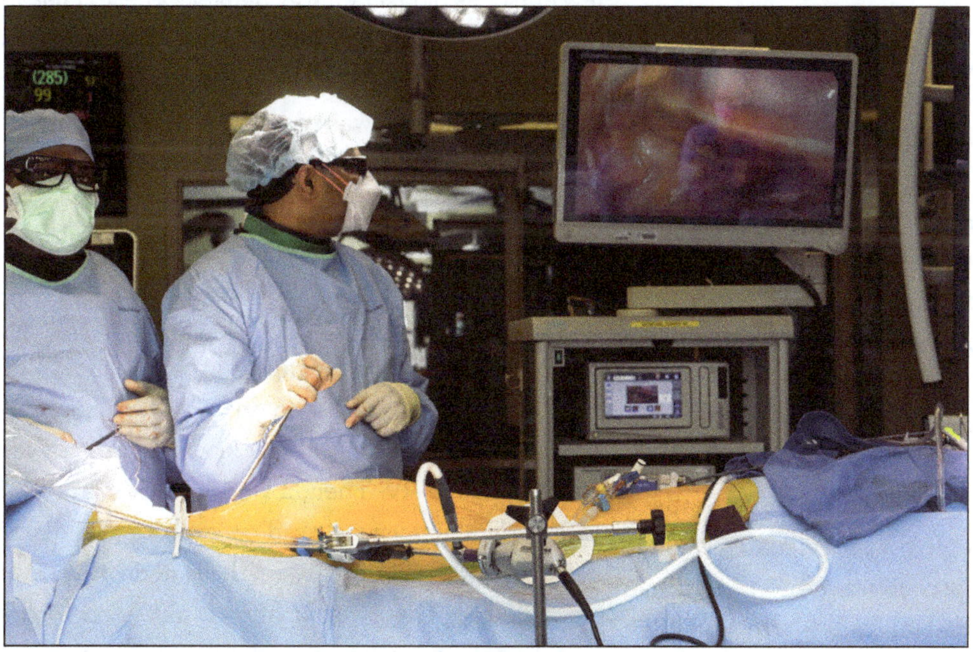

Figure 14.3 The operators can visualize the SVC lateral wall and pericardium on the screen throughout the extraction course.

Difficulty in Extraction and SVC Tear

The left infraclavicular scar was reincised, and the dissection was carried down to the pulse generator, which was freed from the pocket. Device pocket infection was apparent. Cautery was used to achieve hemostasis, and blunt dissection was undertaken to free the leads. The sutures on the sleeves were removed. A stylet was placed into the left ventricular (LV) lead, which had fibrous adhesions in the left subclavian vein. We then proceeded with the components of the laser lead extraction. The lead was prepared, and a locking stylet was placed. A 12-Fr Excimer laser (Philips Medical) was selected and tested for normal function. The LV lead entered the subclavian vein just under the left clavicle, which prevented the laser sheath advancement. At this point, a universal locking stylet was placed in the RA lead and advanced to the tip of the lead. A Prolene suture was used to tie the atrial lead to the locking stylet. The 14-Fr laser sheath was carefully advanced to the innominate vein and SVC junction.

At this location, three leads appeared to be tangled together. The laser sheath around the atrial lead could not be advanced to the SVC. The operator then prepared for extracting the RV high-voltage lead. A stylet was placed in the RV lead, and the active-fixation helix was retracted. The locking stylet was inserted into the lead. The 14-Fr Excimer laser sheath was gradually advanced to the left subclavian area by laser energy delivery and separating the lead from surrounding fibrosis. Apparently, the lead entrance was also just under the left clavicle, giving minimal space for the laser sheath to pass. The laser sheath was switched to the 11-Fr Evolution sheath (Philips Medical). The operator could not make progress passing the Evolution sheath to the innominate vein on the RV lead. The high-voltage lead was transected at this point, and we lost the traction force via the locking stylet. The operator then placed a 14-Fr Excimer laser sheath over the RA lead and advanced the sheath to the innominate vein SVC junction. This was the most challenging portion of the lead extraction due to significant fibrosis, which tangled three leads together. The SVC and RA were visualized by VATS. The laser sheath was advanced to the mid-SVC level to remove the atrial lead, where an SVC tear occurred. Bleeding from SVC to the right thorax was observed (unfortunately, the video was not recorded by error).

Surgical Repair

The SVC tear was small, a pinpoint bleeding with enough extravasation of blood volume that it required surgical suture for correction. Given the need for surgical intervention, we elected at this point to proceed with sternotomy in a control fashion. Therefore, we divided the sternum with a Sarns saw (3M Inc.) and visualized the bleeding source from the SVC into the right hemithorax. We did not open the pericardium and instead opened the right pleural cavity and placed a 4-0 Prolene pledged stitch in a horizontal mattress fashion, which achieved excellent hemostasis. There were no other surgical maneuvers required at this point.

Complete Lead Extraction in the Open Chest

The patient's blood pressure remained stable above 90 mmHg systolic without requiring pressors, and fluid resuscitation to the end as SVC repaired was achieved within 5 minutes of bleeding. We proceeded with the continued extraction of the remaining leads. The operator placed the 14-Fr Excimer laser sheath back to the RA lead. With a few episodes of laser energy delivery, the atrial lead was removed in its entirety. Then, the LV lead was also being removed by laser sheath without further difficulty. Lasering was required only at the subclavian and innominate veins for the LV lead. As the RV lead was transected and retracted into the innominate vein (**Video 14.2**), the operator used the right femoral working station to extract the lead from below. An 8-Fr EPT catheter (Blazer, Boston Scientific) could capture the RV lead from the RA. The lead was pulled down toward the inferior vena cava (IVC), and the lead's distal tip was freed from the RV. Then, a Goose Neck snare (GN 1500, Medtronic) was used to capture the distal end of the RV lead and pulled the lead down to IVC (Video 14.2). There was a fibrotic adhesion to the RA preventing the lead completely free. The operator obtained the left subclavian vein access and tried to use the Goose Neck snare to capture the proximal end (the broken end) in the innominate vein, which was unsuccessful (**Video 14.3**).

Contrast injection from the subclavian vein showed subclavian to innominate vein fibrosis with a contained dissection at the transected RV lead location (**Video 14.4**). At this time, the cardiac surgeon joined and opened the pericardium. Under direct whole-heart visualization and bypass standby, we pulled the lead from the femoral station using the Goose Neck snare with a stronger force pulling towards the IVC. We were successfully pulling the entire lead off the venous and atrial myocardial structure without any hemodynamic consequence or myocardial rupture (**Video 14.5**). The cardiovascular surgeon closed the chest and also did a pocket capsulectomy. A wound VAC was placed. The patient tolerated the procedure well and was transferred to the Surgical Intensive Care Unit.

POSTPROCEDURAL COURSE

The patient recovered well from the surgery. Five days later, a new CRT-D device was implanted on the right side (**Figure 14.4**).

DISCUSSION

One of the riskiest aspects of lead extraction is the adhesions and scarring around the SVC.[1] Due to its thin-walled structure, the SVC is at risk of tear and disruption during extraction. Live TEE examination during extraction can help detect pericardial effusion, but we have introduced a VATS technique to detect significant bleeding much faster and efficiently. Especially in this example, the tear resulted in bleeding into the pleural cavity and not the pericardium. Without VATS direct visualization, the detection of this complication could have been delayed significantly until the patient started showing signs of hypotension and deterioration. The early detection provided by VATS allowed us to intervene quickly before the patient experienced any hemodynamic instability. **Video 14.6** shows a

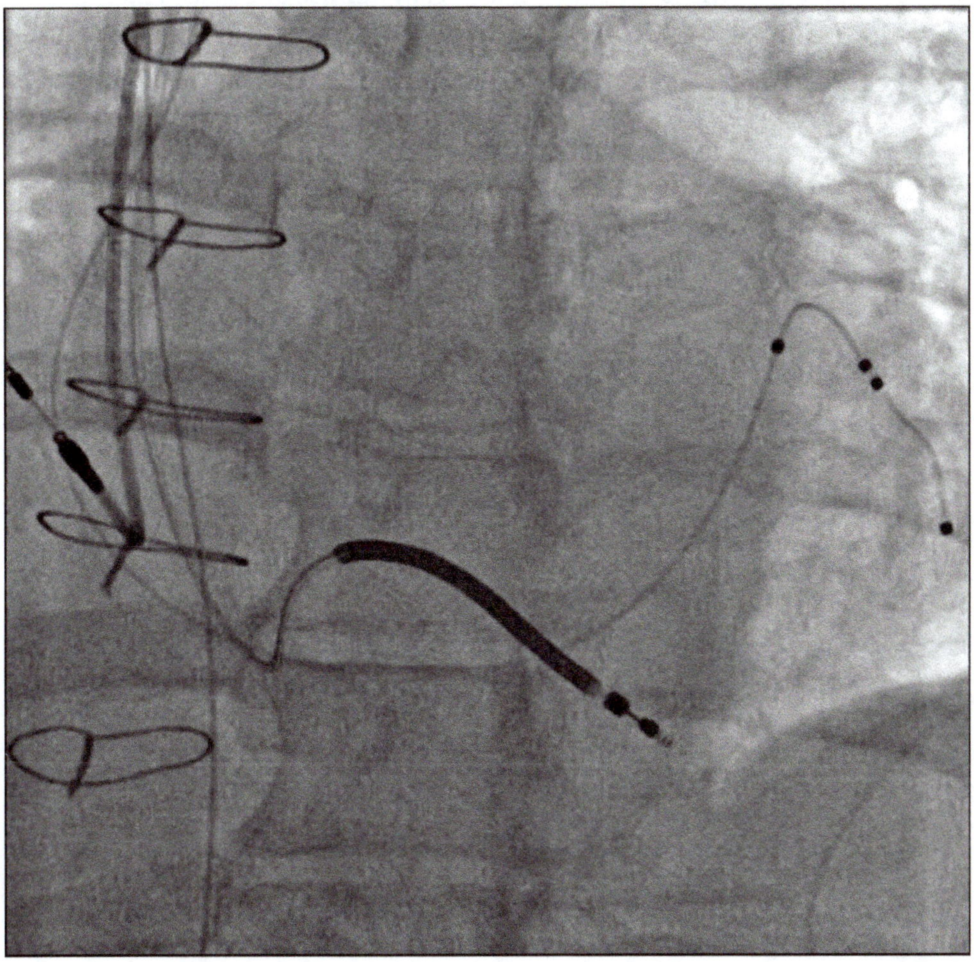

Figure 14.4 A new CRT-D device was implanted on the right side.

different patient who underwent a combined VATS procedure and lead extraction for pacemaker pocket infection. The RA appendage movement is visualized under the pericardium (yellow arrow). Note that the traction force on the atrial lead is pulling the appendage downward until the lead is removed from the appendage. The blue arrow follows the atrial lead tip, which is pulling back along the SVC lateral wall.

We believe in select patients, direct visualization of the pericardial structures, and SVC via the right VATS to help detect complications earlier and provide a safer window of intervention for the patient, resulting in less morbidity. We are working on the techniques to repair the SVC using the VATS approach in the future if such an event is to happen again. This will allow us to spare the patient a sternotomy and expedite their dismissal.

SUMMARY POINTS

- Patient is an immune-compromised host, prone to infection.
- Alternating laser and rotating mechanical sheaths facilitates separating the binding fibrosis in multiple leads.
- SVC tear occurs more often than myocardial rupture during lead extraction.
- VATS is very helpful for early detection of SVC tear and early surgical control of bleeding. The SVC lateral wall can be continuously visualized during the extraction. This patient had timely sternotomy and SVC repair without hemodynamic compromise or consequence associated with bleeding.

REFERENCE

1. Bongiorni MG. Transvenous lead extraction: From simple traction to internal transjugular approach. Milan: Springer-Verlag Mailand, 2011.

VIDEO LEGENDS

Video 14.1 VATS (right side) shows pericardium and the beating right atrium and its junction to SVC under the pericardium. Right-sided phrenic nerve is seen. The right lung is deflated. [00:25]

Video 14.2 Proximal lead is transected and retracted to the innominate vein (red arrow). The distal lead is snared from below and pulled into IVC (blue arrow). [00:01]

Video 14.3 Snaring proximal RV lead from the subclavian vein was attempted but unsuccessful. [00:01]

Video 14.4 Contrast injection shows subclavian to innominate vein fibrosis with dissection at the broken RV lead area. [00:02]

Video 14.5 All 3 leads are removed by extraction from above and below. [00:01]

Video 14.6 A different patient who underwent a combined VATS procedure and lead extraction for pacemaker pocket infection. The right atrial appendage movement is visualized under the pericardium (yellow arrow). Note that the traction force on the atrial lead is pulling the appendage downward until the lead is removed from the appendage. The blue arrow follows the atrial lead tip, which is pulling back along the SVC lateral wall. [01:11]

15 | Percutaneous Management of Superior Vena Cava Tear

Yong-Mei Cha, MD

CLINICAL VIGNETTE

A 55-year-old male has a history of nonischemic biventricular heart failure. He has cardiorenal syndrome, a history of peripherally inserted central catheter infection, left ventricular (LV) thrombus on anticoagulation therapy, atrial fibrillation/flutter, and ventricular tachycardia history on amiodarone. He has been treated with milrinone since 2018. He presented to an outside hospital with chills, nausea, vomiting, headache, and decompensated heart failure. He required vasopressors when he initially presented, which were later weaned during his hospitalization. Transthoracic echocardiogram (TTE) on admission showed an ejection fraction of 15%, but no thrombus was noted. However, both of 2 blood cultures drawn on admission grew *Candida albicans* 3 days later. Subsequent transesophageal echocardiogram (TEE) reported a large mobile echo-density (2.1 × 1.6 cm) vegetation that prolapsed into the right atrium (RA) and appeared to be attached to the ICD lead. (**Video 15.1**) There were no reported vegetative lesions on the mitral or aortic valves. There was moderate tricuspid valve regurgitation (TR). CT chest showed bilateral ground-glass opacities, concerning for multifocal pneumonia of possible fungal etiology. There was also a concern for necrotizing lymphadenitis and aortic and iliac artery aneurysm with thrombus. His peripherally inserted central catheter has been removed due to a concern for it being the source of candidemia.

Device Details

Device Component	Manufacturer/Model	Implant Date
CRT-D generator	Boston Scientific G 158 Dynagen	12/7/2015
RA lead	Cardiac Pacemakers Inc 4469 Fineline II Sterox EZ	
RV lead	Boston Scientific 0696 Reliance 4-Front G	
LV lead	Boston Scientific 4677 Acuity x4 spiral Long	

PREPROCEDURAL PLANNING

The patient had a *Candida albicans* bloodstream infection and large vegetation on one of the device leads. *Candida* is a relatively rare cause of mycotic aneurysms, but more aggressive treatment is needed in this setting. The other etiologies, including *Histoplasma*, *Blastomyces*, and *Cryptococcus*, were excluded. The patient has persistent candidemia despite intravenous caspofungin therapy. Lead extraction and device removal were strongly considered by infectious disease and heart rhythm services.

CASE 15

Cardiovascular Surgery Consultation

The lead extraction was undertaken in the device lab as the patient was not a candidate for sternotomy. Note that the cardiovascular surgeon did not consider the patient to be a sternotomy candidate, should the patient developed massive bleeding event, due to his advanced stage of heart failure. The chest CT without contrast shows one of the leads is in contact to the SVC lateral wall (**Figure 15.1**).

 ISBN: 978-1-942909-54-5

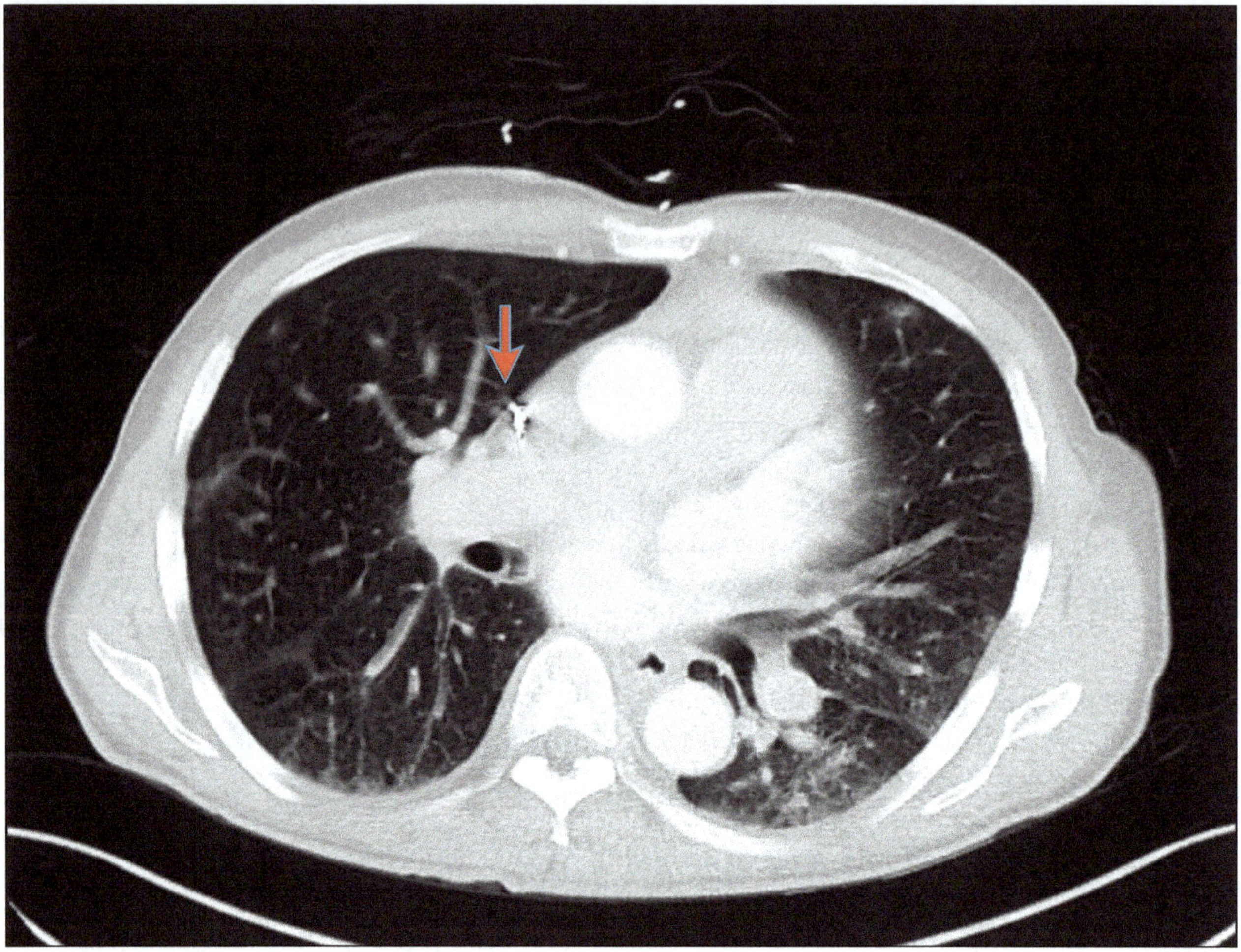

Figure 15.1 Noncontrast chest CT: **Red arrow** points to transvenous leads against the wall of SVC.

PROCEDURAL DETAILS

Anesthesia

The patient was intubated and ventilated throughout the procedure.

Venous Access

Two venous accesses were obtained from the left-side femoral vein for fluid resuscitation and intracardiac ultrasound catheter placement. Two venous accesses were also obtained from the right-side femoral vein for a 16-Fr workstation and 12-Fr Bridge Occlusion Balloon placement (Philips Medical). An Amplatz wire was placed in the right jugular vein from the right femoral vein. The Bridge Occlusion Balloon catheter was tested and placed in the inferior vena cava (IVC) to be ready.

Device Pocket Dissection

The device pocket was dissected, and 3 leads were freed from the pocket. There was no sign of pocket infection. Stylets were placed in each individual leads. RA lead body was counterclockwise rotated to free the Sweet Tip lead. RV lead active fixation was able to be retracted. However, all 3 leads were unable to be removed by gentle pulling.

Extraction

A universal locking stylet was inserted into the RA lead lumen and advanced to the lead tip. One-Tie (Cook Medical) was used to fix the locking stylet to the lead body. Traction is thus transmitted more effectively to the lead distal end. Initially, an 11-Fr TightRail rotational mechanical sheath (Philips Medical) was considered. Due to the concern of

TightRail sheath and 5-Fr lead mismatch, the 14-Fr Excimer laser sheath was selected. The laser sheath passed over the lead. At points of resistance, a circumferential laser beam with a penetration depth of 80 μm is delivered to vaporize adhesions from the left subclavian to the RA (**Videos 15.2–15.4**). The RA lead tip was freed from the RA appendage after the countertraction, and the lead was removed in its entirety. Next, the coronary sinus (CS) lead was prepared, and a universal locking stylet was inserted into the lead tip and the lead locked in place by using One-Tie. The laser sheath was slowly advanced over the CS lead by episodes of lasing energy (**Video 15.5**). When the laser sheath was advanced to SVC–RA junction, the CS lead was removed from CS and completely extracted back into the laser sheath by gentle pulling (**Video 15.6**).

SVC Tear and Management

The locking stylet was placed into the last RV ICD lead. At this point, the operator noticed a small pericardial effusion, which was gradually increasing, on intracardiac echocardiography (ICE). **Video 15.7** shows a moderate size of pericardial effusion. ICE also revealed a severely reduced LV systolic function, a chronically organized and calcified LV endocardial thrombus. The patient required epinephrine from the beginning of the procedure for hemodynamic support. His blood pressure remained to be stable at 85/60 mmHg. A tear in the lower part of the SVC was suspected. The Bridge Occlusion Balloon was advanced to the SVC and inflated with 40 cc of mixed contrast/saline in a 1:4 ratio. There was no further increase in pericardial effusion. Pericardiocentesis was the next step. The subxiphoid area was sterilized. A 14-Fr Tuohy needle was inserted from the subxiphoid (2 cm below and 1 cm left to the sternum tip) toward the anterior pericardium guided by fluoroscopy in lateral view. When tested using a small amount of contrast injection, pericardium tenting was observed, and the needle was advanced into the pericardial space, which was confirmed by contrast injection. **Video 15.8** shows agitated saline injection through the Tuohy needle to confirm it at pericardial space. A 0.035-inch wire was located in the pericardial space using cinegraph in RAO and LAO views. A 7-Fr sheath was advanced into the pericardial space over the wire. Then, a pigtail catheter was placed into the pericardial space via the Safesheath. Approximately 350 cc dark blood was removed from the pericardial space and sent to a cell saver for reinfusion. The patient was hemodynamically stable during this pericardiocentesis process. The pericardial effusion was under control at this point. The SVC balloon was deflated, and the operator then continued extraction to remove the last RV lead. The 14-Fr laser sheath was advanced to the subclavian vein over the lead. Two laser episodes were required to advance the laser sheath to the innominate vein, yet laser energy was not needed to advance from the innominate vein to the RA. The RV lead tip came off from the RV apex and the lead was then removed in its entirety. However, after the RV lead removal patient had a blood pressure drop, and reaccumulation of pericardial effusion was visualized. Contrast injection at SVC did not show clear contrast extravasation (**Video 15.9**). The Bridge Occlusion Balloon was reinflated in the lower SVC, which controlled the bleeding (**Video 15.10**). This confirmed that the SVC tear was the source of bleeding causing pericardial effusion. As the patient was not a candidate for open-chest SVC repair, we consulted a vascular surgeon for consideration of placing a covered stent (Gore Aortic Extender, Gore Medical) in the SVC to close the opening (**Figure 15.2**). This self-expanding stent is 3 cm in length and 23 mm in width. After the covered stent placement, the patient had no further accumulation of pericardial effusion. The final ICE image showed no further pericardial effusion, and the pigtail catheter was dry. We injected 10 cc lidocaine into the pericardial space and stabilized the pigtail catheter in place. The left chest device pocket was washed, and the incision was closed.

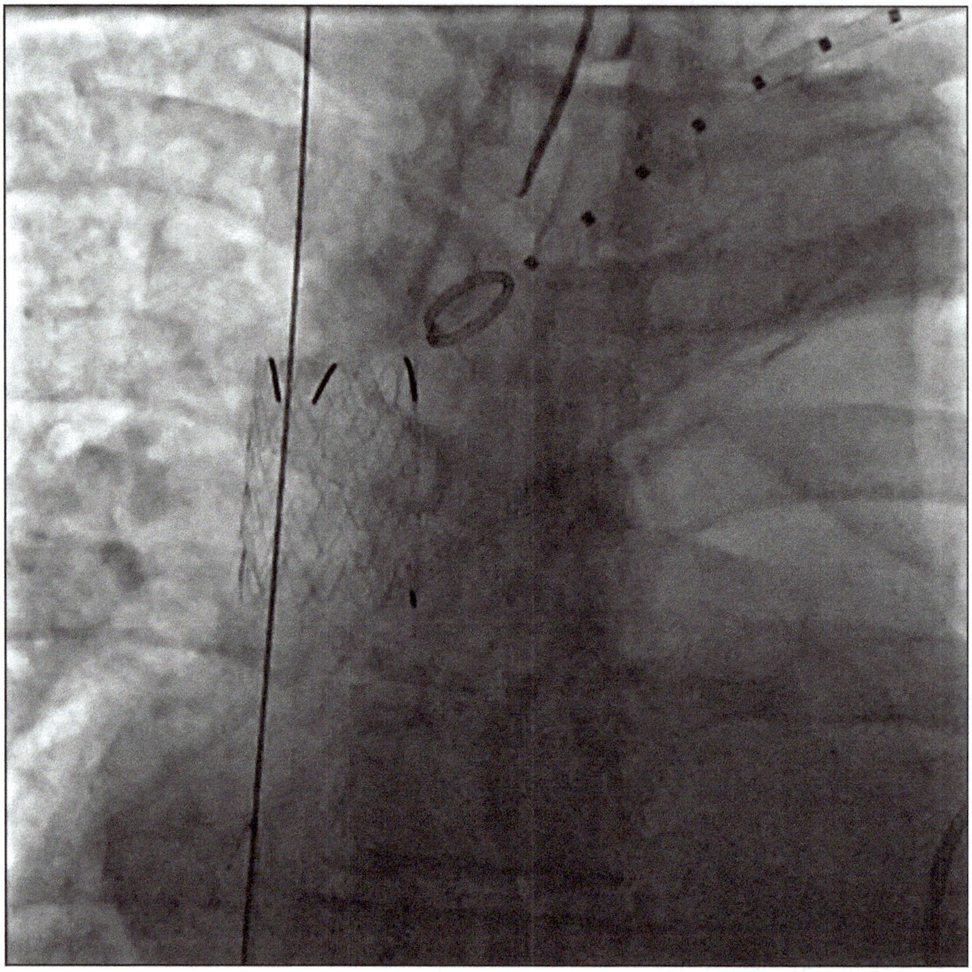

Figure 15.2 Covered stent is placed at lower SVC and RA junction.

POSTPROCEDURAL COURSE

The patient remained to be intubated and transferred to the CICU. The patient continued to require hemodynamic support for advanced heart failure and septic shock in the intensive care unit. After much deliberation, the family decided to withdraw life support according to the patient's prior wishes.

AUTOPSY

The patient underwent an autopsy, which revealed nonischemic dilated cardiomyopathy and severe cardiac hypertrophy. The heart weighs 1,191 grams (approximate expected, mean 367 g). Marked endocardial fibrosis of the LV was associated with multifocal organized and recent mural thrombus (**Figure 15.3**). Clinical history was torn SVC during lead removal, and status post-stent-graft placement in SVC. Focal defect of SVC at the junction with RA was seen, 0.6 × 0.2 cm, with surrounding soft-tissue hemorrhage (**Figure 15.4**).

Cause of death was mixed cardiogenic and septic shock related to ICD infection and nonischemic cardiomyopathy. Manner of death: natural.

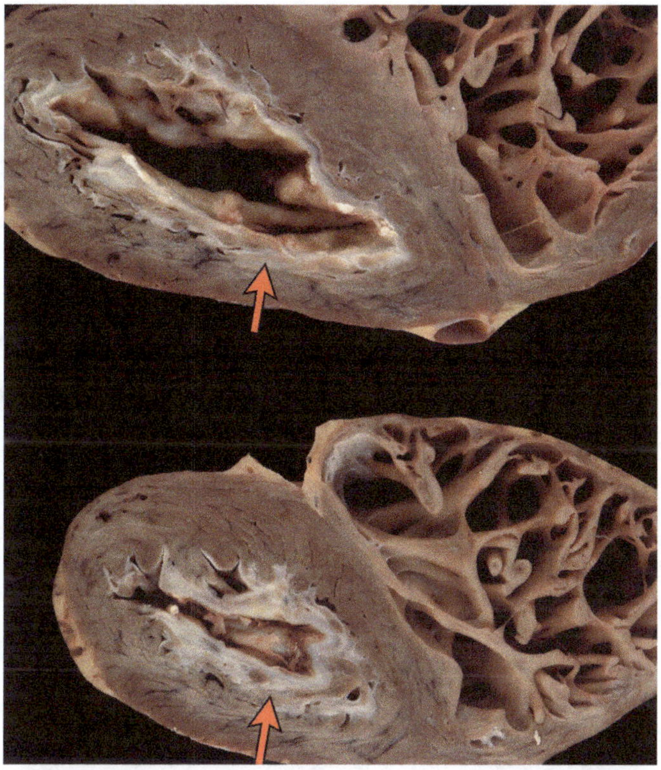

Figure 15.3 Autopsy shows organized thrombus and fibrosis at left ventricular apex (**red arrows**).

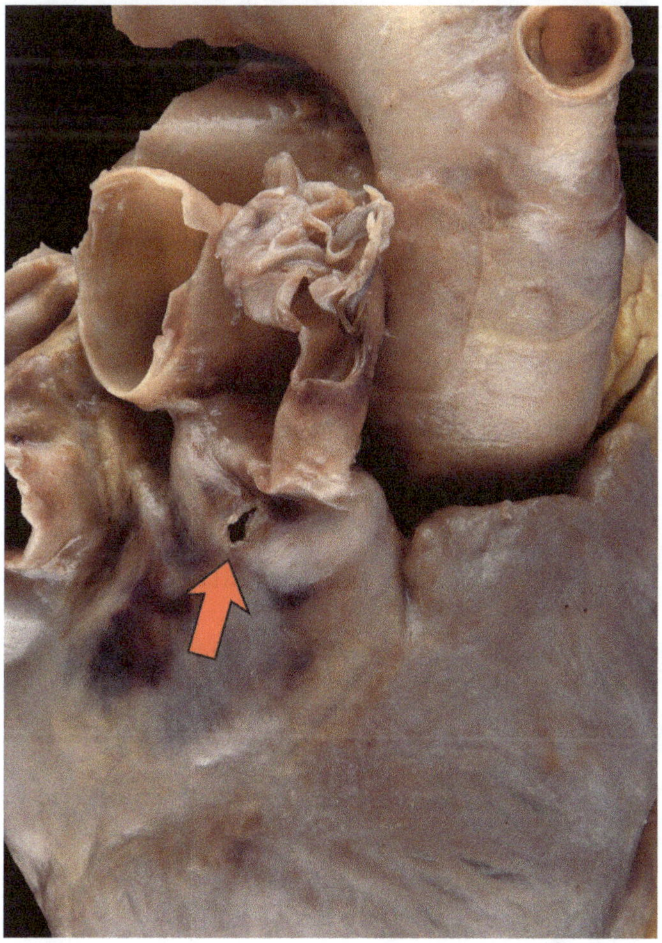

Figure 15.4 Autopsy shows stented SVC tear opening (**red arrow**) and surrounding soft tissue hemorrhage.

SUMMARY POINTS

Potential risk factors for SVC tear and how to prevent it:

- SVC intimal dissection during lead placement.
- Lead is against and fibrosed on the SVC wall.
- During lead extraction, consider mechanical (non-laser) sheath first.
- Sheath and lead French size mismatch, giving rise to a gap between the sheath and the lead.

SVC tear managment:

- Transcatheter covered stent placement. This is nonsurgical approach, a good alternative to sternotomy.
- Consult with vascular surgery or interventional radiology for stent placement.
- Open chest repair is challenging in patients with previous sternotomy. Patient may not be a candidate for redo sternotomy, such as in this case.
- Cardiovascular surgery standby is critical.

REFERENCES

1. Kusumoto FM, Schoenfeld MH, Wilkoff BL, et al. 2017 HRS expert consensus statement on cardiovascular implantable electronic device lead management and extraction. *Heart Rhythm.* 2017 Dec;14(12):e503–e551.
2. Kancharla K, Acker NG, Li Z, et al. Efficacy and safety of transvenous lead extraction in the device laboratory and operating room guided by a novel risk stratification scheme. *JACC Clin Electrophysiol.* 2019 Feb;5(2):174–182.

VIDEO LEGENDS

Video 15.1 TEE report large mobile echo-density (2.1 × 1.6 cm) consistent with vegetation prolapses into the right atrium and appears to be attached to the ICD lead. [00:04]

Video 15.2 14-Fr Excimer laser sheath is advancing over the RA lead at subclavian vein region. [00:06]

Video 15.3 14-Fr Excimer laser sheath is advancing over the RA lead at SVC. [00:05]

Video 15.4 14-Fr Excimer laser sheath is advancing over the RA lead at SVC and RA region. Outer sheath is supporting the laser sheath, which is in alignment to the lead. [00:37]

Video 15.5 14-Fr Excimer laser sheath is advancing over the LV lead at subclavian vein region. [00:05]

Video 15.6 The laser sheath is at SVC and LV lead is removed by pulling back without laser energy application at this point. [00:05]

Video 15.7 Pericardial effusion was present. Note organized and calcified apical thrombus in the left ventricle. [00:02]

Video 15.8 Pericardial effusion. During pericardiocentesis, agitated saline is injected to confirm the needle in the pericardial space (red arrow). Note left ventricular systolic function is severely reduced. [00:02]

Video 15.9 Contrast injection through the pigtail catheter, which is located at innominate vein (A) and SVC [00:06]. (B) shows that contrast flows into right atrium without apparent extravasation into the pericardium. [00:05]

Video 15.10 SVC Bridge Occlusion Balloon inflation to control the bleeding after all leads are removed. [00:01]

16 | Tools and Techniques for the Extraction of Leadless Pacemakers

Gurukripa N. Kowlgi, MBBS; Paul A. Friedman, MD

INTRODUCTION

Leadless pacemakers have created a revolution in cardiac pacing, improving the ease of implant, and minimizing conventional lead-related complications.[1] Presently, the Micra transcatheter pacing system (TPS; Medtronic) is the only commercially available leadless pacemaker in the United States. Over 2800 patients have undergone successful implantation of the Micra TPS in clinical trials.[2] The multicenter Micra Investigational Device Exemption (IDE) trial reported a successful implant in over 99% of patients and a 4% complication rate at 1 year.[3]

The manufacturer recommends turning off and abandoning leadless pacemakers that are malfunctioning or at the end of their usable life. However, conditions such as infection, device-induced pericarditis, and device dislodgement may mandate extraction. While leadless pacemaker revisions during implants are not infrequent, there is a paucity of data on the delayed retrieval of the Micra TPS (at least 1 day after implant).[4,5] In this chapter, with the help of case examples, we will describe the various tools and techniques available to extract the Micra TPS successfully.

CLINICAL VIGNETTE #1

A 77-year-old male with persistent atrial fibrillation with slow ventricular response on anticoagulation with rivaroxaban, history of a first-degree atrioventricular (AV) block, Mobitz type I AV block, hypertension, and benign prostatic hypertrophy was evaluated in the heart rhythm clinic. The symptoms reported by the patient included lightheadedness and occasional shortness of breath. It was ascertained that the symptoms were predominantly due to slow heart rates, which were as low as 34 beats/minute during awake hours. After a discussion, the patient opted to undergo a leadless pacemaker implant. The patient underwent a Micra TPS implant in the right ventricular apical septum that was uneventful. Postprocedure, he complained of sharp chest pain that was worse with inspiration and lying down. The symptoms worsened overnight, and a transthoracic echocardiogram (TTE) revealed a small to moderate pericardial effusion, with no evidence of tamponade physiology (**Video 16.1**). The device was located at the right ventricular (RV) apex, and no tines were visibly protruding into the pericardial space. The patient had persistent symptoms despite an anti-inflammatory regimen consisting of colchicine and nonsteroidal anti-inflammatory drugs. The treatment team and the patient engaged in shared-decision making and mutually decided to extract the leadless pacemaker and reimplant a new leadless pacemaker higher on the septum.

CASE 16

PREPROCEDURAL PLANNING

Serial echocardiograms were obtained to ensure that the pericardial effusion was stable. Anticoagulation was suspended. Blood type and cross-match were performed. Informed consent was obtained, and the patient was brought to the pacing lab. Two large-bore peripheral intravenous accesses were established. A wide epicardial chest preparation was performed, and bilateral femoral sites and right neck were cleaned and prepared. A standard preprocedural time-out was performed. Antibiotics were administered.

 Cardiotext Publishing. ISBN: 978-1-942909-54-5

PROCEDURAL DETAILS

A radial arterial line was established for invasive blood pressure monitoring. Bilateral femoral venous sites were accessed after lidocaine infiltration in the skin and subcutaneous tissue. An intracardiac echocardiogram (ICE) catheter was inserted into the heart via the left common femoral vein. We used lidocaine to anesthetize the subxiphoid region and obtained pericardial access with a 17-G Tuohy needle (Epimed Inc.) using left lateral fluoroscopy and gentle contrast injections. We advanced a guidewire into the pericardial space, and through that, placed a 65-cm pigtail drain. Subsequently, 160 cc of blood was aspirated, and the drain was left in the place for the remainder of the procedure.

Subsequently, we placed a stiff wire into the superior vena cava (SVC) through the right common femoral venous access. We performed serial dilations and eventually advanced the Micra delivery system into the right atrium (RA). We placed a 16-Fr Cook sheath inside the Micra TPS delivery sheath to prevent back bleeding due to a lumen diameter step-down. Through this sheath, we passed a large-curve steerable 8.5-Fr Agilis sheath (Abbott Vascular Devices Inc.) across the tricuspid valve (**Figure 16.1**, Panel A).

A 25-mm Amplatz Goose Neck snare (Medtronic) was advanced through the steerable sheath into the RV and was maneuvered using biplane fluoroscopy and ICE. The snare was used to grasp the proximal retrieval knob of the Micra leadless pacemaker (Figure 16.1, Panels B and C and **Video 16.2**). Gentle, steady traction was applied to free the tines from the myocardium with back support from the steerable sheath. Once the device was free, it was withdrawn slowly into the Micra TPS delivery sheath. The steerable sheath and the Goose Neck snare, and the Micra leadless pacemaker were removed as a unit. ICE imaging was utilized to ensure no increase in pericardial effusion. The delivery sheath was used to implant a fresh Micra leadless pacemaker into the RV apical septum (**Video 16.3**A and B). The total procedure time was 90 minutes, and the fluoroscopy time was 20.1 minutes.

POSTPROCEDURAL CARE

The patient was transferred to the cardiac intensive care unit. He remained asymptomatic and hemodynamically stable. Postprocedure echocardiogram showed resolving pericardial effusion. The patient was discharged the day after the procedure. He continued to do well with stable device parameters at the 3-month follow-up.

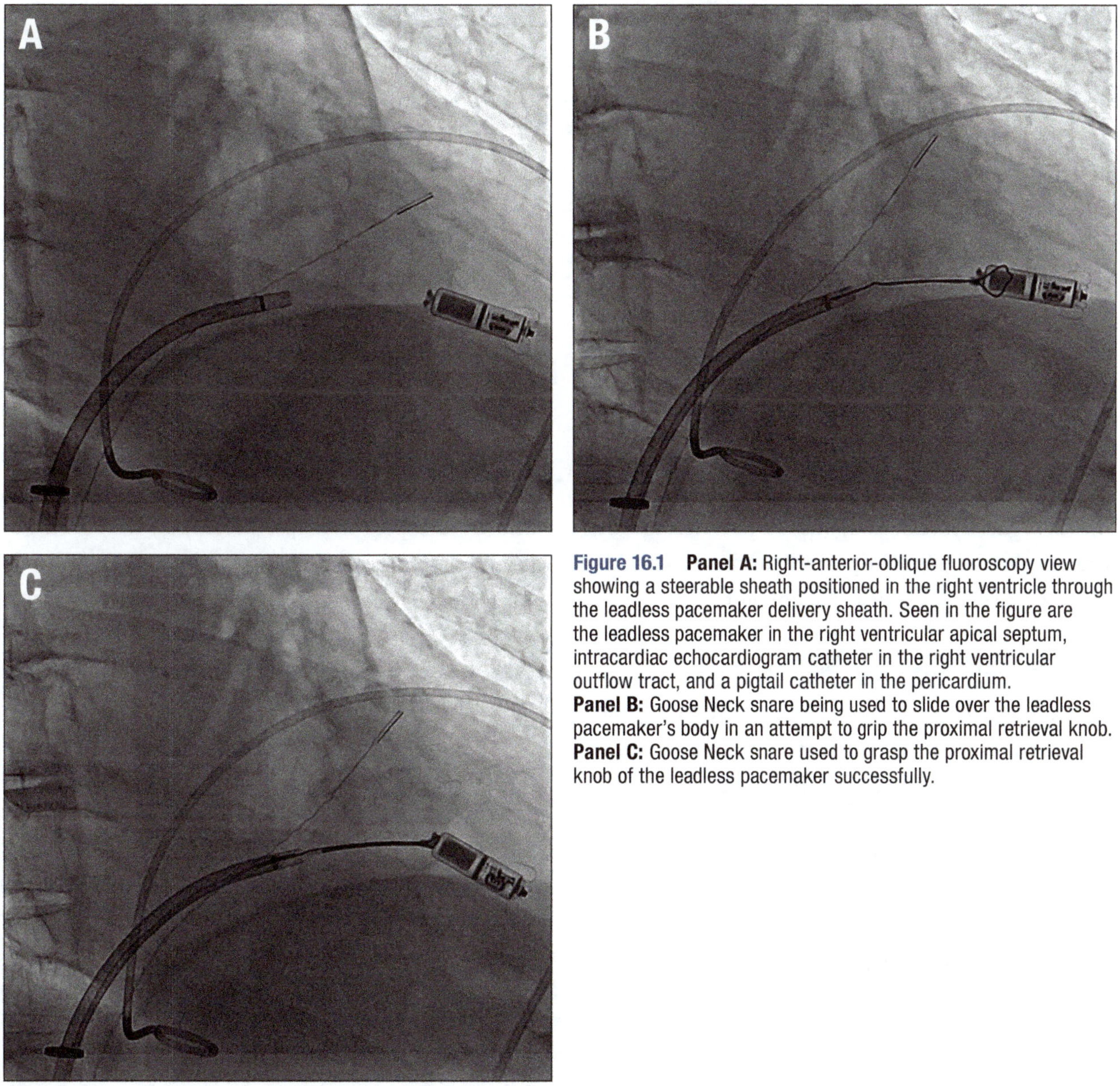

Figure 16.1 **Panel A:** Right-anterior-oblique fluoroscopy view showing a steerable sheath positioned in the right ventricle through the leadless pacemaker delivery sheath. Seen in the figure are the leadless pacemaker in the right ventricular apical septum, intracardiac echocardiogram catheter in the right ventricular outflow tract, and a pigtail catheter in the pericardium.
Panel B: Goose Neck snare being used to slide over the leadless pacemaker's body in an attempt to grip the proximal retrieval knob.
Panel C: Goose Neck snare used to grasp the proximal retrieval knob of the leadless pacemaker successfully.

SUMMARY POINTS

- The Micra TPS was extracted due to acute pericarditis and pericardial effusion likely from RV apical microperforation. The subsequent reimplantation was performed higher (more proximal) on the apical septum.
- The Micra TPS delivery sheath was used along with a steerable sheath and a Goose Neck snare. Extraction was facilitated by the recent implant date and relatively apical position so that the proximal aspect of the Micra was readily accessible without valvular interference.
- Prophylactic pericardial access is an infrequently used but useful adjunct when concern regarding effusion enlargement exists.

CLINICAL VIGNETTE #2

A 61-year-old male with a history of rheumatic heart disease and type 2 diabetes mellitus was admitted for acute endocarditis secondary to methicillin-resistant *Staphylococcus aureus*. His medical status includes mechanical mitral and aortic valve replacements, single-vessel saphenous vein bypass graft to the first obtuse marginal artery for coronary artery disease, atrial fibrillation with 2 prior ablations, and AV node ablation with placement of a Micra leadless pacemaker. His hospital course was complicated with sepsis, thrombocytopenia, and acute kidney injury. In the setting of severe sepsis with multi-organ dysfunction, shared decision making was conducted with the patient, and it was decided to extract to the leadless pacemaker.

PREPROCEDURAL PLANNING

A transesophageal echocardiogram (TEE) was obtained, which demonstrated normal left ventricular ejection fraction. There was evidence of mitral prosthetic valve endocarditis (**Video 16.4**A and B). Informed consent was obtained, and the patient was brought to our pacing lab. Two large-bore peripheral intravenous accesses were established. Bilateral femoral sites and right neck were cleaned and prepared. A standard preprocedural time-out was performed. Antibiotics were administered.

PROCEDURAL DETAILS

The setup, including vascular access and sheath use, was similar to the prior case. As the patient was pacemaker-dependent, we advanced a 5-Fr RV quadripolar catheter (Boston Scientific) into the RV apex for backup pacing. ICE catheter was used for visualization. The 27-Fr Micra delivery sheath, 16-Fr Cook workstations, and an 8.5-Fr Agilis large-curve steerable sheath (Abbott Vascular Devices Inc.) were placed in the heart as described previously. We used the 25-mm Amplatz Goose Neck snare (Medtronic) and attempted to grasp the proximal retrieval knob of the Micra leadless pacemaker (**Video 16.5**A and B). Despite multiple attempts, we could not get the snare to latch on to the retrieval knob. Instead, we were able to get the snare securely around the mid-body of the Micra leadless pacemaker. Gentle, steady traction was applied to free the tines from the myocardium with back support from the steerable sheath. Once the device was free, it was withdrawn slowly towards the Micra delivery sheath. At this point, we could not pull the device into the Micra sheath because it was not co-axial due to the site of our grip (**Figure 16.2**). We attempted to use an 8-Fr steerable standard curve Blazer II XP (Boston Scientific) from the right femoral vein to straighten the Micra leadless pacemaker, but the effort was unsuccessful (**Video 16.6**A and B). Subsequently, we obtained access from the right internal jugular vein. Through this access, we advanced a 25-mm Goose Neck snare from the top and were able to grasp the retrieval knob (**Video 16.7**A). This action allowed the device to become more co-axial with the Micra TPS sheath (see Video 16.7B).

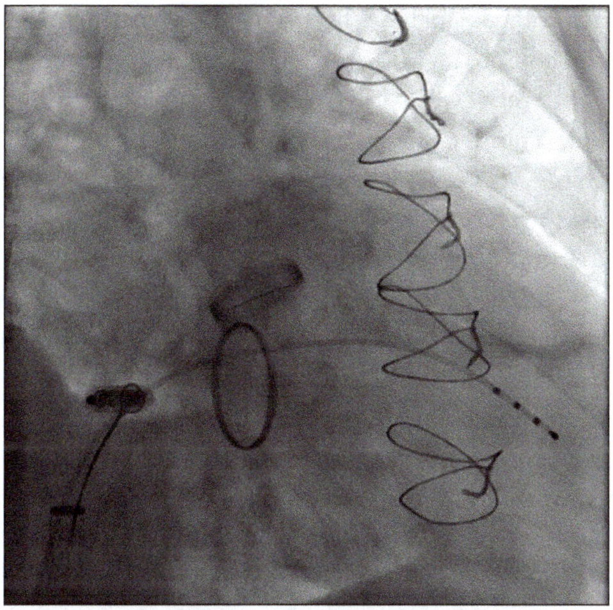

Figure 16.2 Right-anterior-oblique fluoroscopy view showing the leadless pacemaker being held by the Goose Neck snare at the body and not the proximal retrieval knob. With this orientation, the device is not co-axial with the delivery sheath and cannot be pulled into it.

The steerable sheath, the Goose Neck snare, and the Micra leadless pacemaker were removed as a unit. ICE imaging was utilized to ensure no pericardial effusion. A permanent-temporary RV pacemaker was implanted. The total procedure time was 118 minutes, and the fluoroscopy time was 28 minutes.

POSTPROCEDURAL CARE

The patient was transferred to the cardiac surgical intensive care unit. He remained hemodynamically stable. The blood cultures cleared up over the following checks. After a multidisciplinary team discussion, it was decided to hold off on the high-risk mitral valve replacement. The patient was treated with a range of broad-spectrum antibiotics. After an inpatient course of almost a month, the patient recovered to baseline. He had a transvenous dual-chamber pacemaker implanted prior to discharge.

SUMMARY POINTS

- Micra TPS was extracted due to acute endocarditis and bacteremia that persisted despite antibiotic therapy. In many cases of bacteremia, leadless pacemaker extraction is not required.
- The Micra delivery sheath was used along with a steerable sheath and a Goose Neck snare. Micra capture in the ventricle may be challenging due to interference from the subvalvular apparatus, valve leaflets, fibrous capsule, or limitations with reach.
- Multiple vascular access sites permit the deployment of several tools simultaneously to manage the device and avoid embolization.

DISCUSSION

Indications for Retrieval

After the advent of leadless pacemaker systems, it was envisioned that the device would get encapsulated at the end of its usable life and hence be abandoned, with a new one implanted adjacent to it.[6,7] The typical longevity of Micra TPS is about 10 to 12 years. Since it has only been about 5 years for Micra TPS implants, retrievals in the current era are pursued for alternate reasons. These include elevated pacing thresholds, device dislodgement, upgrade to an implantable cardioverter-defibrillator/cardiac resynchronization therapy, or device infection.[5] Over the next few years, the incidence of Micra TPS extractions is predicted to escalate significantly.[8]

Preprocedural Imaging

A plain radiograph should be obtained before any leadless pacemaker explant. For suspected infection, echocardiography (TTE and/or TEE, including 3D echocardiography when available) will add crucial information regarding other structures involved. If the device were implanted many years ago, an echocardiogram might help determine whether the device is encapsulated or not. Furthermore, it can help confirm the thickness of the RV wall, the presence of pericardial effusion, and ease of access to the pacemaker due to surrounding anatomic structures and distance from the tricuspid valve. A contrast-enhanced computed tomography scan may add value in cases where dislodgement or protrusion of the tines is suspected.

Extraction Approaches

There are 2 described techniques for the extraction of the Micra leadless pacemaker (**Figure 16.3**).[5,8] In one approach, the Micra TPS sheath can be used along with the delivery catheter. In this approach, up to 10-mm snares can be backloaded into the central lumen. The snare can then be used to capture the retrieval knob. This technique's advantages include better countertraction with the cup of the Micra delivery catheter and convenient retrieval of the device into the sheath and out. The disadvantage is the catheter's unidirectional curve, which may make it challenging to grasp the retrieval knob as it moves with the cardiac motion in space.

The second approach involves using a steerable sheath within the Micra delivery sheath, as described in our cases. The advantages include better maneuverability and the potential to use larger-diameter snares. Due to the step down from the Micra sheath 24-Fr lumen to the 8.5-Fr Agilis large-curve steerable sheath (Abbott Vascular Devices Inc.), there could be back bleeding. To mitigate this, a short 16-Fr Cook sheath can be used. Once the device is freed from the RV myocardium and pulled into the Micra TPS sheath, caution must be observed to remove the unit as a whole. Because the Micra TPS has a larger diameter than the Agilis inner lumen, the device will not fit inside the steerable sheath. Cases have been described where the Micra leadless pacemaker has been dislodged while pulling it out of the delivery sheath's hemostatic valve.[5] Intraprocedural ICE can be a useful guide when the device is difficult to snare, and more importantly, to continuously monitor for potential complications.

Complications

Operators must be aware of the potential complications of leadless pacemaker extraction. There is a possibility of bleeding, hematoma, pseudoaneurysm, arteriovenous fistula, or venous thrombosis with large-bore access.[9] Ultrasound guidance should be used to obtain access over the common femoral vein and minimize complications.[10] Other complications include acute pericarditis, myocardial perforation, mechanical damage to the tricuspid valve apparatus, device dislodgement, and pulmonary embolism. A surgical backup must be considered for complex cases, especially when the

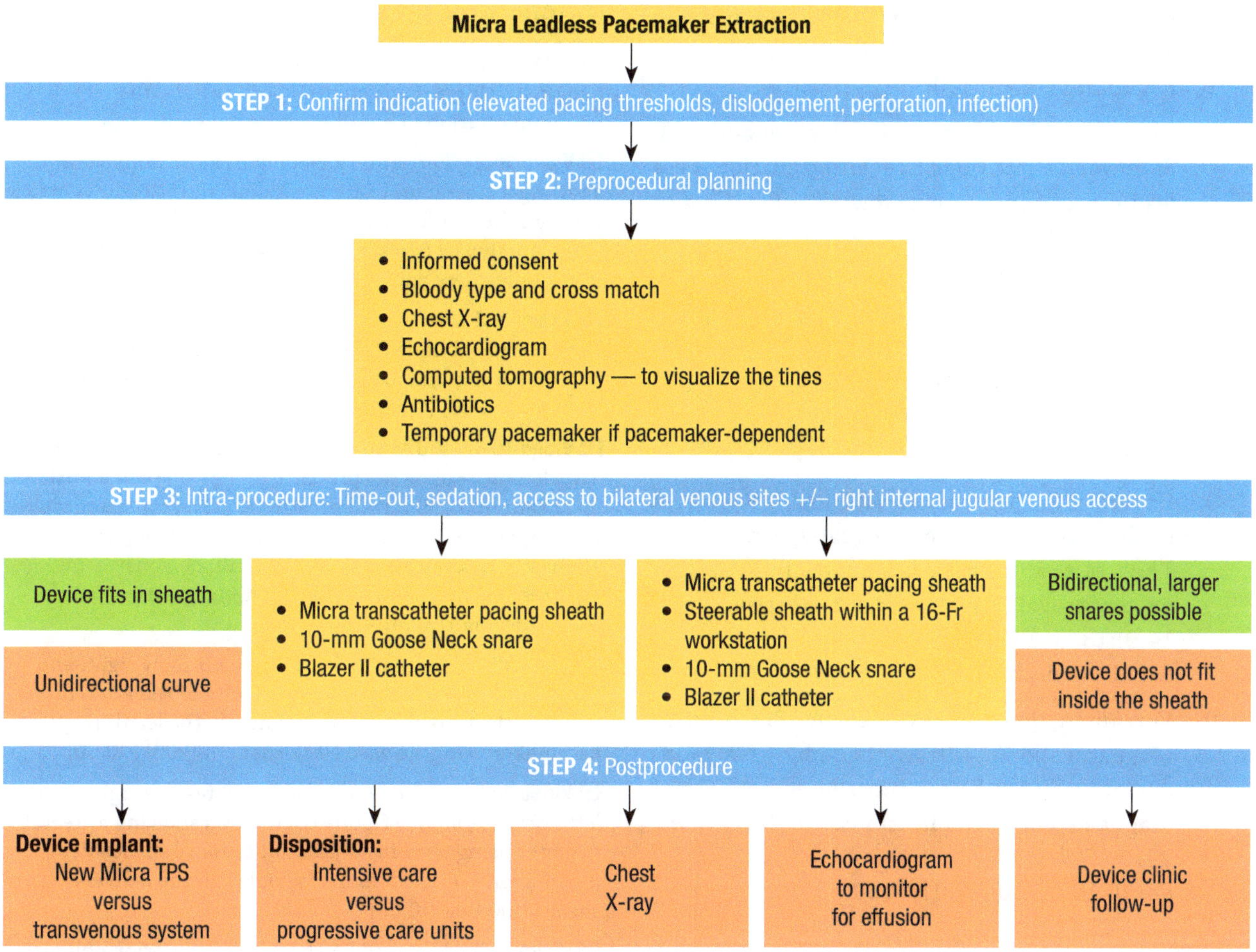

Figure 16.3 A flowchart summarizing the steps and approaches of leadless pacemaker extraction. *Abbreviation*: TPS, transcatheter pacing system.

tines are visualized in the pericardial space during preprocedure evaluation.

REFERENCES

1. Reddy VY, Exner D V., Cantillon DJ, et al. Percutaneous implantation of an entirely intracardiac leadless pacemaker. *N Engl J Med*. 2015;373(12):1125–1135. doi:10.1056/NEJMoa1507192
2. Garg A, Koneru JN, Fagan DH, et al. Morbidity and mortality in patients precluded for transvenous pacemaker implantation: Experience with a leadless pacemaker. *Heart Rhythm*. 2020;17(12): 2056–2063. doi:10.1016/j.hrthm.2020.07.035
3. Reynolds D, Duray GZ, Omar R, et al. A leadless intracardiac transcatheter pacing system. *N Engl J Med*. 2016;374(6):533–541. doi:10.1056/NEJMoa1511643
4. Grubman E, Ritter P, Ellis CR, et al. To retrieve, or not to retrieve: System revisions with the Micra transcatheter pacemaker. *Heart Rhythm*. 2017;14(12):1801–1806. doi:10.1016/j.hrthm.2017.07.015
5. Afzal MR, Daoud EG, Cunnane R, et al. Techniques for successful early retrieval of the Micra transcatheter pacing system: A worldwide experience. *Heart Rhythm*. 2018;15(6):841–846. doi:10.1016/j.hrthm.2018.02.008
6. Vamos M, Erath JW, Benz AP, Bari Z, Duray GZ, Hohnloser SH. Incidence of cardiac perforation with conventional and with leadless pacemaker

systems: A systematic review and meta-analysis. *J Cardiovasc Electrophysiol*. 2017;28(3):336–346. doi:10.1111/jce.13140

7. Kypta A, Blessberger H, Lichtenauer M, Steinwender C. Complete encapsulation of a leadless cardiac pacemaker. *Clin Res Cardiol*. 2016; 105(1):94. doi:10.1007/s00392-015-0929-x
8. González Villegas E, Al Razzo O, Silvestre García J, Mesa García J. Leadless pacemaker extraction from a single-center perspective. *Pacing Clin Electrophysiol*. 2018;41(2):101–105. doi:10.1111/pace.13242
9. Roberts PR, Clementy N, Al Samadi F, et al. A leadless pacemaker in the real-world setting: The Micra transcatheter pacing system post-approval registry. *Heart Rhythm*. 2017; 14(9):1375–1379. doi:10.1016/j.hrthm.2017.05.017
10. Vezzani A, Manca T, Vercelli A, Braghieri A, Magnacavallo A. Ultrasonography as a guide during vascular access procedures and in the diagnosis of complications. *J Ultrasound*. 2013;16(4):161–170. doi:10.1007/s40477-013-0046-5

VIDEO LEGENDS

Video 16.1 Apical 4-chamber view of a TTE demonstrating circumferential pericardial effusion postimplantation of a leadless pacemaker. [00:08]

Video 16.2 Left-anterior-oblique fluoroscopy view showing a steerable sheath positioned in the right ventricle through the leadless pacemaker delivery sheath. The orthogonal view helps in directing the Goose Neck snare over the leadless pacemaker. [00:07]

Video 16.3 Videos 16.3 A and 16.3B feature right and left anterior-oblique fluoroscopic views of the new leadless pacemaker implanted in the right ventricular apical septum. [00:06] [00:06]

Video 16.4 Video 16.4A shows 4-chamber view of a TEE demonstrating the presence of a mobile echodensity on the mechanical mitral prosthetic valve, consistent with vegetation in the clinical scenario. [00:06] Video 16.4B shows a short-axis view of a TEE demonstrating the presence of a mobile echodensity (vegetation) on the mechanical mitral prosthetic valve. [00:06]

Video 16.5 Videos 16.5 A and 16.5 B show right, and left anterior-oblique fluoroscopic views of the attempt to grasp the proximal retrieval knob of the leadless pacemaker using a Goose Neck snare. [00:06] [00:06]

Video 16.6 Video 16.6A and 16.6B feature right, and left anterior-oblique fluoroscopic views showing a steerable catheter being used in an attempt to move the leadless pacemaker to make it more coaxial with the delivery sheath. [00:06] [00:06]

Video 16.7 Video 16.7A shows a left-anterior-oblique view showing the use of a Goose Neck snare from access obtained in the right internal jugular vein to help make the leadless pacemaker more co-axial with the sheath. [00:06] Video 16.7B shows a right-anterior-oblique fluoroscopic view of the leadless pacemaker being successfully withdrawn into the delivery sheath. [00:06]

17 | Femoral Device Extraction

Siva K. Mulpuru, MD, MPH

CLINICAL VIGNETTE

An 80-year-old male patient presented to the hospital with chronic drainage from the right inguinal region (**Figure 17.1**). He had complete heart block necessitating implantation of a right-sided, pectoral dual-chamber pacemaker in 1995. He developed device site infection in 2011 after pulse generator replacement. The right-sided, dual-chamber pacemaker was extracted, and the patient underwent implantation of a dual-chamber pacemaker from the right inguinal region. The most recent device details are as follows.

Device Details

Device Component	Manufacturer/Model	Date of Implant
Pulse generator	Medtronic Adapta	10/2011
Right atrial lead	Medtronic 5076	
Right ventricular lead	Medtronic 5076	

His other pertinent past medical history included persistent atrial fibrillation, hypertension, depression, and mild cognitive impairment. He presented to the hospital with purulent discharge from the femoral pacemaker site for 4 months. He denied local trauma or redness of skin before the onset of discharge. He denied fever, chills, rigors, although he complained of malaise and more than 5-lb weight loss during the preceding 3 months. Echocardiogram revealed an ejection fraction of 45% with moderate tricuspid regurgitation (TR). His hematology panel and electrolytes were within normal limits. Chest X-ray (CXR) and abdominal X-ray are shown in **Figures 17.2** and **17.3**, respectively. Operative reports from the prior pacemaker extraction and reimplantation procedure could not be obtained due to the previous healthcare facility's closure.

PREPROCEDURAL PLANNING

The patient was evaluated by cardiac surgery, plastic surgery, vascular surgery, and infectious diseases teams before the procedure. After blood cultures were drawn, broad-spectrum antibiotics were initiated. A transesophageal echocardiogram (TEE) before the procedure did not reveal any evidence of valvular vegetations. A careful review of the X-rays revealed 3 leads in the femoral vein with additional lead (ring electrode) in the femoral region (Figure 17.3). A lead tip fragment was noted in the heart separate from the 2 intravascular leads (Figure 17.2). A preprocedure planning CT scan of the chest, abdomen, and pelvis was obtained, looking for vascular lesions, pelvic abscess, and understanding the leads' course. Tight stenosis of the right subclavian vein and complete occlusion of the superior vena cava (SVC) below the azygous vein was noted on the CT scan. Pelvic reactive lymphadenopathy was noted on the abdominal CT scan. In summary, the patient presented with an inguinal pacemaker pocket infection without bloodstream infection.

PROCEDURAL DETAILS

A preprocedure huddle was performed with all teams in attendance. The patient was taken to the hybrid operating room and was prepped from the neck to the groin in a sterile manner. General anesthesia was administered, and a TEE probe was placed for monitoring during the procedure. Four units of blood cross-matched, packed red cells were available in the room for the procedure. He was given intravenous vancomycin 1 hour before the procedure. Venous and arterial accesses were obtained using ultrasound guidance and

 Cardiotext Publishing. ISBN: 978-1-942909-54-5

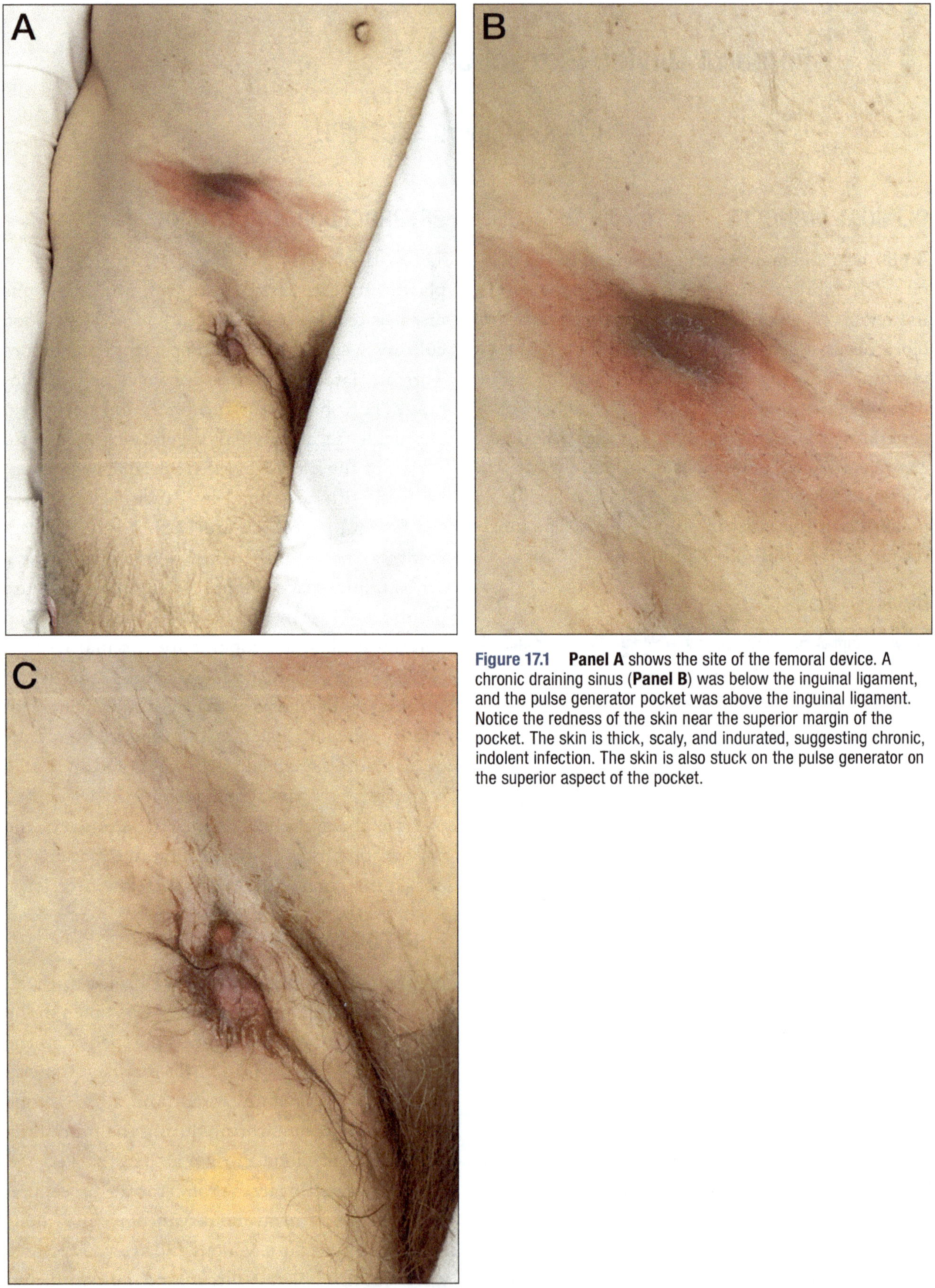

Figure 17.1 **Panel A** shows the site of the femoral device. A chronic draining sinus (**Panel B**) was below the inguinal ligament, and the pulse generator pocket was above the inguinal ligament. Notice the redness of the skin near the superior margin of the pocket. The skin is thick, scaly, and indurated, suggesting chronic, indolent infection. The skin is also stuck on the pulse generator on the superior aspect of the pocket.

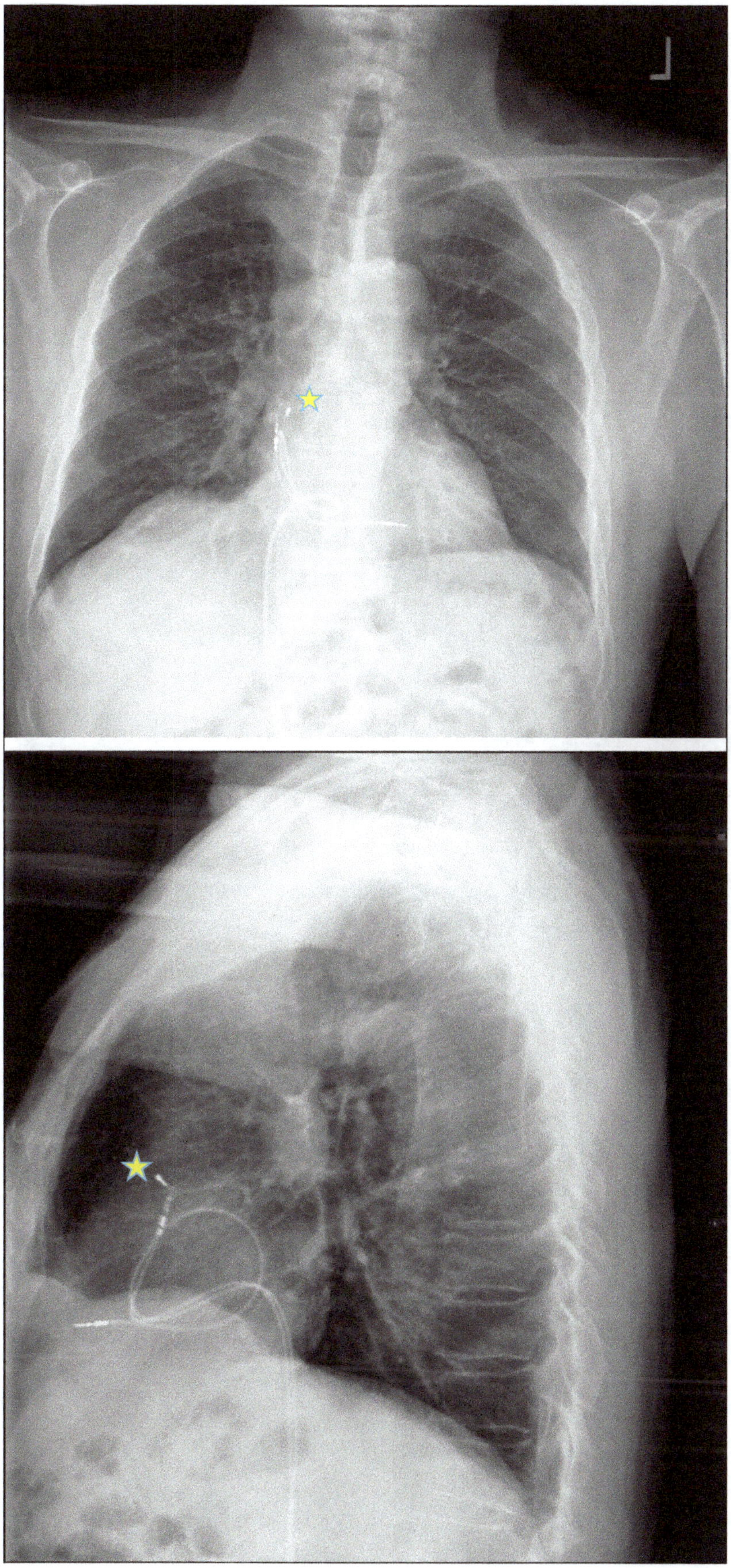

Figure 17.2 Posteroanterior (PA) and lateral views of the patient's CXR. Atrial and ventricular active fixation leads were noted. A separate passive fixation tip electrode was noted in the chest, denoted by a **yellow star**.

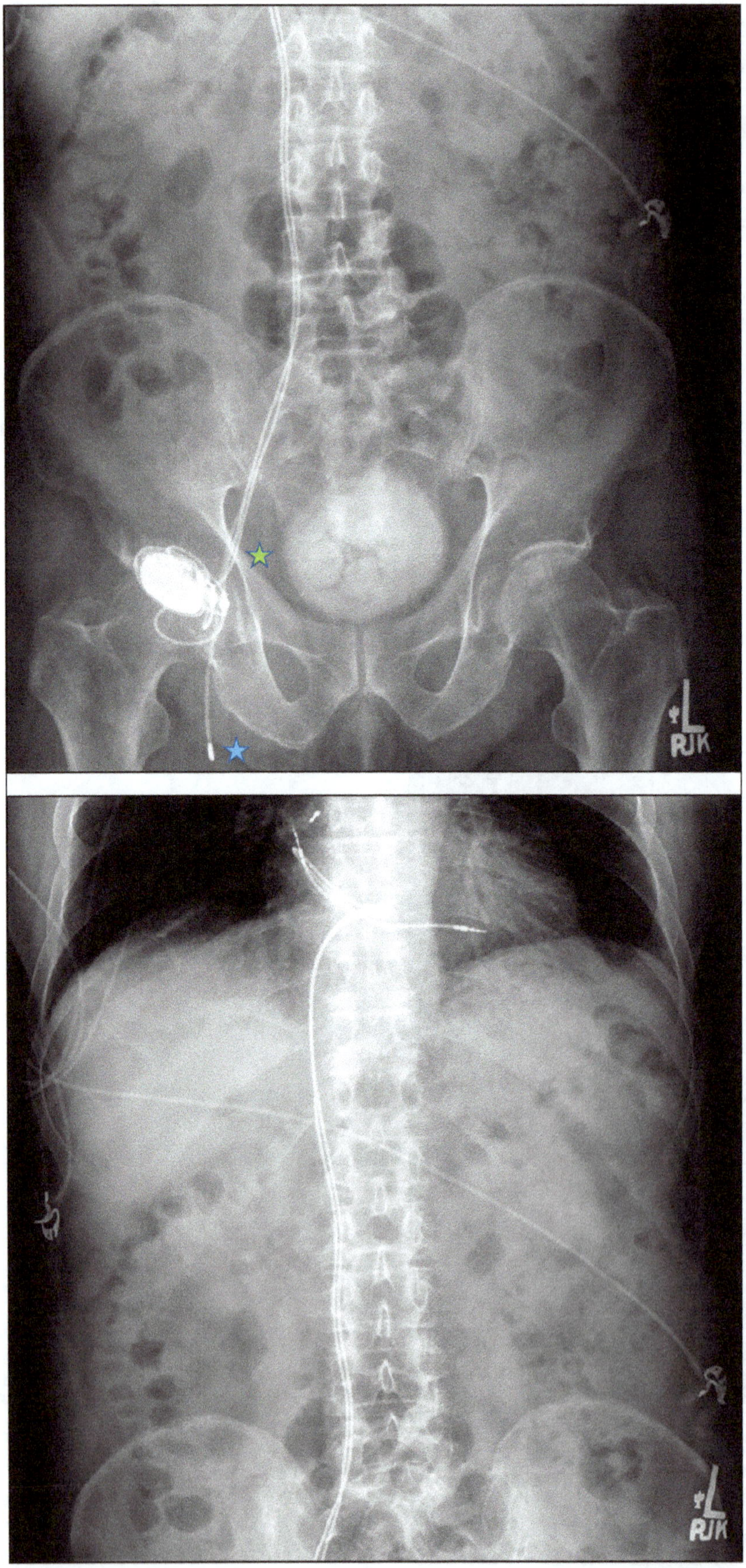

Figure 17.3 Abdominal and pelvic X-rays: Pulse generator was noted to be an inguinal region connected to 2 leads. Three leads in the femoral vein can be appreciated on closer inspection (**green star**). The third lead with ring electrode can be seen at the level of the lesser trochanter.

modified Seldinger's technique. A 9-Fr sheath was placed in the left common femoral vein for high-volume crystalloid or blood product infusion. A 5-Fr sheath was placed in the left femoral artery for hemodynamic monitoring. A 6-Fr sheath was also placed in the left common femoral vein for temporary right ventricular (RV) pacing catheter as the patient was pacemaker dependent without a reliable underlying rhythm. A 9-Fr and 6-Fr sheaths were also placed in the right internal jugular vein for superior vascular access. Selective venography using 5-Fr Terumo Glidecath (Terumo Interventional Systems) showed complete occlusion of the SVC with a prominent azygous vein (**Video 17.1**). The teams felt that reliable superior access is needed for resuscitation in a vascular catastrophe. Using a vein finder (Worley vein selector, Merit Medical) and a medium-support 0.15-inch wire, the occlusion was crossed, and the wire was eventually advanced to the inferior vena cava (IVC; **Video 17.2**). The wire was exchanged for a stiff 0.35-inch wire for adequate support. Venoplasty was performed using a 4- × 40-mm Mustang balloon (Boston Scientific) (**Video 17.3**). An active fixation pacing lead was placed through the right internal access site for stable RV pacing during the case.

The femoral pocket site was then opened, and the leads were disconnected from the pulse generator. The sutures were cut, and the suture sleeves were mobilized. A second incision was made in the region of the chronic draining sinus. Exploration of the site showed the exposed ring electrode of the retained lead fragment. The retained lead was grabbed by the ring electrode and gently pulled out with manual traction. The helices of the active fixation leads could not be retracted even with many turns. The leads were prepared using locking stylets (Lead Locking Device EZ, Philips Medical). Due to the suprainguinal entry of the leads into the vasculature, there were concerns about the need to avoid creating a larger entry site due to the potential for retroperitoneal bleed. A mechanical extraction tool (Tightrail, Philips Medical) without the outer sheath was used to free up the leads from the surrounding adhesions (**Videos 17.4** and **17.5**). A lot of tortuosity was noted around the leads, and the leads were noted to be entangled with one another. Both the leads were freed to the IVC–right atrial (RA) junction using traction-countertraction techniques. The leads could not be pulled back into the mechanical extraction sheath due to entanglement of leads and "snowplowing" of the scar tissue (**Video 17.6**). The mechanical sheath was exchanged for a 14-Fr laser extraction sheath (Glidelight, Philips Medical). The laser sheath's metal tip provided support to advance the sheath over the lead and push the lead back to the RA and disentangle the leads. The lead and snowplowed scar tissue were pulled inside the outer sheath, and the lead was taken out of the body (**Video 17.7**). The second (atrial) lead came after simple manual traction as all the lead-to-lead bindings sites were already broken. After the leads were taken out, the hemodynamics were stable without any evidence of retroperitoneal bleed. The pocket was debrided by vascular surgery, and a vacuum-assisted suction device was applied to the incision site (**Figure 17.4**). All the necrotic tissue at the infrainguinal site was debrided, and the wound was packed with iodoform gauze. The retained lead tip was embedded in the tissue by echocardiography and could not be accessed. A decision was made to abandon the lead fragment. All sheaths were removed from the groin, and the hemostasis was achieved with manual compression. The temporary permanent pacing lead was secured to the skin at the right internal jugular venous access site.

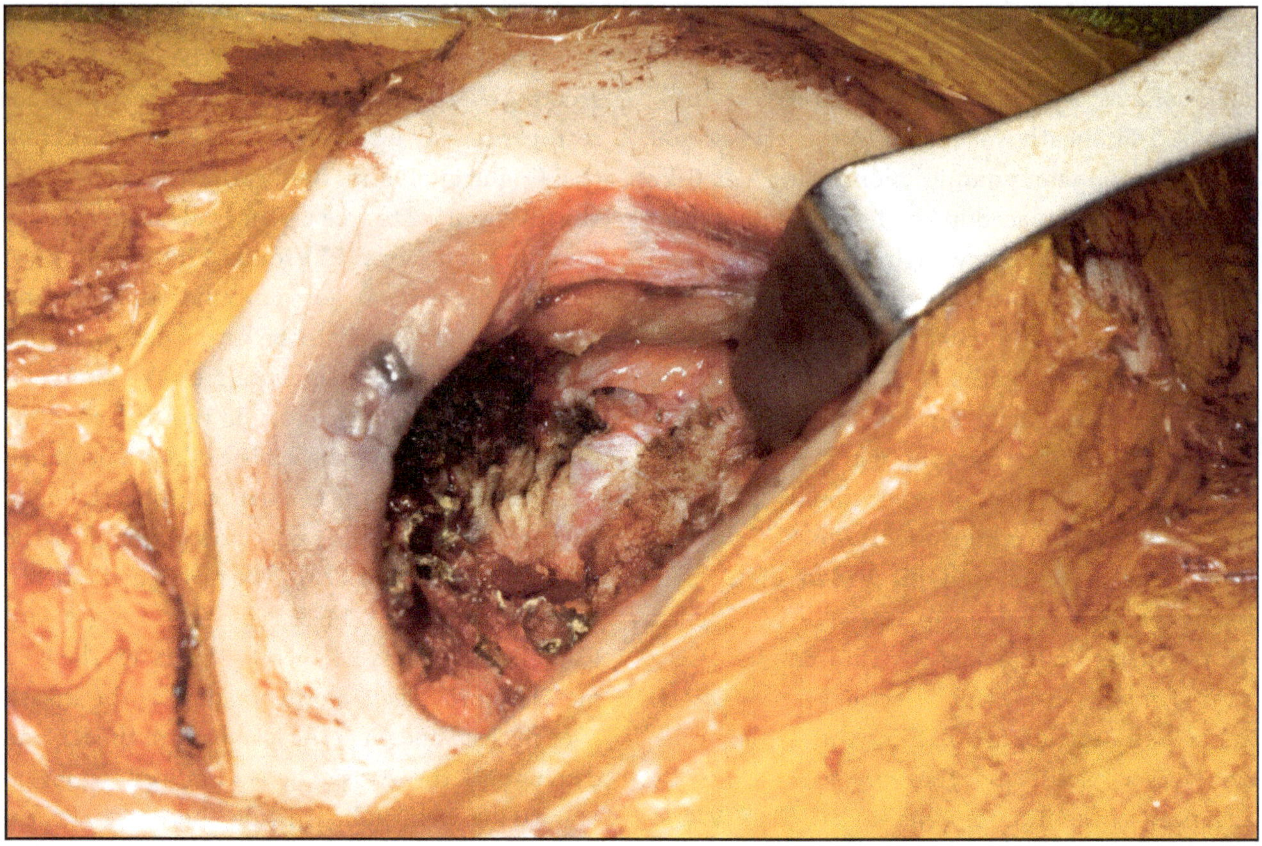

Figure 17.4 Suprainguinal pocket after debridement of the necrotic tissue and excision of the capsule.

POSTPROCEDURAL COURSE

The patient was extubated in the recovery room and was transferred to the floor service. The vacuum-assisted suction device was removed on day 3, and the wounds were allowed to heal by secondary intention (**Figure 17.5**). Blood cultures remained persistently negative. He underwent placement of a leadless cardiac pacemaker (Micra VR, Medtronic) as he was in persistent atrial fibrillation and complete heart block. The temporary permanent pacemaker was removed at the time of the leadless pacemaker implant. His wound culture grew *Actinomyces europaeus* and *Cutibacterium acnes*. Both microbes were sensitive to penicillin, and he completed a 2-week course of amoxicillin/clavulanic acid. He remained infection-free during follow-up.

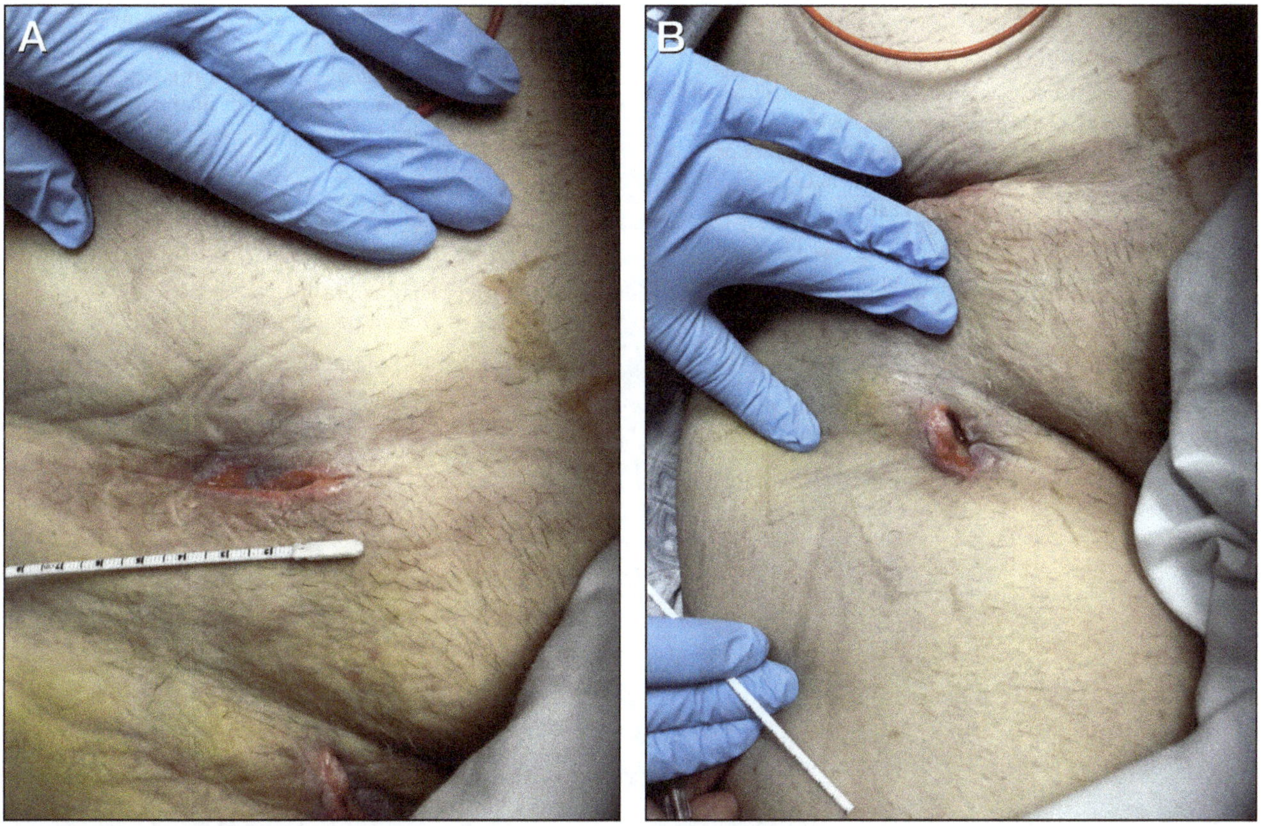

Figure 17.5: **Panel A** (suprainguinal pocket) and **Panel B** (infrainguinal pocket) illustrate wound healing by secondary intention on day 5 after the lead extraction procedure.

SUMMARY POINTS

- Femoral site for device implantation is less favored site especially with the advent of tools and techniques for venoplasty.
- Care should be taken to remove all retained leads at the time of extraction. Retained leads may erode and may develop into chronic draining sinus.
- Venoplasty techniques are utilized to open up chronic venous occlusions to establish superior access for resuscitation and ventricular pacing.
- As the leads enter the vasculature above the inguinal ligament, consider the possibility of retroperitoneal bleed with hemodynamic collapse during the extraction procedure. Superior venous access is essential for resuscitation.
- Lead entanglement with other leads or wires can occur during femoral extraction.
- A combination of mechanical and laser sheaths were used for successful device extraction.
- Extractions sheaths are not long enough to cross the tricuspid valve from the femoral region and to break adhesions on the ventricular leads.

VIDEO LEGENDS

Video 17.1 Selective venography from the catheter confirms complete occlusion of the SVC. Note the massively dilated azygous vein that serves as a conduit to deliver the venous drainage from the superior part of the body to the RV through azygous system that eventually drains to the right atrium through the IVC. [00:07]

Video 17.2 The SVC occlusion was crossed using a vein-finder catheter and a medium support 0.15-inch wire. [00:04]

Video 17.3 After a stiff wire was exchanged with its tip in the IVC, venoplasty was performed to open the SVC occlusion. [00:05]

Video 17.4 Mechanical extraction sheath over one of the pacemaker leads was used to break the adhesions. [00:08]

Video 17.5 As the mechanical sheath was advanced, we can notice the lead rotating in the vasculature. It points to the inadequate engagement of the scar tissue. The mechanical sheath has to be pulled back and advanced coaxially over the lead to engage the adhesion binding sites. [00:04]

Video 17.6 The presence of multiple loops, temporary pacemaker wires, and 0.35-inch wire from the SVC increases the risk of lead entanglement. The mechanical extraction sheath is currently on the ventricular leads, which is looped around the other wires. [00:14]

Video 17.7 A 14-Fr laser sheath (GlideLight, Philips Medical) was advanced over the lead to push it back to the right atrium to disentangle the loops. The lead, along with the inner sheath, was pulled back into the outer sheath. [00:02]

18 | Lead Extraction Through the Femoral Venous Route

Pierce J. Vatterott, MD

INTRODUCTION

The extraction physician takes advantage of the device lead insertion route for lead removal. The cardiac implantable electronic device (CIED) leads track through the right or left subclavian vein, superior vena cava (SVC), and the heart from the insertion site. Leads and the locking stylet deployed together are used as the rail by which extraction tools are advanced. Few extractors routinely use the femoral approach but rather consider the approach a "bailout" when failing with a superior approach. Nothing could be farther from the truth. A robust extraction program includes the routine use of a femoral approach.

In understanding the benefits of femoral extraction, one must first start with extraction goals and understand the tools available to accomplish that goal. Situations where femoral extractions are beneficial are listed in **Table 18.1**. One must understand the tools and their strengths and weakness. Some of those tools are listed in **Table 18.2**. Whether it is snaring for lead stability, snaring a lead end or lead fragment, attempting to remove a lead, or protecting the SVC fully, all require an understanding of the right tool most appropriate for the situation. The greatest benefit of using the femoral snaring approach is stabilizing the extraction rail for extraction tools to be advanced safely and successfully from a superior approach. Such an example is the need to remove a lead for vascular access. Femoral snaring can also be used to stabilize and preserve leads that one does not wish to extract. The image in **Figure 18.1** shows us a commonly used technique involving an ablation catheter and Goose Neck snare. The catheter and snare are advanced from the femoral approach. The ablation catheter is looped over the lead of interest, and then the end of the ablation catheter is snared with the Goose Neck snare. **Video 18.1** is a corresponding case example of a successfully ensnared ICD lead protected against dislodgement while an attached nonfunctioning Select Secure Model 3830 (Medtronic) lead was removed.

Table 18.1 Benefits of the femoral approach

1. Gaining access through an occluded subclavian or innominate vessel. A femoral snared lead is stabilized, allowing an extraction tool's advancement over the lead through the occlusion.
2. Stabilizing a lead with lead-to-lead interaction during extractions. This is helpful when concerns over dislodging leads intended to be preserved.
3. When the superior approach's forces are greater than the tensile strength of the lead, snaring the lead and locking stylet within provides a strong rail for extraction.
4. Inability to advance the extraction tool safely from the superior approach as the extraction rail has failed.
5. Lead is firmly adhered to the SVC.
6. Retrieving lead fragments.
7. When a very large vascular sheath is needed for removal of hardware, attached clot, or vegetations.

CASE 18

Table 18.2 Tools for extraction through the inferior access sites

1. Femoral Workstation or other sheaths a. transcatheter aortic valve replacement sheaths, cryoballoon catheter sheaths, Agilis deflectable sheath (Abbott Medical)
2. Needle's Eye snare (Cook Medical)
3. Goose Neck snare (Medtronic)
4. Steerable ablation catheter in conjunction with a Goose Neck snare
5. EnSnare Basket (Merit Medical)
6. Biopsy tools
7. Cardiac or gastrointestinal Raptor tool (Steris Health Care)
8. Angioplasty guide
9. Angiography catheters

 Cardiotext Publishing. ISBN: 978-1-942909-54-5

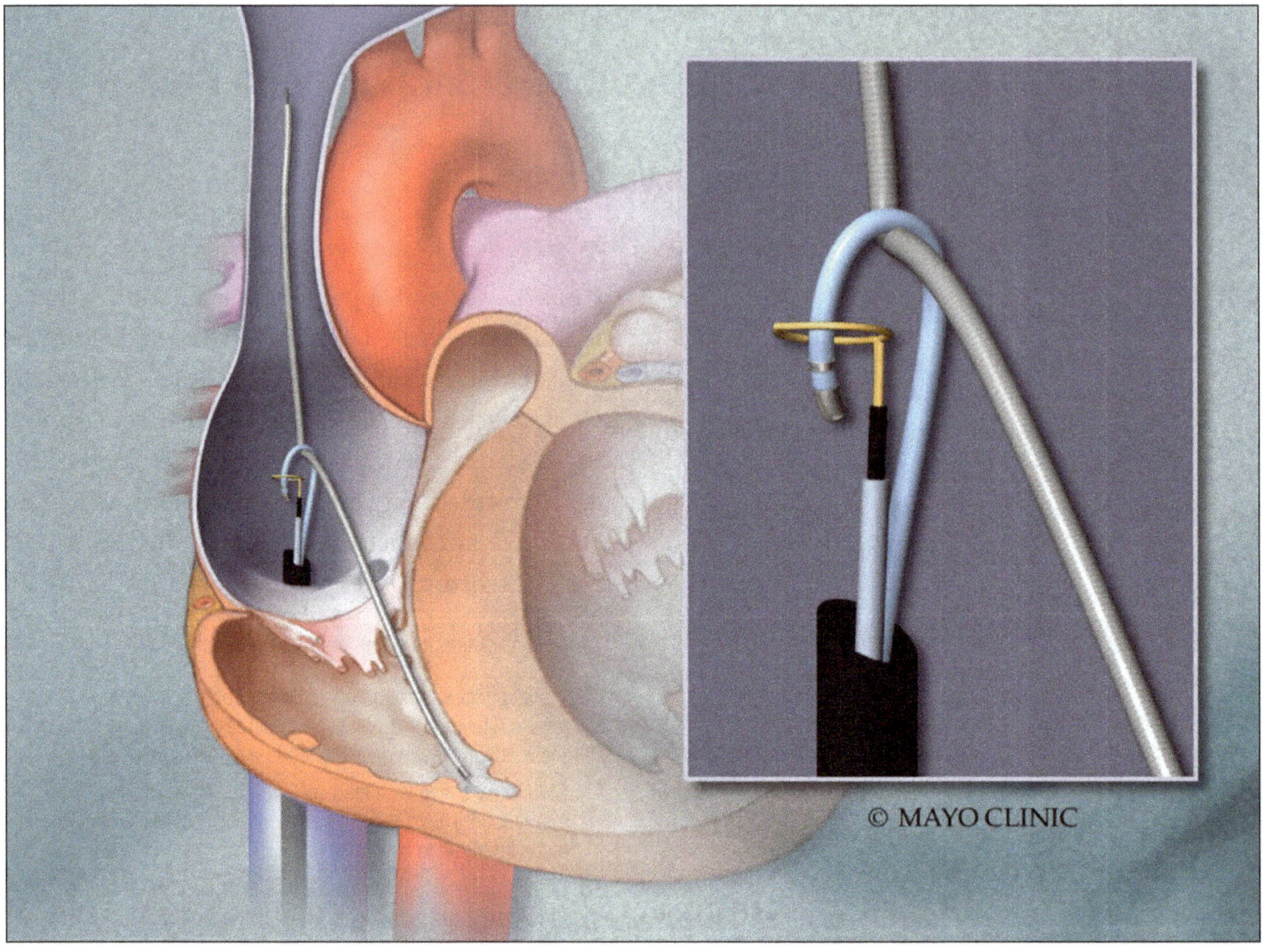

Figure 18.1 Pictorial image of how to use an ablation catheter in conjunction with a Goose Neck snare.

Leads can also be removed from a femoral approach. This allows extraction tools to be in line with leads in the right atrium and the SVC, permitting excellent traction force and a more direct advancement of those tools. This direct approach may be safer for removing leads adhered to the SVC. **Figure 18.2** is taken from a case of a 25-year-old male with an ICD system placed 11 years earlier for hypertrophic cardiomyopathy. Intracardiac echocardiogram (ICE) images demonstrated significant lead adherence to the SVC (**Video 18.2**). A thoracoscope was placed for monitoring the SVC for a possible tear during extraction. **Video 18.3**A and 18.3B illustrate a comparison of traction on the adhered lead from a left subclavian versus femoral approach. A greater localized concentration of traction force is transmitted to the SVC wall from a subclavian versus femoral approach. Finite element modeling was used to quantify the vascular wall stresses in a 3D model (**Video 18.4**). A wall stress model in traction force applied from a simulated subclavian approach resulted in 2–3 times higher maximum vascular stress than the same traction forces from a femoral approach.[1] For leads attached to the wall of the SVC, extracting from a femoral approach may be safer. However, no comparative clinical study has been completed.

A major weakness of the femoral approach is the inability to apply adequate traction and countertraction to remove leads adhered to the right ventricle. The ability to transfer traction force to a lead tip diminishes when the traction force deviates from direct in-line traction. **Figure 18.3** is a pictorial representation of how a minimal amount of traction force is applied to a lead tip when using the femoral approach. One can see how difficult it

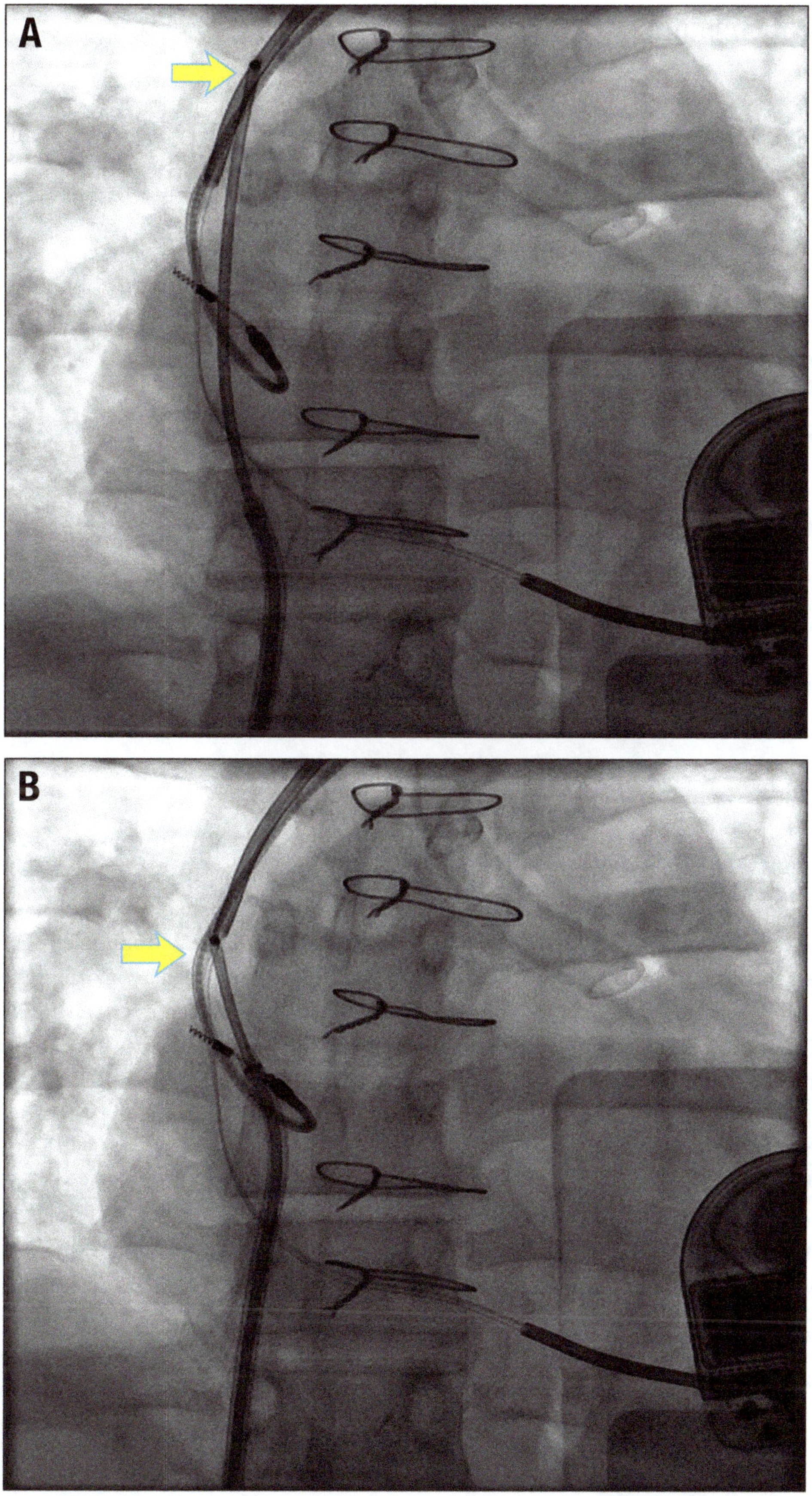

Figure 18.2 Panels A and B: The pulldown of a rotational intracardiac ultrasound catheter (**yellow arrows**) with the corresponding image shown in Video 18.2.

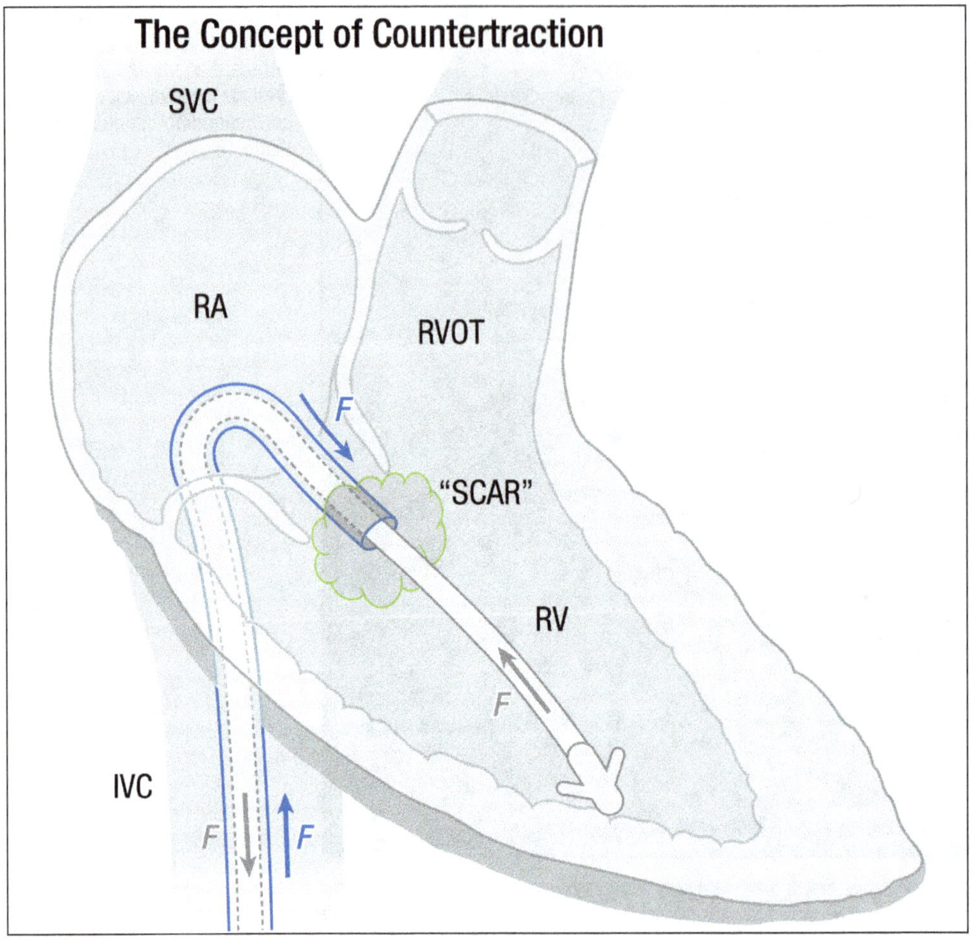

Figure 18.3 Pictorial imaging depicting the loss of traction force (**Gray F**) with deviation from a direct traction line. In addition, countertraction (**Blue F**) with a non-powered sheath can fail to disrupt thickened or calcified scar. *Abbreviations*: SVC, superior vena cava; RA, right atrium; RVOT, right ventricular outflow tract; IVC, inferior vena cava; RV, right ventricle.

is to apply traction around an angle, such as the entrance into the right ventricle. The gray force (arrows) is minimal, and now the extractor is dependent on advancing a non-powered sheath to dissect the lead free. These sheaths often cannot disrupt thickened and possibly calcified scar. It is easily understood why this bailout method fails.

For lead remnants within the right ventricle, returning to a superior approach is recommended. This allows the use of direct traction forces and also powered sheaths. **Video 18.5**A and 18.5B show us the platform of tools that can be used to snare a lead remnant from a superior approach and then advance a powered sheath. An 18-Fr Gore Dry Seal introducer sheath (Gore) is placed over a stiff wire in the subclavian vein and advanced toward the SVC. An EnSnare catheter (Merit Medical) is placed within an 8.5-Fr Agilis sheath (Abbott Medical). The Agilis sheath is within a large powered sheath. In this case, the Agilis was placed within a 16-Fr laser sheath (Philips Medical). The Agilis sheath is then used to guide EnSnare for snaring the proximal end of the lead remnant. Once the lead is snared, the powered sheath is then advanced over the Agilis sheath and its new rail to complete the extraction (Video 18.5B).

A unique benefit of femoral snaring is improving the extraction rail by stabilizing a lead with low tensile strength. When the extraction forces exceed the tensile strength of a lead, the extraction rail can come apart as lead components fail. Such an example is the Fineline lead (Boston Scientific). The construction of a Fineline lead is shown in **Figure 18.4**. The cathode and anode are constructed of a single filar wire 0.005 OD with an ethene-co-tetrafluoroethylene (ETFE) coating 0.002 inches thick.

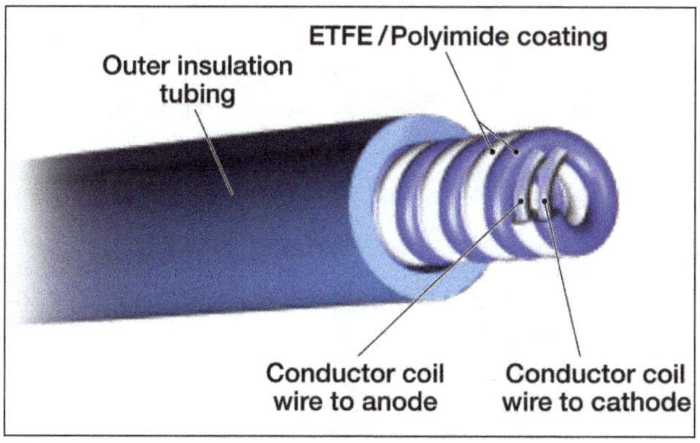

Figure 18.4 The design elements of a Fineline pacemaker lead. (Image courtesy of Boston Scientific.)

In comparison, industry-standard coaxial leads are 3–4 filars for each anode and cathode. Each Fineline filar is coated with a .002 inch coating of ETFE and locking stylets have difficulty locking within this channel, which is coated with a Teflon-like substance. Under the typical traction forces of extraction, these leads tend to undergo coil unraveling and insulation break. In **Video 18.6**, a locking stylet fails to lock within the Fineline successfully, and with the traction, the stylet slides back within the lumen. Subsequently, the traction load is transferred to the coils, which unravel and stretch, as shown in **Figure 18.5**. A corresponding case example is shown in **Figure 18.6**. This is a poor extraction platform to advance extraction tools safely. **Figure 18.7** is the same lead after removal demonstrating the locking stylet that failed to lock in the distal lead, broken outer coil, and stretched inner coil.

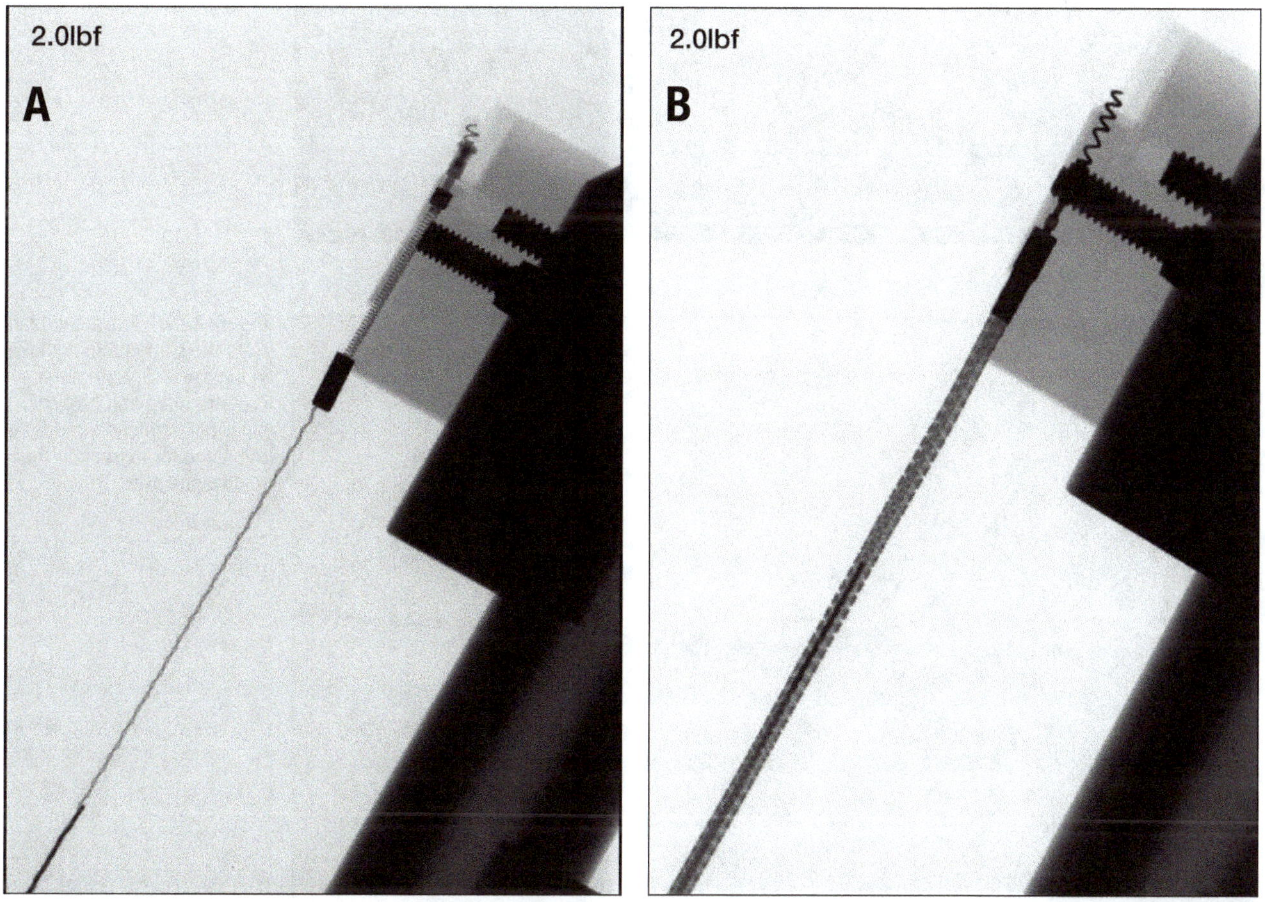

Figure 18.5 A comparison of the single filar Boston Scientific Fineline lead (**Panel A**) and an industry-standard three filar lead (**Panel B**) undergoing 2 lbs of traction. Note with the Fineline lead the significant coil unwinding and subsequent stretching. (Figures courtesy of Medtronic.)

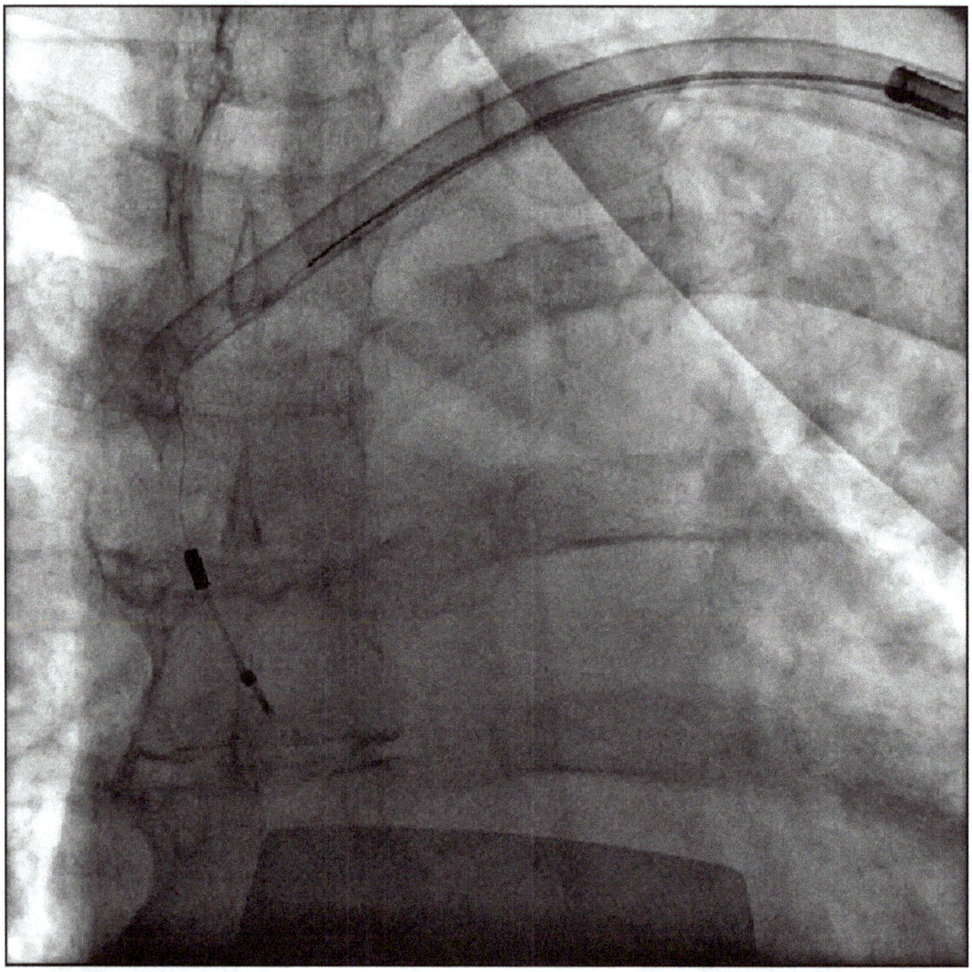

Figure 18.6 Clinical example of Fineline (Boston Scientific) lead coil unwinding and stretching with loss of the extraction rail.

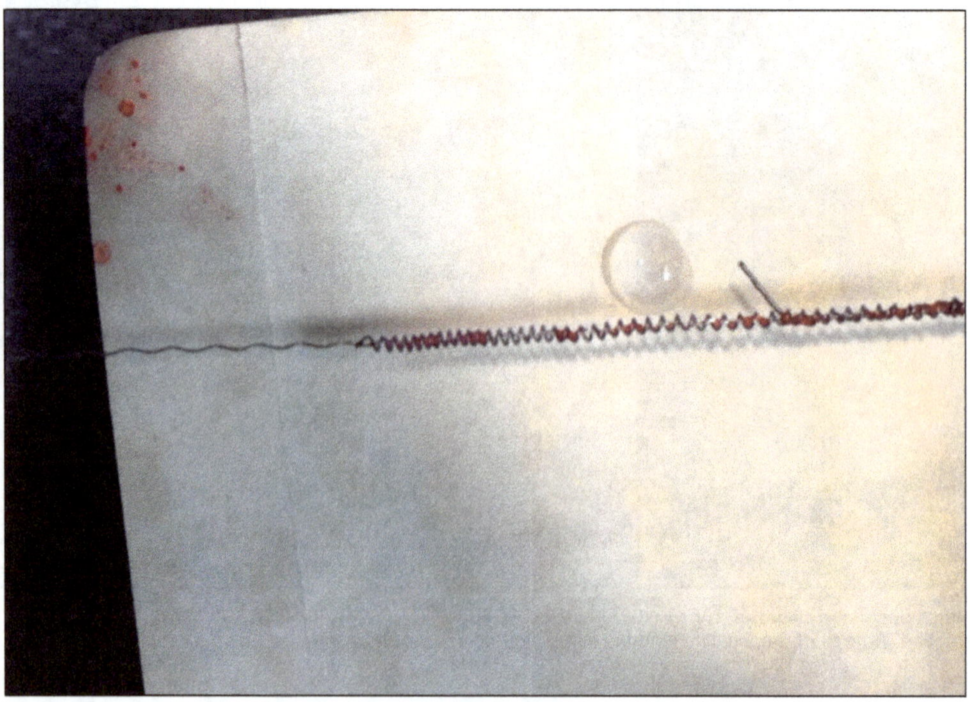

Figure 18.7 Extracted lead from the same patient shown in Figure 18.5. Note outer coil stretched and broken inner coil stretched and little remained for extraction tool to advance over.

CLINICAL VIGNETTE

A 72-year-old female is referred for extraction because of lead endocarditis. She has a history of hypertension, hyperlipidemia, asthma, rheumatoid arthritis, and obesity. Cardiac issues include coronary artery disease with 2 prior stent placements and ischemic cardiomyopathy (ejection fraction < 35%). Nine and a half years before admission, she underwent placement of a dual-chamber pacemaker for the tachy-brady syndrome. After an episode of sustained ventricular tachycardia, the pacemaker was upgraded to an ICD 1 year before extraction. Roughly 10 months later, the patient was admitted to the home hospital with fever, confusion, and blood cultures positive for methicillin-sensitive *Staphylococcus aureus* (MSSA). Treatment with IV cefazolin for 2 weeks, but 1 month after treatment ended, the patient returns with sepsis, confusion, fever. Once again, blood cultures were positive for MSSA. The patient was referred for extraction due to persistent positive blood cultures.

Device Details

Device Component	Manufacturer/Model	Date of Implant
	Original implant	
Atrial lead	Boston Scientific 4469 Fineline	12/22/10
Ventricular lead	Boston Scientific 4470 Fineline	12/22/10
	Upgrade to ICD	
ICD lead	Medtronic 6935	4/10/18
ICD generator	Medtronic Evera	4/10/18

Chest X-ray (CXR) is shown in **Figure 18.8**.

PREPROCEDURAL PLANNING

All patients are admitted to hospitalist service and seen in consultation by an extraction physician. Subspecialist physicians are asked to assist in care depending on patient issues (i.e., infection). All patients undergo a PA and lateral CXR, extraction CT scan, and echocardiogram (See Chapter 3). Type and crossmatch for 4 units of blood is performed along with basic metabolic profile, hematology, and coagulation profiles.

PROCEDURAL DETAILS

All extractions are performed in a hybrid room capable of performing extractions and, if needed, cardiac surgery. Procedures are done under general anesthesia with a single-lumen endotracheal tube. Preparation for possible urgent cardiac surgery is performed. Deep venous thrombosis prevention wraps are placed on the lower extremities. A 5-Fr sheath is placed in the femoral artery for arterial BP monitoring and potential need for conversion to bypass lines. Four large-bore venous sheaths (two right and two left femoral vein) are placed for (1) use by the anesthesia service and possible need for femoral snare; (2) intracardiac echo; (3) potential need for an SVC balloon; and (4) possible need for a temporary pacemaker. Our standard procedure includes ICE with an examination of the individual leads.

The ICE catheter was advanced within a deflectable sheath from the femoral approach to the upper SVC at the innominate vein level. From here, the ultrasound catheter was pulled down to the right atrium looking for any lead binding to the SVC, lead-to-lead binding, and any vegetations. In this patient, a small (0.7 cm) vegetation was noted on the atrial lead. All leads moved independently of the SVC wall. The two Fineline leads were noted to adhere to one another in the SVC.

All lead preparations are performed to create a strong rail for extraction sheaths. Each lead is cut and prepped with an EZ locking stylet (Philips Medical), One-Tie (Cook Medical), and a fiber wire (nonabsorbable suture). However, please note recent research suggests that maintaining the terminal pin may be of benefit. A Bulldog (Cook Medical) is used to secure ICD lead cables.

A cardiovascular surgical team was present at the initiation of the extraction procedure. The team remained till 10 minutes after the last lead is removed and the patient clinically stable. The

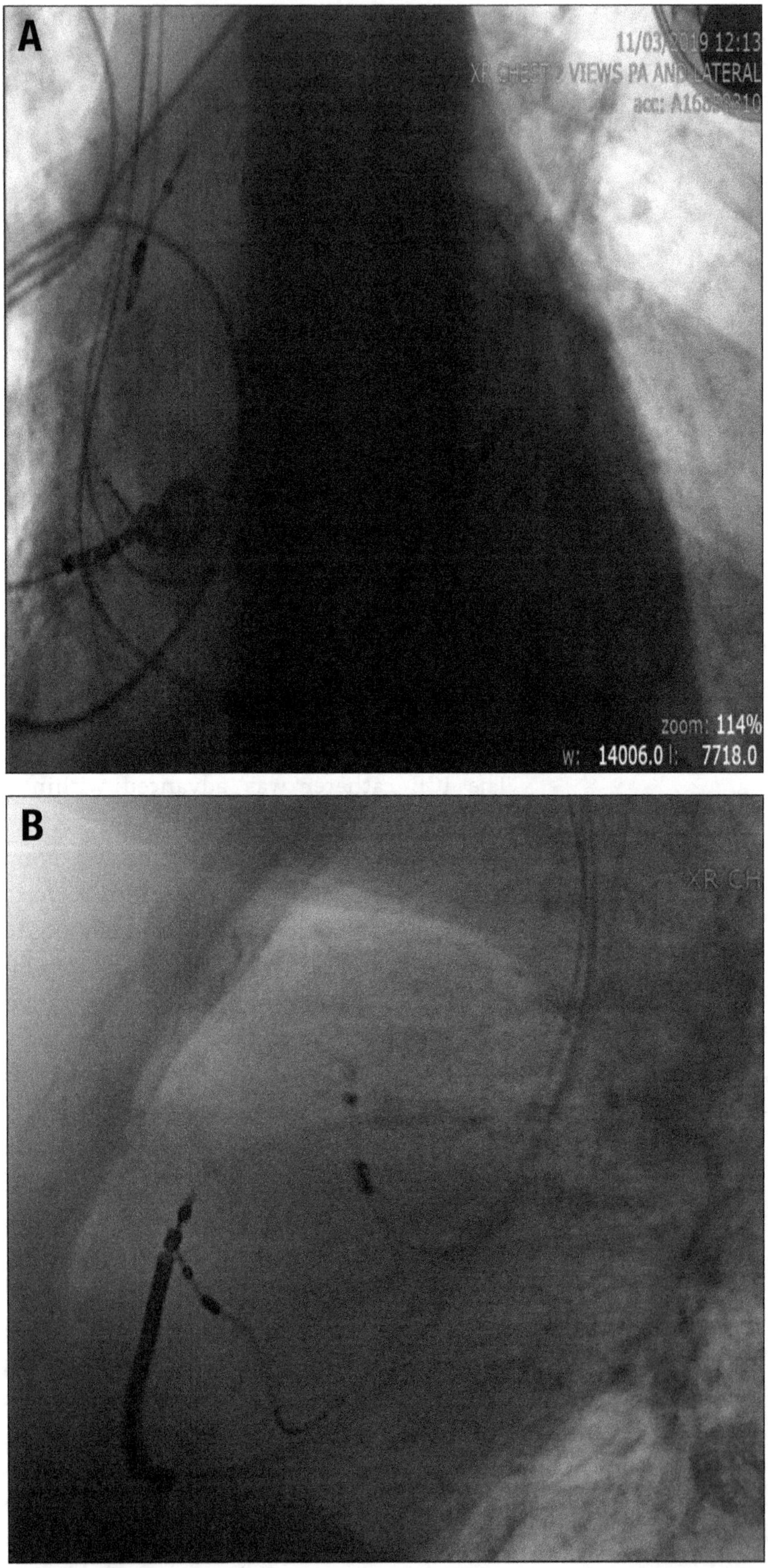

Figure 18.8 Preprocedure PA and lateral CXR demonstrate Medtronic ICD lead, and the two Boston Scientific Fineline leads. These leads are more easily seen on the lateral film. Both ventricular leads are fixed in the right ventricular outflow tract.

recently placed ICD lead was removed with tension alone. To provide a better rail for removing the Fineline leads, the decision was made to snare the leads and the locking stylet within it. A Cook femoral workstation was chosen with a 16-Fr outer sheath, 12-Fr inner curved sheath, and a 13-mm Needle's Eye Snare. During the procedure, first the atrial lead and later the ventricular leads were snared. However, an important difference existed. The atrial lead was snared and the lead easily unscrewed with a counterclockwise rotation, as seen in **Video 18.7**A. Please note the distal end of the locking stylet is visible between the anode and cathode. The atrial lead was folded into the workstation sheath, kinking (crimping) the locking stylet and firmly binding the snare and the locking stylet. Now the strength of the extraction rail is the locking stylet's strength (the breaking point for a Philips or Cook locking stylets is more than 15 lbs, and the snare more than 20 lbs). In Video 18.7B, we see the removal of the atrial Fineline lead intact. Under fluoroscopy, the end of the locking stylet remains visible between the cathode and anode.

An example of the incomplete application of the snaring tool is the removal of the ventricular lead. In **Video 18.8**, the femoral lead appears snared, and 13-mm Needle's Eye Snare is snug against the lead body. Without pulling the lead into the 12-Fr inner femoral sheath, the locking stylet is not kinked, and the snare does not have adequate control of the locking stylet. As seen in **Video 18.9**, traction locking stylet easily slipped within the ETFE-coated coradial wires, and the extraction platform was lost. The coil stretched and insulation broke. Although this lead was successfully removed, the rail was once again poor, could have easily broken, and patient complications could have become higher.

DISCUSSION

It is critical to understand the advantages and disadvantages of the femoral approach. With a superior approach, leads with poor tensile strength come apart during extraction. The case example above demonstrates the benefit when used in combination with a superior approach. A similar situation is shown in **Figure 18.9** with 2 Boston Scientific Ingevity leads extracted successfully and fully intact utilizing this technique. Note the kink present that bounded the locking stylet and lead, more proximal on the ventricular lead.

In summary, a complete extraction program includes active use of the femoral approach. This approach can augment the superior approach by stabilizing leads to gain access through vascular occlusions, stabilize individual leads during extraction to prevent dislodgement, and help extract fragile leads that cannot tolerate the traction forces necessary for a superior approach. Femoral extraction of leads adhered to the SVC may also be safer.

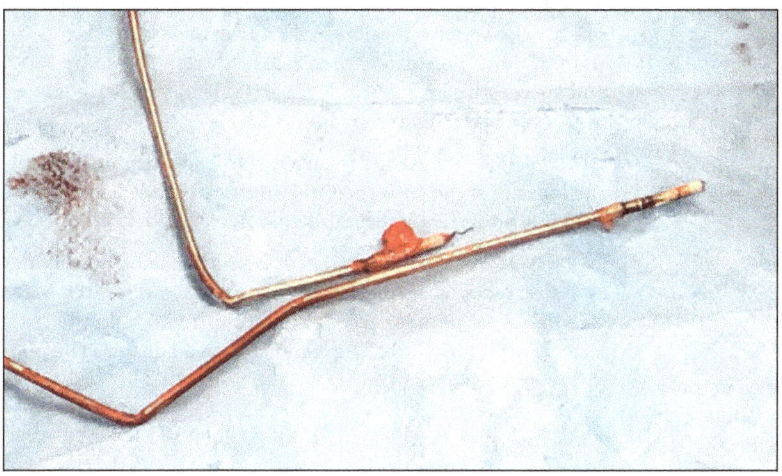

Figure 18.9 Two Boston Scientific Ingevity leads are removed from a superior approach with a femoral snare used for stabilizing the leads. Note leads are fully intact, and the kinking that occurs when lead and locking stylet within are retracted into the Cook inner sheath.

SUMMARY POINTS

- Routine use of a femoral approach is part of a robust extraction program.
- Femoral snaring can be used in many situations including helping with reimplant through occluded vessels, retrieving lead remnants, stabilization of leads intended to be preserved during the extraction procedure, improving lead rail strength and as a primary method of lead extraction.
- Traction and counter traction forces created during the process of femoral snaring are optimal for leads within the right atrium and superior vena cava. Lead remnants in the RV are best extracted from a superior approach.
- When the forces of extraction from a superior approach are greater than the lead's tensile strength, consider stabilizing the lead with a femoral snare.
- To stabilize those leads, the locking stylet must be effectively snared and become the extraction rail. Such a rail has a strength of 15–18 lbs.

REFERENCE

1. Toloui M, Marshall M, Vatterott P, Zhang P, Lahm R, Lulik T, Harris M. Numerical modeling of vascular stresses during lead extraction: Subclavian vs. femoral. Proceedings of the Design of Medical Devices Conference, Minneapolis, MN, April 6–9, 2020. https://doi.org/10.1115/DMD2020-9003

VIDEO LEGENDS

Video 18.1 A Clinical case where a combination of ablation catheter and Goose Neck snare used to stabilize ICD lead during the extraction of the nonfunctioning pacing lead, Model 3830 (Medtronic) attached to the ICD lead. [00:01]

Video 18.2 Intracardiac echo (open rotational) showed that the ICD and atrial leads are firmly embedded in the SVC wall. [00:06]

Video 18.3 Images are taken through a thoracoscope during the extraction of an ICD lead. The SVC is imaged while traction is applied to lead/locking stylet from the left subclavian lead entry site (Video 18.3A) [00:18] and then with the lead snared through a femoral approach (Video 18.3B) [00:20]. With subclavian traction, force is concentrated in a discreet area. With femoral traction, force is dispersed over a larger area of tissue. This difference, likely helps to preserve tissue integrity.

Video 18.4 Animation of the results of Finite element wall modeling. Vascular wall stresses subclavian (Video 18.4A) versus femoral pull (Video 18.4B). The highest stress points are denoted in white.[00:05]

Video 18.5 Technique to extract lead fragment from superior approach. Video 18.5A demonstrating 16-Fr laser sheath advanced (non powered mode) over a wire through a 18-Fr dry gore sheath. [00:01] In Video 18.5B, the lead fragment has been snared with an EnSnare. An Agilis sheath (visible within the 16-Fr laser sheath) was used to guide the EnSnare (see text). [00:29] Lead successfully removed.

Video 18.6 The effects of traction on deployed locking stylet within a Fineline lead. Deployed stylet unable to bind within ETFE coated lumen. [00:45]

Video 18.7 (A) Cine of snaring Fineline lead and locking stylet within. After snaring, the snare is first used to unscrew the lead tip from its atrial attachment. The lead and locked locking stylet are then pulled into the Cook femoral workstation inner sheath with kinking of the stylet. This snared locking stylet provides a strong rail for extraction tools to be safely advanced from above. [00:14] (B) Cine demonstrating the removal of an atrial Fineline lead. The snared locking stylet provides a safe and stable rail for the lead extraction tool's advancement to the right atrium. The lead is then released from the snare and successfully removed. Note atrial lead structure is preserved is during removal. [00:53]

Video 18.8 Snaring of ventricular lead without pulling the locking stylet into the Cook inner sheath. The lead is held but not effectively stabilized. [00:07]

Video 18.9 Without a firm grip on the lead, the locking stylet retracts with traction, coils unwind and stretch. Needle's Eye Snare is removed after failing to hold the locking stylet in place. The lead is removed despite the poor rail from the snare. [00:42]

19 | Coronary Sinus Lead Extraction of a Starfix Lead

Pierce J. Vatterott, MD

INTRODUCTION

On August 15, 2008, Medtronic released its Attain Starfix (model number 4195) over-the-wire cardiac resynchronization therapy (CRT) lead. It is a unipolar lead with a 5-Fr diameter with the tip electrode 5.3 Fr. The design includes 3 soft, pliable lobes that can be deployed up to 24 Fr and enable stable lead placement in a target location. Although successful in lead stability, the deployed lead lobes create an extraction challenge. **Figure 19.1** illustrates Starfix lobe deployment. **Video 19.1** shows these lobes fixating within a vessel. It is easy to foresee the challenges of Starfix extraction if one considers scar formation (**Figure 19.2**) around the deployed 24-Fr lobes adhered to the vessel wall. In addition, there is an inability to undeploy the lead lobes due to intravascular scar formation along the length of the lead and the blue tubing deployment mechanism.

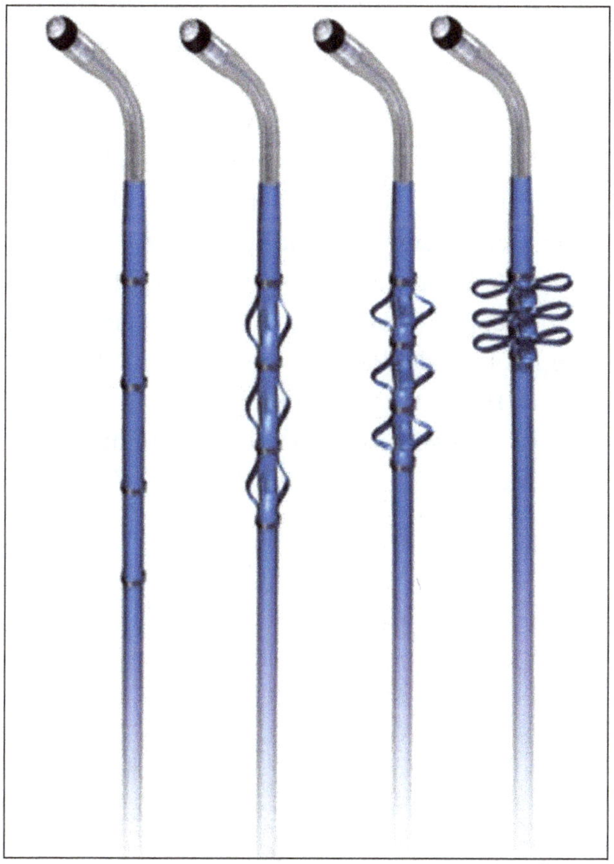

Figure 19.1 Demonstration of Starfix lobe deployment mechanism by advancing the blue-colored hydrophilic-coated polyurethane tubing over the main body of the polyurethane lead. The fully undeployed Starfix lead is shown on **far left**; the fully deployed Starfix lobes are shown on the **right**. (Courtesy of Medtronic.)

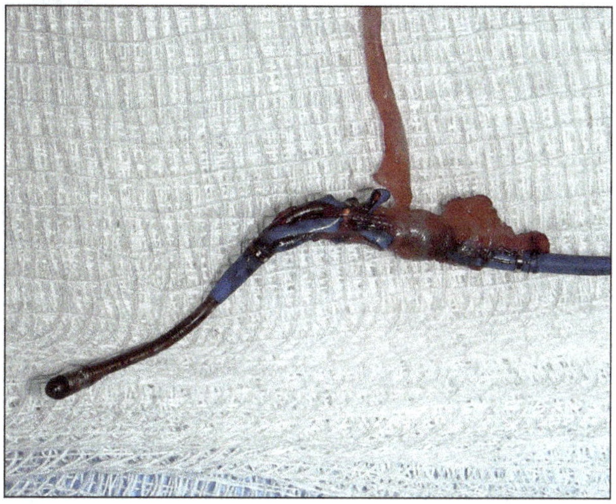

Figure 19.2 Extracted Starfix lead demonstrating scar tissue bound to deployment lobes.

Our experience in chronically implanted Starfix leads is that full undeployment of the lead lobes is not possible. In response to these findings, the following Starfix lead preparation method was developed. The goal is the undeployment of the proximal lead lobes. Partial undeployment presents the lobes' proximal end during lead removal as a narrow end of a cone (**Figure 19.3**). This is theoretically easier to retract through scar binding sites. Fundamental to this approach is a preparation of the Starfix deployment mechanism separately from the main lead body. The Starfix has an outer blue

 Cardiotext Publishing. ISBN: 978-1-942909-54-5

hydrophilic-coated polyurethane tubing that acts as the lobe deployment mechanism. This moves freely over the lead body of standard 55D polyurethane. Removal of the lead scar by a powered sheath allows engagement of the lobe deployment mechanism (blue tubing).

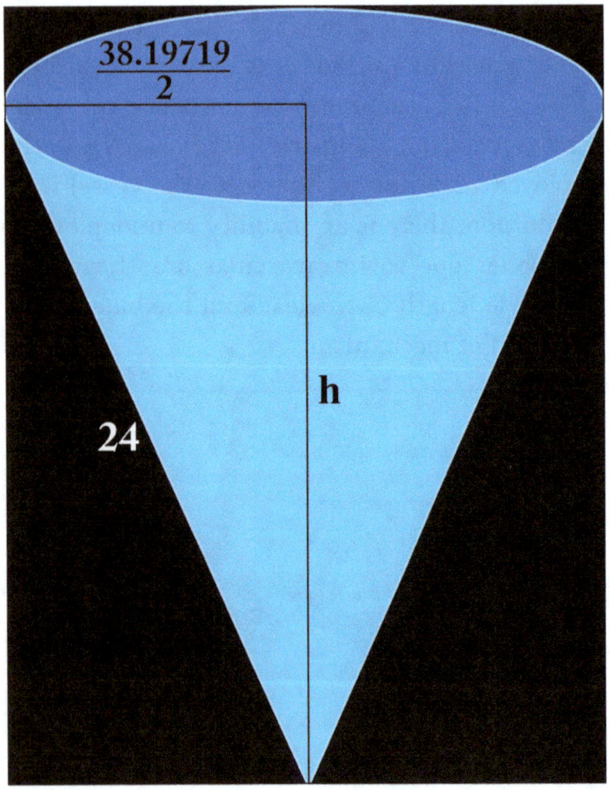

Figure 19.3 Illustration of the goal of Starfix lead prep. The described lead prep results in partial undeployment. This presents more of a cone shape with the proximal lobes collapsed. As one retracts the lead back through the vessel, the cone's narrow portion has less tendency to interact with scar tissue than fully deployed lobes.

In our lab, we do not attempt lobe undeployment until the extraction sheath is approaching the coronary sinus (CS) os. The goal is to not engage the undeployment mechanism until as much scar tissue as possible is removed. Otherwise, one is pulling against the most proximal lead scar attachment and damaging the deployment mechanism. The following figures are taken from a lead prep outside the human body. **Figure 19.4**, Panel A is of a Starfix lead with fully deployed lead lobes. The retention sleeve, which is used for lobe deployment, has a single suture; Panels B–D show initial prep with the removal of the proximal lead end, retention suture, and a locking stylet placement. **Figures 19.5** and **19.6** illustrate how to independently control the blue polyurethane tubing (used for lobe deployment) from the main lead body. In Figure 19.5, the white retention sleeve and the proximal blue hydrophilic polyurethane tubing are separated from the lead body (Panels A and B) and cut proximally to accommodate the tube stretching with traction (Panel C). A 1 silk suture is attached only to the blue tubing to allow traction independent of the main lead body (Panel D). Figure 19.6 illustrates the final prep with a standard prepped main lead body and separately prepped blue deployment mechanism (Panel A). During the extraction, process traction can be applied independently to the blue tubing or the main lead body, or both (Panel B).

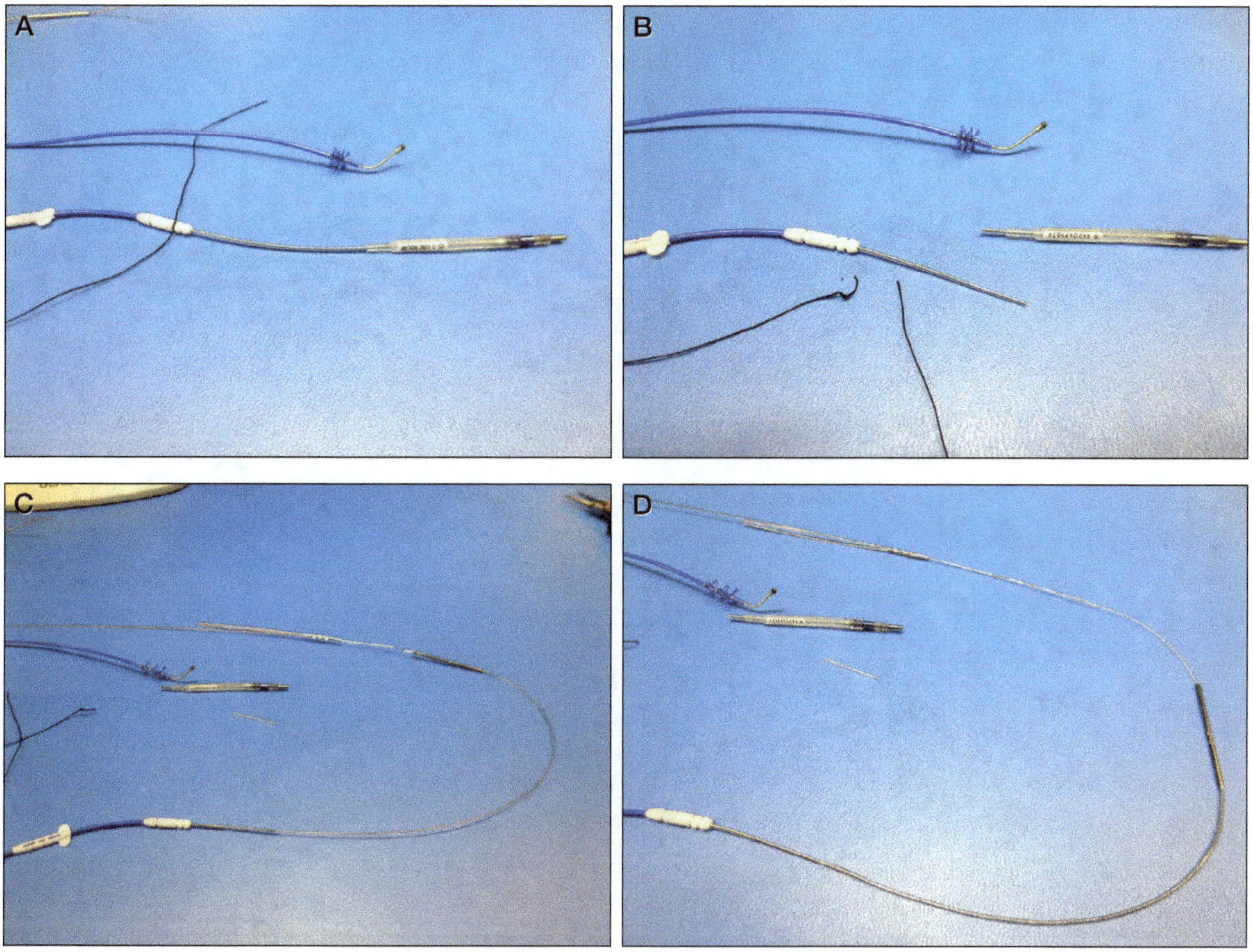

Figure 19.4 **Panel A:** Fully deployed Starfix lead with suture attachment on retention sleeve (deployment mechanism). **Panel B:** Proximal lead end has been removed and retention lead suture removed. **Panel C:** Lead locking stylet placed. **Panel D:** Locking stylet deployed.

An example from a patient referred to an infected biventricular system is shown in **Video 19.2**. Our approach is to remove the "most vulnerable" lead last, and in this case, that lead is the Starfix. Removal of other leads often decreases scar binding sites encountered during the removal of subsequent leads. After extracting other leads, the extractor advances the powered sheath over the Starfix lead to the orifice of the CS. Now traction is applied to the blue deployment tubing (**Video 19.3**). This typically results in a collapse of the most proximal 1 or 2 lobes, resulting in pulling the narrow end of a cone back through the vasculature. If needed, the extraction sheath is advanced in a nonpowered mode into the CS (**Video 19.4**) to break up bindings sites gently. **Video 19.5** is a CS venogram demonstrating occlusion of the prior target vein after Starfix removal.

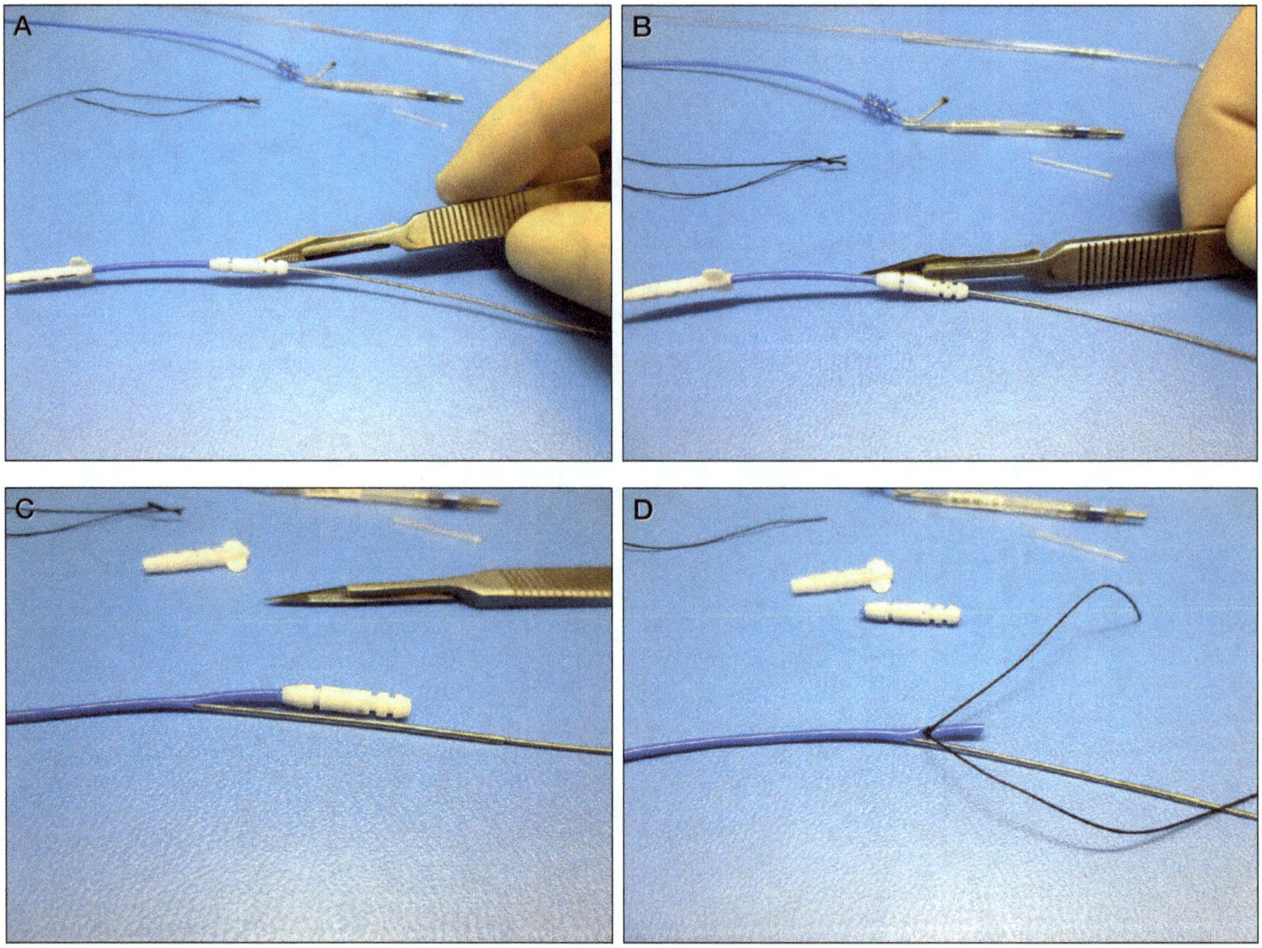

Figure 19.5 **Panel A:** Retention sleeve removal. **Panel B:** Proximal hydrophilic blue tubing removed. **Panel C:** Retention sleeve and blue tubing removed from the lead body. Additional tubing can be removed to accommodate for a stretch during traction. **Panel D:** Retention sleeve removed. A 1 silk suture attached to blue polyurethane tubing allows traction independent of the main lead body.

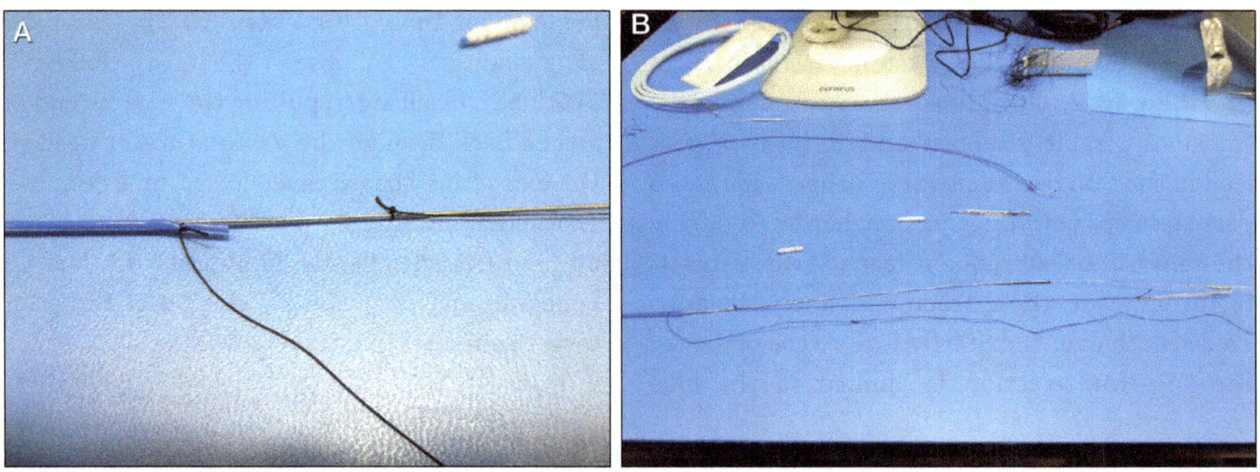

Figure 19.6 **Panel A:** Prepped lead illustrating independent control of blue polyurethane deployment lobes separate from the lead body. **Panel B:** More extensive view of proximal lead end demonstrating capabilities to independently apply traction to either lead body or blue polyurethane tubing.

CLINICAL VIGNETTE

This 67-year-old male was referred for *Enterococcus faecalis* endocarditis. Prior history of ischemic cardiomyopathy, coronary bypass surgery, chronic systolic heart failure, and paroxysmal atrial fibrillation with a rapid ventricular response. In 2012, he underwent a cardiac resynchronization therapy/pacemaker (CRTP) implant with AV node ablation and, 1 year later, an upgrade to a CRT-defibrillator (CRT-D) for ventricular tachycardia. The prior placed Medtronic 5076 ventricular lead was removed. In March 2018 the patient underwent a CRT-D generator replacement. Six months later he was admitted to an outside hospital with recurrent fevers. Multiple blood cultures positive for *Enterococcus faecalis*, and transesophageal echocardiogram (TEE) demonstrated lead vegetations. Patient was transferred for system removal.

Device Details

Device Components	Manufacturer/Model	Date of Implant
CRT-D	Medtronic Claria MRI CRT-D	3/27/2018
RA lead	Medtronic 5076	11/16/2012
RV lead	Medtronic 6947	5/24/2013
LV lead	Medtronic 4195 Starfix	11/16/2012

PREPROCEDURAL PLANNING

For lead extraction, the patient is seen in consultation by an extraction physician. The patient undergoes device evaluation for current thresholds, checking underlying pacing dependence, sensing characteristics, and any prior rhythm abnormalities. Preprocedure PA and lateral chest X-ray (CXR) are obtained, as well as a lead extraction CT scan with contrast and a 3D echocardiogram (please see Chapter 3 on lead extraction imaging).

PROCEDURAL DETAILS

The hybrid room offers quality fluoroscopy and the ability to convert to an open chest cardiac procedure. The patient was placed under general anesthesia with intubation. Sequential leg wraps were used to decrease venous thrombosis incidence. Cine images in the AP, RAO, and LAO views were taken of the leads to evaluate lead-to-lead binding and possible calcified scar visible on the leads. The extraction physician was given time to study these images before scrubbing.

The patient was prepped and draped from the neck to the groin for possible open chest procedure. Ultrasound-guided access to the right femoral artery and bilateral femoral veins was obtained. A 5-Fr arterial sheath was placed for precise blood pressure monitoring and, if needed, for conversion to bypass. The right femoral venous sheaths were set for a femoral snare device's possible use and through an 8.5-Fr deflectable sheath, intracardiac echocardiogram. Two left-sided femoral vein sheaths were placed: a 6-Fr for a temporary pacer wire in this pacemaker-dependent patient and a second 12 Fr for a possible superior vena cava (SVC) rescue balloon deployment. A stiff wire was guided through a multipurpose catheter with the distal end placed in the right internal jugular vein. This wire can be used as a rail for rescue balloon advancement in the event of an SVC tear, and it should always be done before extraction.

Intracardiac ultrasound examination from the SVC–innominate junction demonstrated no evidence that any of the 3 leads were adhered to the vessel wall or each other.

Lead Prep

After surgical incision of the device pocket, cautery was used to free up the device and leads. Anchoring sleeves were removed. With standard stylets, we undeployed both fixation mechanisms on the 5076 lead and the ICD 6947 lead. All leads were then prepped, with special attention played to the Starfix. For the atrial lead, we used a Philips EZ locking stylet, a Cook One-Tie, and a fiber wire suture (attached from the lead body to locking stylet). For the ICD lead, a Philips EZ locking stylet was placed and deployed in the inner lumen. A Cook Bulldog combined with a One-Tie was used to engage the ICD cables in the traction platform. Fiberwire placed from the insulation to the locking stylet. The Starfix lead was prepped as described above.

Lead Extraction

A 14-Fr laser (internal diameter [ID] 10.2-Fr) was chosen for the 7-Fr and 9-Fr atrial and ICD leads. It is important to avoid both undersizing, and risk damaging the lead, or oversizing, and risk engaging the vessel wall. Lasering across the subclavian to the innominate, the Medtronic 5076 atrial lead came free from its binding sites and was removed without difficulty. Attention was then focused on the ICD lead. Advancing slowly with the laser, the lead binding sites in the subclavian were freed up. Further advancement of the laser was difficult, and consideration for switching to a cutting tool was made. However, by advancing the outer sheath over the laser, the ICD lead was freed from its innominate binding sites and removed. Attention was then turned to the Starfix. Using a 12-Fr laser (ID 8.3-Fr), binding sites were freed up in the subclavian and innominate veins. In a non-powered mode, the sheath was advanced down the SVC to the CS. Using the suture attached to the blue tubing, traction was applied to undeploy the proximal electrode while maintaining lead body traction. No binding sites were found at the CS, and the extraction sheath was advanced in a nonpowered mode into the CS. The successful lead removal is shown in **Video 19.6**.

SUMMARY POINTS

- The extraction physician should understand the lead construction of their patient's leads and the unique challenges those leads present for removal.
- The implanted Starfix lead has fixation lobes that present a challenge for removal.
- A prep technique that individually engages the Starfix deployment mechanism allows partial undeployment of the fixation mechanism, potentially benefitting the process of Starfix removal.
- If other leads are to be extracted, remove those prior to Starfix lead removal. This decreases the scar burden encountered with the removal of the Starfix lead.
- Do not attempt to undeploy the Starfix lobes until the extraction sheath is approaching the CS ostium. Decreasing scar burden on the lead allows engagement of the undeployment mechanism.

VIDEO LEGENDS

Video 19.1 The deployment of a Starfix lead with lobe attachment to the vessel wall. [02:08]

Video 19.2 RAO 30 [00:03] and LAO 30 [00:04] images from a patient with device infection referred for extraction. Leads present are Medtronic 6947 dual-coil ICD lead, Medtronic 5076, and Medtronic 4195 Starfix lead.

Video 19.3 ICD lead and atrial lead have already been removed prior to attempt to remove the Starfix lead. As the powered sheath advances on the CS, traction is applied independently to the blue polyurethane tubing. This results in a partial collapse of the proximal lobes with a more favorable physical structure for removing the narrow end of a cone. [00:01]

Video 19.4 With traction applied to both the lead and blue tubing, a powered sheath is advanced in a nonpowered mode into the CS. This disrupts binding sites and allows effective traction delivery. [00:04]

Video 19.5 Coronary sinus venogram after removal of the Starfix lead demonstrating venous branch occlusion after the Starfix removal. [00:03]

Video 19.6 Video of Starfix removal. Atrial pacing and ICD lead have been removed. Temporary pacing lead in place. The laser was advanced in a non-powered mode from the innominate to the CS os and into the CS. Traction is applied to the blue tubing for lobe undeployment as the extraction sheath approaches the CS while also independently applying traction to the main lead body. [00:15]

20 | Extraction of Coronary Sinus Lead

Olurotimi Mesubi, MD, MBBS, MPH; Charles J. Love, MD

CLINICAL VIGNETTE

A 63-year-old female presented with a history of coronary artery disease status post multiple percutaneous coronary interventions, ischemic cardiomyopathy (left ventricular ejection fraction [LVEF] of 30%–35%), and chronic left bundle branch block. She had her initial implant of a Boston Scientific CRT-D device in May 2010 (8 years and 7 months prior to the present presentation). She subsequently had a cardiac vein (CV) lead revision in September 2012 (6 years and 5 months before the current presentation) for a poor pacing threshold, with the abandonment of the previously placed CV lead. Her history also included documented ventricular tachycardia that terminated with antitachycardia pacing. Other comorbid conditions included type 2 diabetes mellitus, a chronic obstructive pulmonary disease requiring chronic supplemental oxygen, and stroke with some residual right-sided weakness.

She developed methicillin-sensitive *Staphylococcus aureus* (MSSA) bacteremia, and endocarditis with vegetations noted on the leads June 2018 prior to presentation to our healthcare facility (8 years following initial implantation). In 2018, she underwent attempted CRT-D system extraction elsewhere, successfully extracting the right atrial pacing lead and right ventricular defibrillation lead. However, the 2 CV leads were not able to be removed entirely. One CV lead was cut and allowed to retract into the subclavian vein. The other lead had been pulled apart with a large fragment retained despite various maneuvers attempted at the time. She was placed on chronic suppressive antibiotic therapy with oral cephalexin and used a wearable defibrillator since the attempted extraction. She subsequently developed deep vein thrombosis in both upper extremities and was on chronic anticoagulation with rivaroxaban. Attempts to stop antibiotics resulted in recurrent fever and bacteremia. She was referred to our facility for extraction of the retained coronary sinus (CS) leads.

Her most recent LVEF was 30%–35% by echocardiogram done in June 2018. Her physical exam was unremarkable other than a well-healed incision in the left prepectoral area. The basic metabolic panel was within normal limits other than elevated glucose of 317 mg/dL. CBC had a normal WBC but a low hemoglobin/hematocrit of 9.5/30.1. Blood culture was negative (noting that she was on chronic cephalexin suppressive therapy). Extraction was felt to be necessary due to the persistence and recurrence of the bacteremia. The only other option for management would be continued life-long suppressive therapy with antibiotics.

PREPROCEDURAL PLANNING

As is typical in our electrophysiology lab, the patient was prepped according to our protocol following the Heart Rhythm Society guidelines.[1] The patient was placed under general anesthesia (endotracheal intubation) by our cardiac anesthesiology team. Intra-arterial pressure monitoring was established. Sterile preparation and draping from the neck to the mid-thigh level were performed. Our cardiac surgeon was fully informed of the procedure and patient history and was immediately available, as was the perfusion team. Four units of cross-matched, packed red blood cells were in the room. We decided not to deploy an occlusive balloon or to place a stiff rescue wire in the superior

 ISBN: 978-1-942909-54-5

vena cava (SVC) given that (1) the leads were not adherent to the venous wall based on fluoroscopic imaging; (2) we were planning only a femoral approach; and (3) we did not anticipate using either mechanical or laser sheaths in the SVC.

PROCEDURAL DETAILS

Transesophageal echocardiogram (TEE) at the beginning of the procedure showed no vegetations, the presence of a small pericardial effusion adjacent to the right ventricle, trivial tricuspid valve insufficiency, no evidence of left-to-right shunt. It confirmed the compromised LV function of 15%–20%. Initial fluoroscopy showed the retained fragments from the two LV leads. One lead extended from the left subclavian vein (with proximal tip cut) to the CS and into a coronary vein tributary. The second lead had the proximal portion in the inferior vena cava (IVC) and the distal portion in the CS. There was apparent calcification around the CS os. (**Video 20.1** and **Video 20.2**).

Two venous vascular access sites were established under fluoroscopic and ultrasound guidance; one in the right femoral vein and one in the left femoral vein. The left femoral venous access was used for a 9-Fr high-volume central venous catheter with high-volume tubing, available for rapid volume or blood infusion if necessary. The right femoral venous access site had a 6-Fr sheath inserted through which 2 guidewires were placed. The first was a standard short J wire clamped to the sterile drape for retained access if needed. We have found this to be very useful during femoral extractions should there be a need to remove the extraction sheath and re-enter the vein. The second guidewire was 150 cm and was advanced to the right atrium. The 6-Fr sheath was removed, and a 16-Fr Byrd femoral workstation sheath (Cook Medical) was placed over the long wire to the right atrium. The long guidewire and dilator were then removed, and the workstation was aspirated and flushed with saline.

The first lead that was addressed (lead #1) was an Acuity lead (model 4554, Boston Scientific), which was initially implanted in 2010 (8 years, 7 months prior to this extraction procedure). This lead's distal end was in a posterolateral vein and the proximal/free end in the IVC. A 24-mm to 45-mm EnSnare endovascular snare system (Merit Medical) was placed through the workstation and utilized to snare the proximal end of lead #1 in the IVC. The lead was quite challenging to grasp. However, once the lead was snared, manual traction was applied. It was noted that not only was the lead adherent to the adjacent tissue, it also traversed a large mass of calcification at the CS os (**Video 20.3**). The lead would not pull free with simple traction, and the Byrd sheath could not be advanced through the dense calcification. Next, the torque device was removed from the EnSnare, and the 16-Fr femoral workstation sheath was removed, leaving the snared and the lead in place, and an 11-Fr TightRail mechanical sheath (Philips) was advanced over the shaft of the snare into the IVC (**Video 20.4**). The torque device was then placed back on the EnSnare, which was then used to maintain traction on the lead; however, the lead broke and had to be snared again (**Video 20.5**). The TightRail was then advanced through the calcified CS os and ultimately into the CS (**Video 20.6**). Though the lead was free within the CS body, it would still not pull out of the target vein as the lead was completely encased by scar and calcium within the vein. As we were applying traction to the lead to advance the TightRail further into the CS, the lead broke, and a portion was removed from the TightRail, leaving the TightRail in place, and the distal end of the lead in the target vessel with some of the conductor in the CS. A 15-mm Amplatz Goose Neck snare (Medtronic) was then advanced through the TightRail, and the lead was again snared. The TightRail was advanced just into the opening of the CV branch was the lead was embedded. Still, it could not be advanced further given the size of the target vein, the inability to get good alignment with the lead, and concern for laceration of the vessel. In an attempt to gain better alignment, the TightRail was then exchanged for a more flexible tool; a 12-Fr GlideLight Laser Sheath (Philips), and the lead was snared once again (**Video 20.7**). However, given the location and takeoff of the lead from the CS, an optimal angle on the lead was still challenging to obtain. While using traction on the lead with the laser catheter, the lead broke off at the junction of the CS and the CV (**Video 20.8** and **Video 20.9**). Given the considerable high risk of further attempts in the target vein and the fact that the lead was encased entirely in scar and calcium, a decision was made to abandon the small fragment that remained.

The second lead was then addressed (lead #2), was a Medtronic Attain Ability lead model 4296, which had been implanted at the time of CV lead revision in 2012 (6 years, 5 months prior to this extraction procedure). The distal end was in a high lateral or anterior interventricular CV. As noted earlier, the proximal end had been cut and retracted in the left subclavian vein, and the lead body was noted to be stretched in the region of the right atrium. Working from the femoral venous access once again, a Needle's Eye Snare (Cook Medical) was used to capture the lead, which was then brought into the sheath (**Video 20.10**). With steady traction, the lead's proximal end was pulled out of the SVC in its entirety, and then the distal portion of the lead released from the CV. The lead was removed in its entirety from the patient (**Video 20.11**).

At the end of the procedure, fluoroscopy was satisfactory, with only the small retained fragment of lead #1 noted in a CV (**Video 20.12**).

Postprocedure TEE showed no change in the preexisting pericardial effusion and tricuspid valve function noted at the beginning of the procedure. Interestingly, she was noted to be hypoxemic and hypotensive at the end of the procedure, which was initially deemed due to her congestive heart failure, pulmonary edema, and chronic obstructive pulmonary disease. She thus remained on mechanical ventilation and transferred to the coronary cardiac unit after the procedure.

POSTPROCEDURAL RECOVERY AND FOLLOW-UP

She was extubated the day following her procedure. Her postprocedure course was notable for fever, hypotension requiring pressors, leukocytosis, and lactic acidosis in the first 24 hours. She was thus started on intravenous vancomycin and cefazolin for presumed bacteremia and sepsis. Preliminary microbiology from CS leads showed gram-positive cocci, which was later confirmed to be coagulase-negative *Staphylococcus* (different than the MSSA noted by the referring physician). Her fever resolved. She was weaned off pressors and was transferred out of the coronary cardiac unit within 48 hours. Blood cultures were negative. Her challenging postprocedure course was deemed due to distributive shock secondary to transient bacteremia. She was discharged 5 days after her extraction with a plan to complete a 14-day antibiotic course with linezolid. The plan was for her to get a new CRT-D reimplantation locally. She was discharged with a wearable defibrillator and had not had recurrent sepsis.

SUMMARY POINTS

- Lead management of initial LV lead by extraction would have been easy 2 years post implant.
- Recurrent bacteremia without confirmed other source requires removal of as much intravascular hardware as possible.
- Multiple tools may be needed to successfully complete an extraction procedure.
- Retain a short guidewire when doing femoral access.
- Know when to stop a procedure to avoid serious bleeding event.

REFERENCE

1. Kusumoto FM, Schoenfeld MH, Wilkoff BL, et al. 2017 HRS expert consensus statement on cardiac implantable electronic device lead management and extraction. *Heart Rhythm.* 2017;14(12);e503–551.

VIDEO LEGENDS

Videos 20.1 and 20.2 Scout fluoroscopy showing the two retained CS leads with the pacing electrodes in separate CVs. The leads have been damaged and retained from a previous extraction attempt. The free end of one is in the left innominate vein, and the other is in the inferior vena cava. [00:09] [00:05]

Video 20.3 The first lead (with the free end in IVC) is snared using a multi-loop EnSnare. [00:18]

Video 20.4 A TightRail extraction sheath in advanced up the IVC to the right atrium. Note the calcification at the os of the CS that is visible near the end of this image. [00:13]

Video 20.5 The free end of the lead is again snared with an EnSnare that has been placed through the TightRail extraction sheath. The sheath is then advanced to the calcification at the CS os. [00:56]

Video 20.6 The TightRail is now at the os of the CS, and with traction on the lead, it begins to bore through the calcification. Not shown: The sheath eventually passes through the calcium to the takeoff of the lead into the target vessel, but due to the severe angulation, coaxial alignment could not be maintained. The decision was made to use a laser sheath to attempt to gain a better alignment. [00:18]

Video 20.7 After a laser sheath is placed into the IVC, the lead is again snared. [00:14]

Video 20.8 The laser sheath is advance to the takeoff of the CV, and lasing with gentile traction to maintain alignment is performed. Note the tissue's hazy appearance around the distal end of the lead, consistent with calcium deposition. [00:24]

Video 20.9 The lead breaks at the takeoff point to the vein. The risk of further attempts to extract this fully embedded fragment was deemed to be higher than the risk of leaving it in place. [00:01]

Video 20.10 A Needle's Eye Snare has been placed into the right atrium. This was used to capture the body of the second lead. [00:01]

Video 20.11 The second lead was retracted into the snare, and the entire lead remnant was pulled into the sheath and out of the body. [00:18]

Video 20.12 Final fluoroscopy showing the retained end of the first lead. [00:01]

21 | Azygous Vein Coil and Subcutaneous Array Extraction

Martin van Zyl, MBBCh; Siva K. Mulpuru, MD, MPH

CLINICAL VIGNETTE

A 73-year-old male presents 4 weeks after opening a cupboard door resulted in an accidental abrasion of the skin overlying his device pocket. Over time, the pocket became swollen, red, and tender (**Figure 21.1**) without fevers, chills, or rigors. He received a single dose of intravenous antibiotics in the local emergency department before being transferred to our institution. He had a left-sided dual-chamber pacemaker implanted in 2012 with a right atrial (RA) and coronary sinus (CS) left ventricular (LV) lead for high-grade AV block in the setting of repaired Ebstein anomaly with bioprosthetic tricuspid valve replacement. Due to frequent nonsustained ventricular tachycardia, he underwent an upgrade to implantable cardioverter-defibrillator (ICD) in 2015. A right ventricular (RV) single-coil ICD lead, an azygous vein coil, and a subcutaneous array electrode were added to achieve acceptable defibrillation thresholds. He had no history of device tachyarrhythmia therapies. The most recent device details are as follows.

Device Details

Device Component	Manufacturer/Model	Date of Implant
Pulse generator	St. Jude Medical Fortify Assura	4/2015
Right atrial lead	Medtronic 5086	8/2012
Left ventricular lead	St. Jude 1258T	8/2012
Right ventricular lead	Medtronic 6935	4/2015
Azygous vein coil	Medtronic 6937A	4/2015
Subcutaneous array	Medtronic 6996	4/2015
DF-1 adapter	Medtronic 6726	4/2015

The patient had underlying sinus rhythm with first-degree AV block at 55 bpm with 72% RA pacing and 92% RV pacing. A chest X-ray (CXR) with posterior-anterior and lateral views was obtained (**Figure 21.2**). Transthoracic echocardiogram (TTE) showed severe RV enlargement with severe systolic dysfunction and normal prosthetic tricuspid valve function and LV ejection fraction of 54%. There were no valvular or pacemaker lead vegetations noted by transesophageal echocardiogram (TEE), and no shunt was evident following agitated saline injection. Multiple sets of blood cultures remained persistently negative.

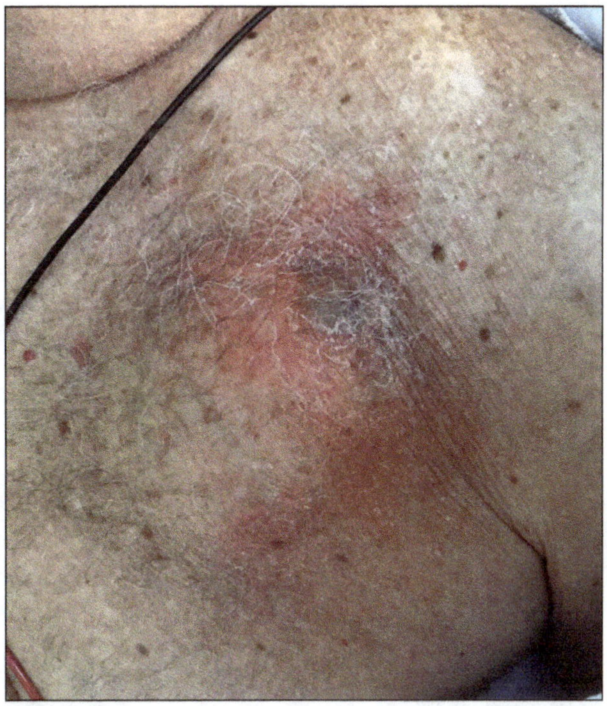

Figure 21.1 Redness, swelling, and a thin scab are noted near the device pocket.

CASE 21

 Cardiotext Publishing. ISBN: 978-1-942909-54-5

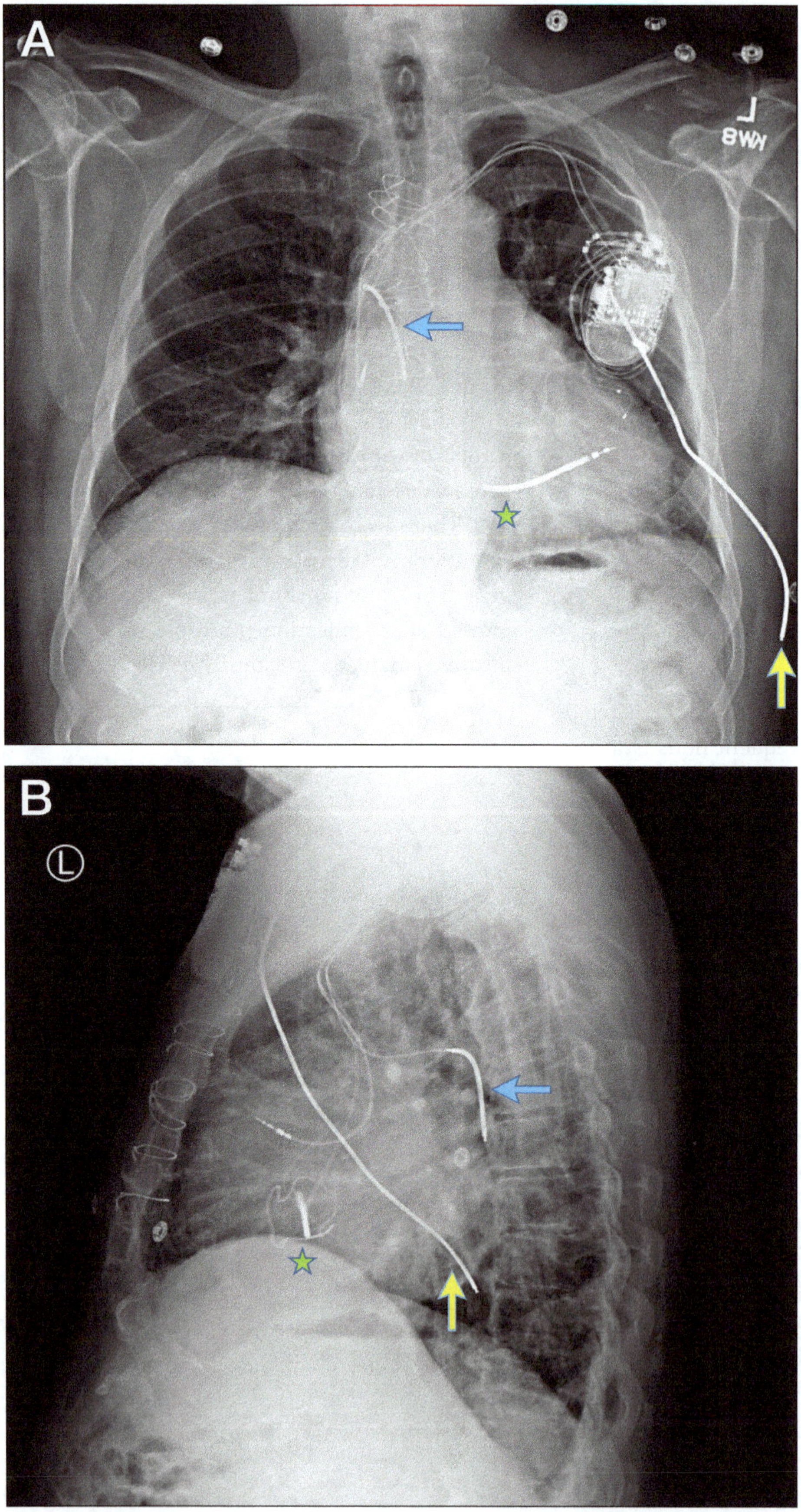

Figure 21.2 CXR AP view in **Panel A**; lateral view in **Panel B** of the patient showing various leads in the chest. Azygous lead (**blue arrow**) is posterior and closer to the spine, while the subcutaneous array courses over the lateral chest wall (**yellow arrow**). A single-coil defibrillator lead is seen through the bioprosthetic valve (**green star**).

PREPROCEDURAL PLANNING

The patient was evaluated by infectious disease, general surgery, and electrophysiology teams. All teams agreed that the clinical picture represented device infection and complete extraction of the device, leads, and the subcutaneous array would be in the patient's best interest. Antibiotics were held pending culture and microscopy from intraprocedural samples.

PROCEDURE DETAILS

A preprocedure huddle was performed with all involved teams in attendance. The patient was taken to the procedural suite and was prepped from the neck to the groin in a sterile manner. General anesthesia was administered, and a TEE probe was placed for monitoring during the procedure. Four units of cross-matched, packed red blood cells were available in the room for the procedure. Venous and arterial accesses were obtained using ultrasound guidance and modified Seldinger technique. A 20G left radial arterial line was placed for monitoring. A 7-Fr peel-away right internal jugular vein sheath was placed, through which a temporary active-fixation pacing lead was placed under fluoroscopic guidance. The exteriorized lead was sutured to the skin and connected to a backup pacing generator. A 12-Fr right common femoral vein sheath was placed to accommodate a stiff 0.035-inch wire and a Bridge Occlusion Balloon (Philips Medical). This was placed in the inferior vena cava after successful test inflation. A second 9-Fr sheath was placed in the right common femoral vein for high-volume crystalloid or blood product infusion. The prior scar was incised over the swollen and erythematous pocket, resulting in an expression of frank purulence. Swab samples were sent for microscopy and culture. Intravenous cefazolin was administered at this point. The leads required extensive dissection to be freed from adhesions and sewing sleeves. The focus was first turned to the azygous vein coil. This was easily explanted with simple traction alone. Attention was then turned to the RV apical ICD lead. After retracting the active fixation helix, a locking stylet (Lead Locking Device, EZ, Philips Medical) was passed into the lead lumen. A 14-Fr laser extraction sheath (GlideLight, Philips Medical) was advanced over the lead. A short burst of laser energy freed the lead at entry into the chest, after which the lead became mobile enough to allow removal. The subcutaneous array was prepared similarly with a regular stylet, and the same laser extraction sheath was advanced over it. The laser was activated, and the sheath was advanced to the mid-chest allowing the lead to be pulled free (**Video 21.1**). The RA lead was also approached with a locking stylet and the laser extraction sheath. With laser energy application for a short distance in the subclavian system, the lead came out with simple traction. Finally, the coronary sinus LV lead was targeted. A lock stylet was placed, and obvious adhesions were noted at the entry and SVC–RA junction site. Laser energy was required intermittently to advance the sheath through the subclavian vein and to the SVC–RA junction. At this point, the lead was able to be removed. No lead remnants were identified by fluoroscopy. Hemostasis was achieved with local pressure at the chest wall. General surgery joined the wound debridement procedure, irrigation, and placement of a vacuum-assisted wound closure device was applied to the incision site. TEE showed stable trivial tricuspid prosthetic valve regurgitation with no pericardial effusion.

POSTPROCEDURAL COURSE

The patient was extubated in the operating room and was transferred to the floor service. He returned to the operating room with general surgery on day 2 for additional wound washout and debridement. The vacuum suction device was removed on day 4, and the pocket was closed with nonabsorbable sutures. Blood cultures and wound cultures remained persistently negative. On day 6, the patient underwent uncomplicated implantation of a Medtronic Evera dual-chamber ICD system on the right side of the chest, and defibrillation threshold testing resulted in effective defibrillation at less than 25 Joules with a dual-coil RV endocardial ICD lead. There was no need to add a subcutaneous array electrode or azygous vein coil. The temporary pacemaker lead was removed at the time of permanent device implantation. The patient was empirically continued on a 2-week course of intravenous daptomycin. He remained infection-free during follow up.

SUMMARY POINTS

- Subcutaneous array electrodes can be challenging to extract due to fibrosis and adhesions in the subcutaneous tissue planes.
- A laser sheath was used to safely and successfully extract a subcutaneous array electrode. Similar principles apply for extraction of ICD leads with significant adhesions.
- Azygous vein ICD coils can be successfully extracted using tools and techniques similar to other transvenous leads.
- Although not an issue in the presented case, the azygous vein joins the posterior superior vena cava at an angle that may be an additional source of adhesions; additional care needs to be taken to keep mechanical and dilator sheaths coaxial with advancement at this site.
- Even if additional coils or arrays were required in the past, modern high-energy biphasic defibrillator systems may achieve acceptable defibrillation thresholds with an endocardial ICD lead alone.

VIDEO LEGEND

Video 21.1 Laser extraction sheath (GlideLight, Philips Medical) is advanced over the subcutaneous coil. The coil is eventually taken out of the tissue plane with traction. [00:02]

22 | Lead Extraction in a Patient with Prosthetic Valvular Endocarditis

Chin Lee, MD; Gordon Ho, MD; Ulrika Birgersdotter-Green, MD

CLINICAL VIGNETTE

A 41-year-old male with a history of a congenital atrioventricular (AV) block with pacemaker placement at birth and upgrade to cardiac resynchronization therapy with pacemaker (CRT-P) for pacing-induced cardiomyopathy, Bentall procedure with mechanical aortic valve replacement for severe aortic insufficiency, and who had a recent generator change, presented with methicillin-susceptible *Staphylococcus aureus* (MSSA) bacteremia. Since the generator change, he noted pocket fluctuance and pain. He developed a recurrent fever and underwent multiple courses of antibiotics for a pocket infection. As part of the cardiac implantable electronic device (CIED) infection workup, a transesophageal echocardiogram (TEE) revealed endocarditis of his prosthetic mechanical aortic valve with mobile vegetation and paravalvular abscess (**Figure 22.1**). Computed tomography (CT) angiography revealed a possible subaortic leak consistent with pseudoaneurysm (**Figure 22.2**). Given the CIED infection findings complicated by prosthetic mechanical valve endocarditis and paravalvular abscess, he was referred for cardiothoracic surgery evaluation. He was turned down for open surgery due to high reoperative risk. Prosthetic valve endocarditis is associated with increased morbidity and mortality. However, in selected patients, a similar rate of long-term freedom from endocarditis could be achieved by medical therapy alone (60%) compared to the surgically treated group (60%).[1] In another study by Huang et al. for patients with prosthetic valves who underwent lead extraction for infection (61% of patients had the lead and valve infection), 95% of patients who survived the infection (no death associated with the extraction procedure) had no evidence of recurrent device-related or valve-related infection.[2] After multidisciplinary team discussion, we decided to proceed with percutaneous lead extraction to decrease his infection burden with a goal of a prolonged course of antibiotic to medically manage the prosthetic valve endocarditis.

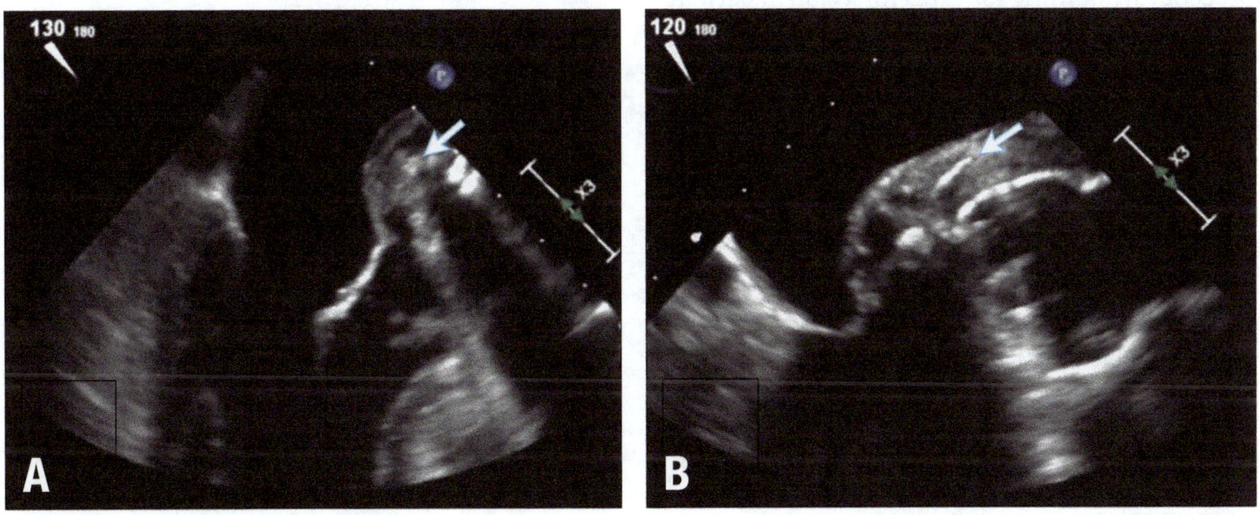

Figure 22.1 TTE revealed a mobile vegetation (0.75 × 0.5 cm) on the mechanical aortic valve and thickening around the aortic valve consistent with perivalvular abscess (**arrow**).

 Cardiotext Publishing. ISBN: 978-1-942909-54-5

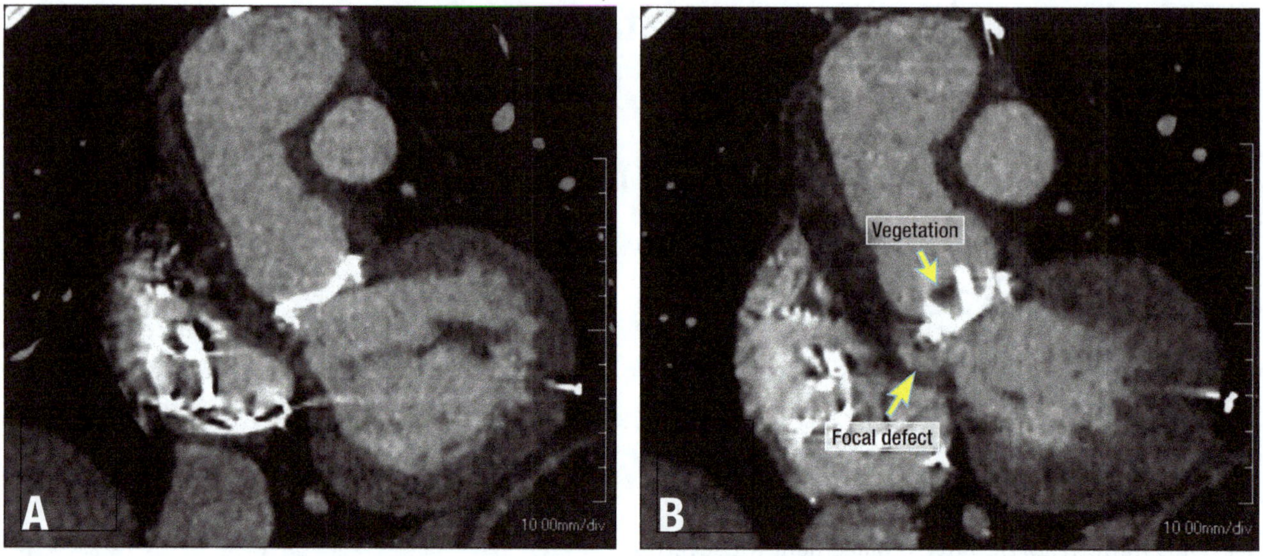

Figure 22.2 Contrast CT angiography showed paravalvular soft-tissue thickening along the aortic root concerning paravalvular abscess formation and graft infection. During the systolic phase, noted 1-cm focal defect along the subaortic left ventricular outflow tract's posterior margin, consistent with a pseudoaneurysm (**long arrow**). Area of low attenuation seen along the mechanical aortic valve leaflets during the cardiac cycle concerning vegetation (**short arrow**).

PREPROCEDURAL PLANNING

For complicated lead extraction, it is important to obtain prior procedural history. Our patient underwent epicardial pacemaker placement since birth via a subxiphoid approach and had multiple abdominal pacemaker generator surgeries throughout his childhood (**Figure 22.3**). Eventually, the device was converted to a prepectoral transvenous system in adulthood, and the epicardial lead was abandoned. A part of the preprocedural planning for CIED infection in patients with epicardial lead is to determine if there is evidence of infection (e.g., fluid collection, abscess) of the intrathoracic portion of the epicardial lead. If there is evidence of infection, then complete removal of the epicardial lead is currently recommended.[3] In patients with multiple thoracic/abdominal surgeries, patency of central access may be compromised, which could affect the prophylactic placement of a Bridge occlusion balloon in high-risk extraction cases for superior vena cava (SVC) tear, or placement of extracorporeal membrane oxygenation cannula if the need for support arises.

His preoperative chest X-ray (CXR) (**Figure 22.4**) revealed a CRT-P system with an abandoned right atrial (RA) lead.

Device Details

Device Component	Manufacturer/ Model	Age of Lead (years)
Subxiphoid amputated epicardial lead	unknown	41 (abandoned)
RA lead #1	Medtronic CapsureFix	18 (abandoned)
RV lead	Medtronic CapsureFix	18
RA lead #2	Medtronic CapsureFix	6
LV lead	Medtronic Attain Ability Straight (passive tines)	6

At our institute, we routinely perform CT angiography for preprocedural planning to evaluate vessel patency, lead-to-lead binding, and severe lead adhesion to vessel wall, which identified high-risk cases for major complication.[4] The patient's CT (**Video 22.1**) showed the abandoned RA and RV lead with fibrotic lead encapsulation bound to the vessel wall obstructing the brachiocephalic

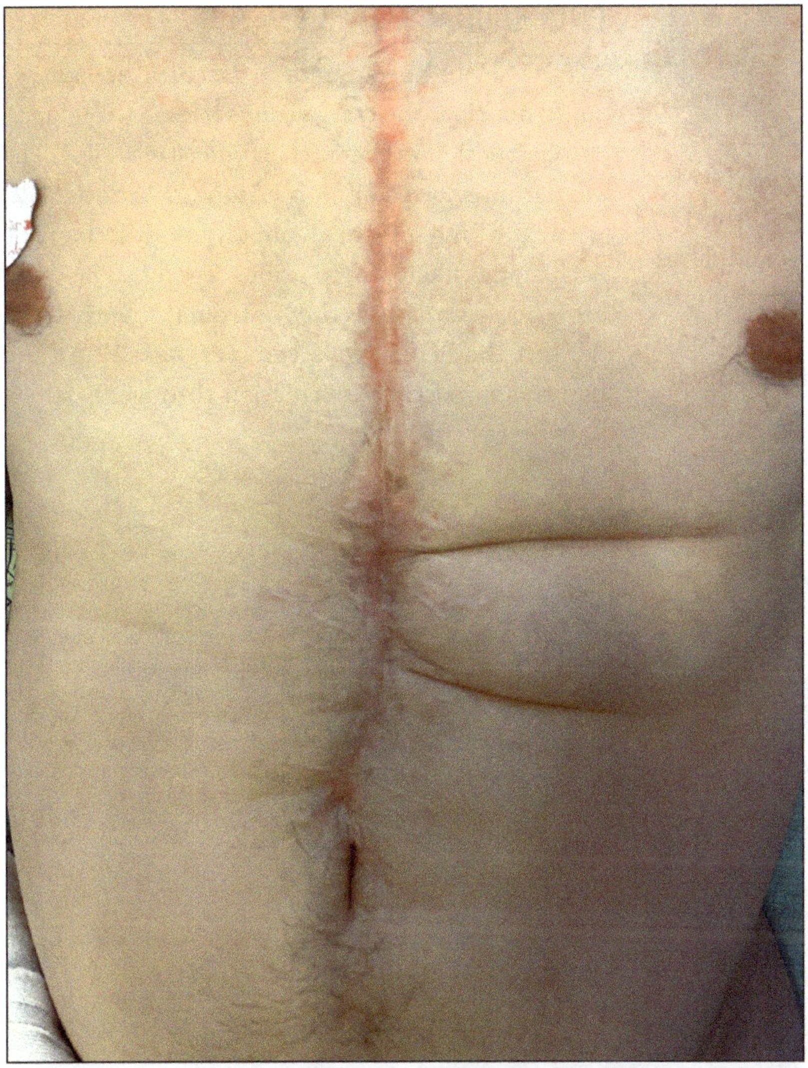

Figure 22.3 Abdominal surgical scars from the patient's prior epicardial pacemaker.

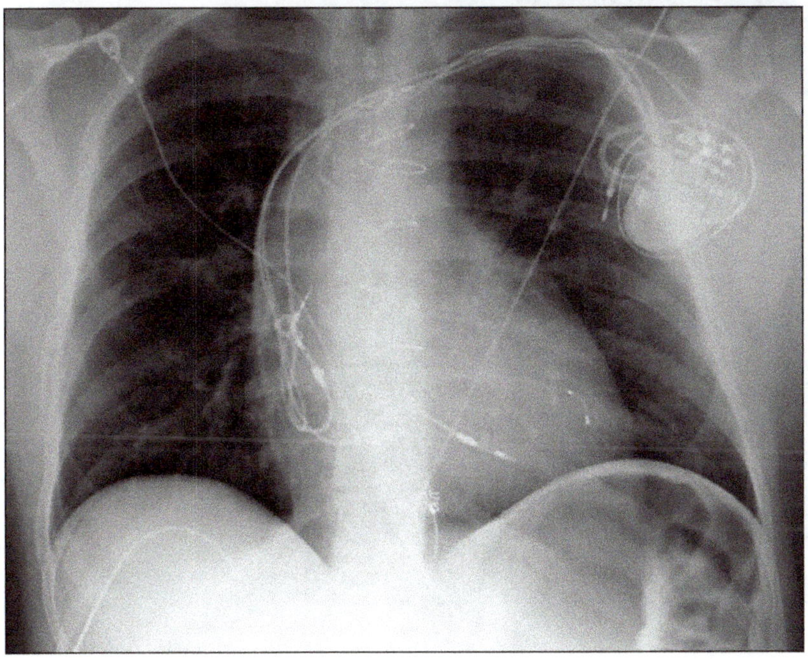

Figure 22.4 CXR revealed his CRT-P system and an abandoned right atrial pacemaker lead.

vein. The remaining leads had significant lead-to-lead binding within the SVC. Preprocedure TEE evaluation is recommended for CIED infection to evaluate for vegetation, valvular dysfunction, and perivalvular abscess, which guide therapy strategy (surgical versus percutaneous extraction).[3,5] Not all patients are suitable surgical candidates due to inherent surgical risk. After the multidisciplinary team discussion, we opted for chronic antibiotic therapy to medically manage his prosthetic valve endocarditis. At the same time, we decided to proceed with percutaneous lead extraction to decrease the nidus for infection.

PROCEDURAL DETAILS

After we obtained femoral vascular access, we could not float the transvenous pacing wire due to an obstruction in the inferior vena cava (IVC). The venogram showed IVC occlusion (**Video 22.2**) with a filling of the hemiazygos system. The occlusion is likely due to prior surgeries. The operators could not access the RA from IVC with glidewire in the hemiazygos vein (**Figure 22.5**) and had to approach the extraction through an alternate access site.

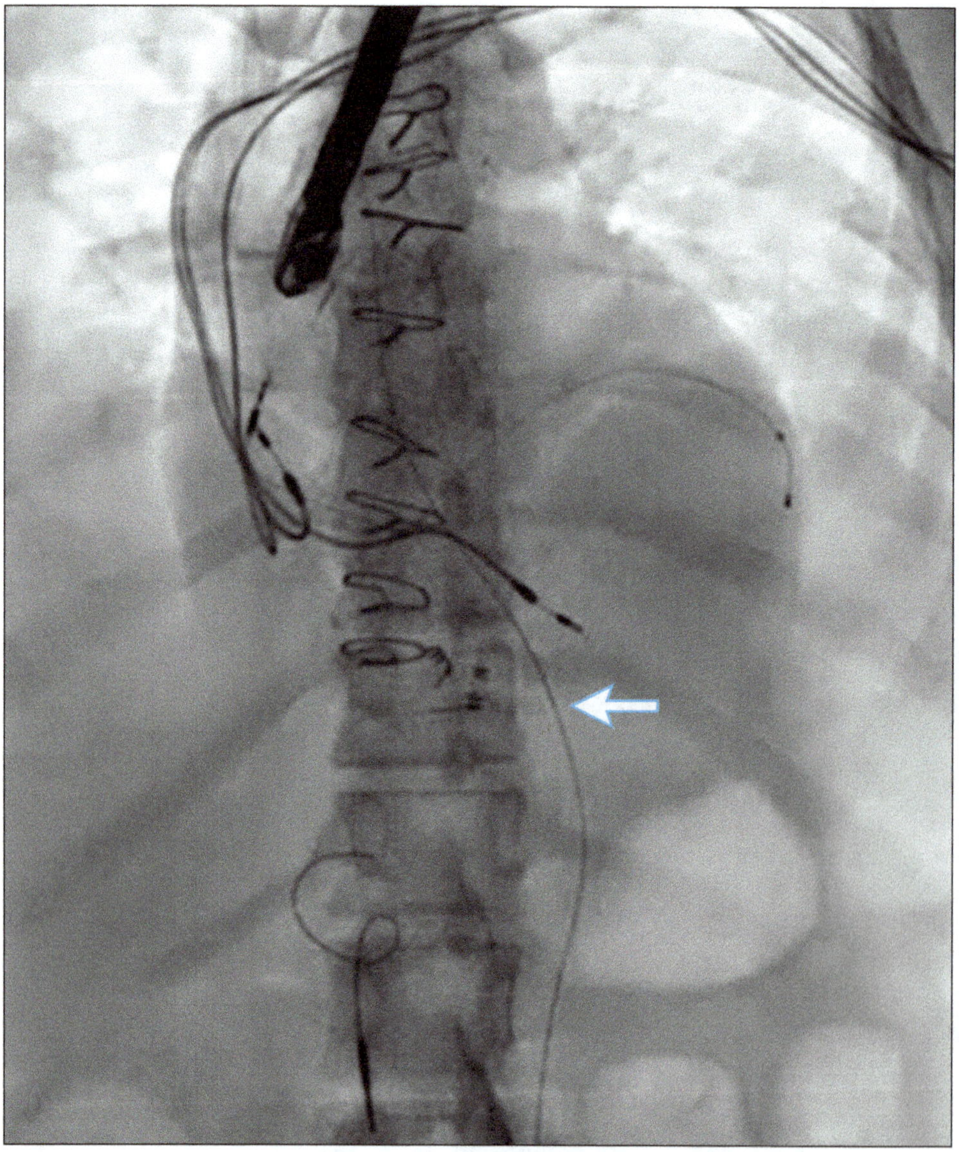

Figure 22.5 An attempt to pass the obstruction with glidewire was unable to access the right atrium. The glidewire is in the hemiazygos vein (**arrow**), which travels on the left side of the vertebral column and crosses the vertebral column before emptying to the azygos vein.

A temporary-permanent pacing lead through the right internal jugular vein was placed. We were concerned about using the right internal jugular vein access for the Bridge Occlusion Balloon because it may dislodge the temporary-permanent lead in a pacemaker dependent patient. Ideally, we would prefer to place the occlusion balloon via the left subclavian vein. However, we noted multiple leads attached to the brachiocephalic vein's posterior wall with significant lead-to-lead binding in the SVC from our preprocedure CT angiography. Thus, there was a concern for occlusion of the brachiocephalic vein that could prevent the occlusion balloon's passing over the wire. Therefore, we planned to remove one of the leads to provide a tract for us to place the occlusion balloon before extracting the remaining leads.

A straight stylet was inserted into the active fixation leads to attempting retracting the helix. Unfortunately, none of the helixes retracted. Next, we inserted Philips EZ locking stylet to the lead to provide stable traction along the lead length during extraction. A 14-Fr Philips laser sheath was used for extracting the coronary sinus (CS) lead. Using short bursts of laser energy, the laser sheath was advanced over the lead. Adhesions and lead-to-lead binding were encountered in the proximal brachiocephalic vein. Laser energy use was minimized at the brachiocephalic–SVC junction to prevent direct injury to this tenuous area. We often only use the inner laser sheath and outer sheath to perform blunt mechanical dissection around the junction. Operators must be cautious when maneuvering the outer sheath by maintaining the sharp bevel tip on the curve's inner side to prevent the vessel's laceration at all time. This successfully freed the binding site in the SVC, and the sheath was advanced to the RA. However, the CS lead remained trapped within the CS, and the locking stylet was starting to retract (**Figure 22.6**). We were unable to further advance the extraction sheath from its RA position without the risk of further retracting the locking stylet and losing distal lead support. When encountering a trapped lead, it may be due to lead-to-lead binding. We then switched the laser extraction sheath to the newer RA lead to free up the lead-to-lead binding, facilitating other leads' extraction. The minimal amount of laser energy was used when close to the brachiocephalic–SVC junction.

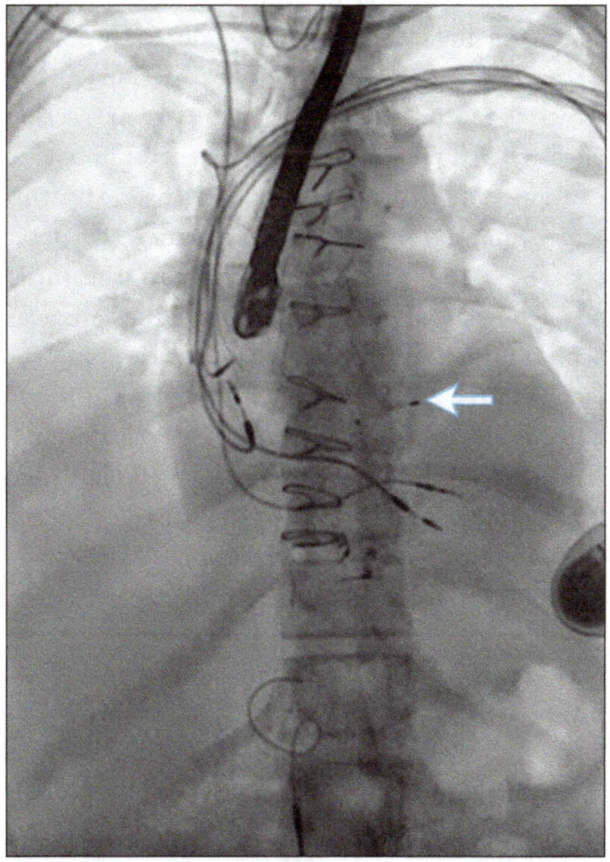

Figure 22.6 Outer extraction sheath freed up the adhesion for the Attain Ability Straight CS lead with passive tines near its distal tip (**arrow**). The lead remained trapped within the CS, and the locking stylet was starting to retract.

When near the junction, we freed up the binding site, including the lead-to-lead binding, using mainly blunt mechanical dissection with the inner laser and outer sheath. We were able to advance both the laser and outer sheath to the RA. Gentle downward traction was applied on the RA lead using the outer sheath but unable to free the RA lead from the right atrial appendage but had passed the CS lead's binding point (**Figure 22.7**). Next, we reloaded the CS lead. After freeing up the lead-to-lead binding, we could advance the extraction sheath to the RA without difficulty. The laser sheath was slowly advanced over the lead to the CS ostium. The outer sheath was then advanced to the CS ostium to provide support for the inner laser sheath. Then, blunt mechanical dissection using the laser sheath at the proximal CS near the lead tip passive tines freed the CS lead (**Figure 22.8**). We avoided using laser energy here due to the risk of CS perforation. We used 14-Fr extraction sheath, which is more flexible than the 16-Fr extraction sheath in tight curves. The extractor must be cautious when using the stiffer 16-Fr sheaths, which may not allow you to advance the outer sheath to the CS ostium to support the inner sheath. A large amount of tissue adhesions was seen on the lead tip contributing to trapping the lead (**Figure 22.9**). The CS lead's removal allowed the passing of a stiff wire and the occlusion balloon through the brachiocephalic vein (▶ **Video 22.3**A and 22.3B). Next, we reload the new RA lead, and gentle downward traction with the laser and outer sheath was used to dislodge the lead from the right atrial appendage (**Figure 22.10**). Next, we load the RV lead for extraction. There was significant lead-to-lead binding that was cleared with laser energy and outer sheath. We had to switch between the abandoned RA and RV lead to pass some of these binding sites. Due to "snowplowing" at the SVC area, we had to upsize to a 16-Fr laser sheath. This allowed the passing of the laser sheath into the RV. Extreme caution was taken to avoid laser energy near the lead tip because of perforation risk. When the lead tip-myocardium interface was reached, countertraction against the myocardium was applied using the laser sheath while gentle traction was applied on the locking stylet, without invaginate the ventricle, until the RV lead was freed from the myocardium (▶ **Video 22.4**). Then, we proceed with extracting the remaining RA lead successfully (**Figure 22.11**). Examining the extracted RA and RV lead showed a significant amount of adhesion at the lead tip and brachiocephalic–SVC junction (**Figure 22.12**).

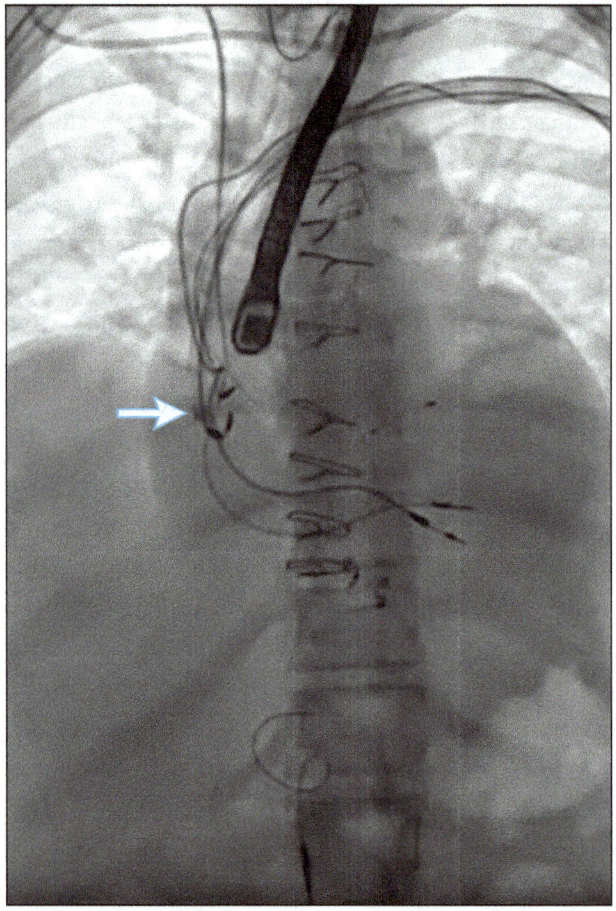

Figure 22.7 Attempt extraction of the newer RA lead to free up the lead-to-lead binding. Gentle downward traction was applied with the outer sheath (**arrow**) but unable to free the RA lead from the right atrial appendage.

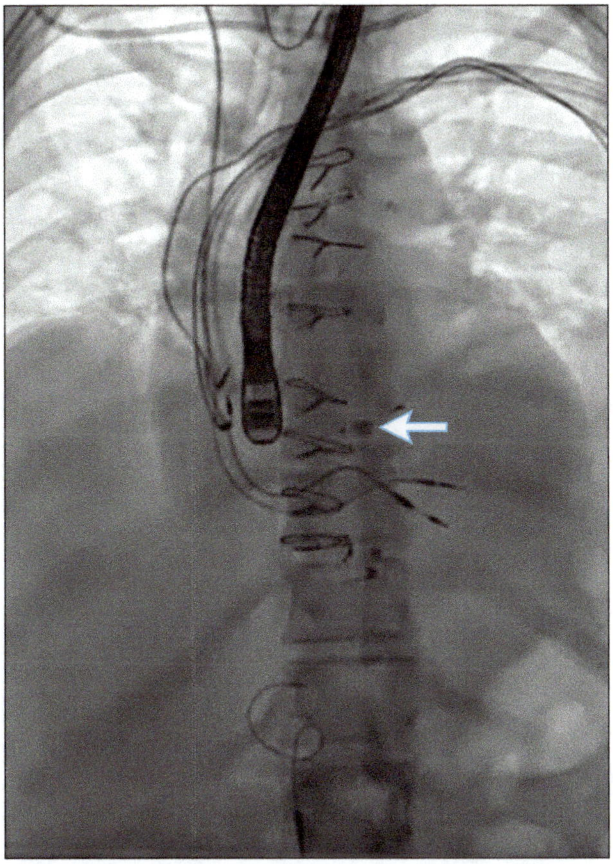

Figure 22.8 After freeing up lead-to-lead binding on the RA lead, we could advance our outer sheath (**arrow**) on the CS lead further to the CS ostium. Blunt dissection with the laser sheath was successful in freeing the CS lead.

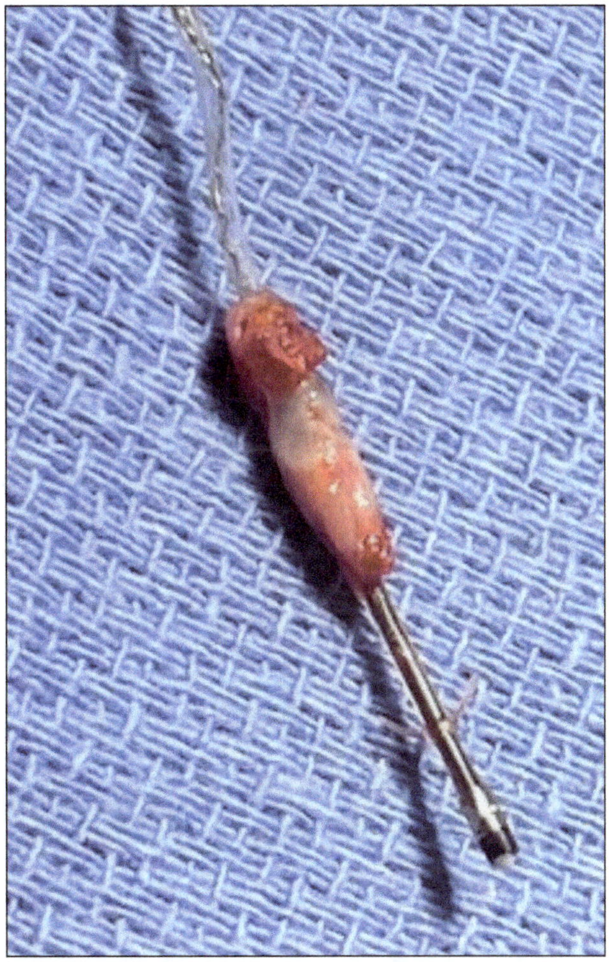

Figure 22.9 Medtronic Attain Stability Straight Lead with passive tines extracted from the patient. Noted the large amount of tissue adhesions that trapped the CS lead.

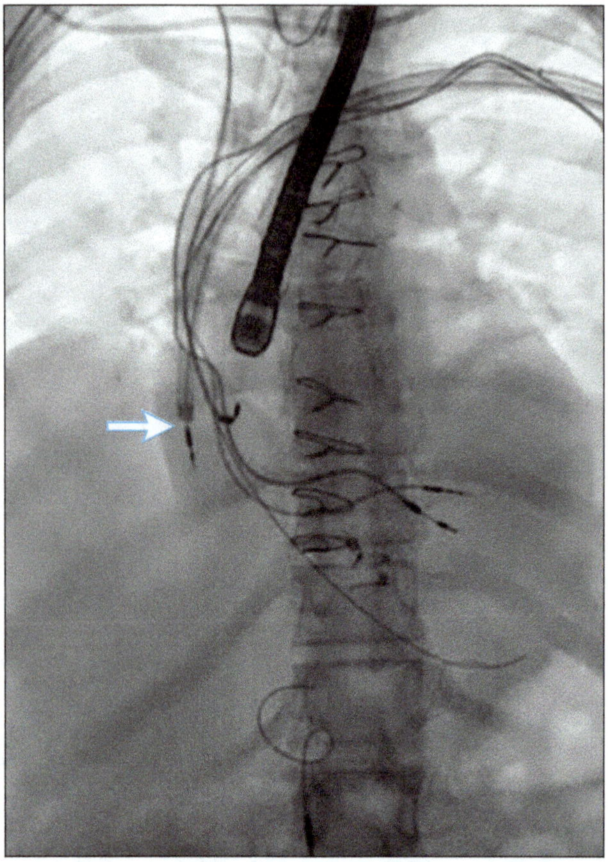

Figure 22.10 Gentle downward traction with the laser and outer sheath (**arrow**) was used to dislodge the RA lead from the right atrial appendage.

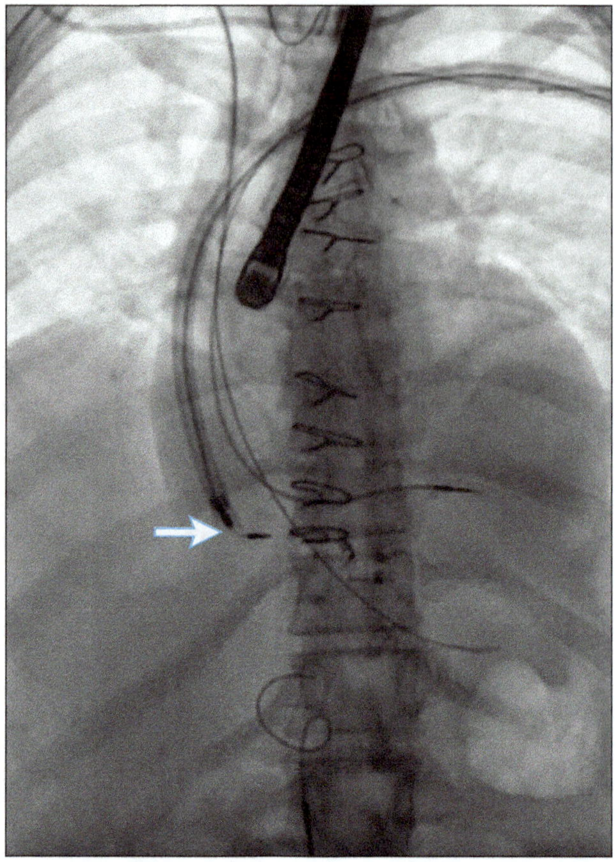

Figure 22.11 The extraction sheath (**arrow**) was used to create downward traction on the lead toward the IVC to dislodge the lead from the right atrial appendage.

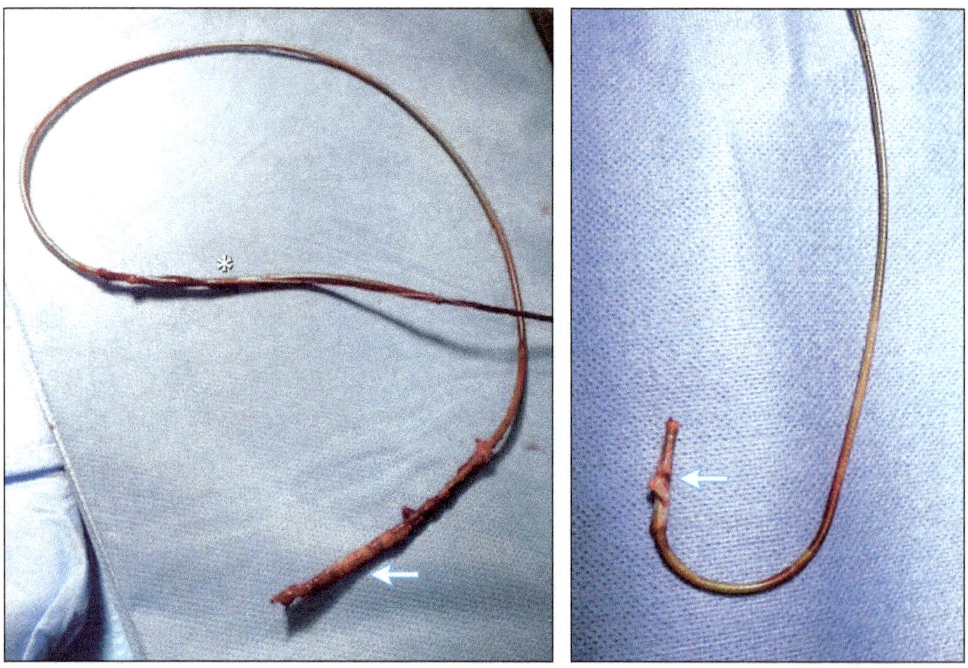

Figure 22.12 Extracted RV and RA leads show a significant amount of adhesions at the lead tip (**arrows**) and near the brachiocephalic vein–SVC junction (*).

POSTPROCEDURAL FOLLOW-UP

A follow-up echocardiogram showed stable prosthetic valve position with mild, paravalvular regurgitation. The patient completed 8 weeks of intravenous antibiotics and started on long-term oral suppressive antibiotic therapy. He cleared the MSSA bacteremia with negative blood cultures 2 days after CIED extraction. After he completed the intravenous antibiotics, the right internal jugular vein temporary-permanent pacemaker was removed, and a new CRT-P system was implanted. The patient remained stable and doing well at 5 months follow-up. Although leadless pacemaker has been associated with low device-related infection[6] and successfully used in patients with prior CIED infection,[7] we decided to reimplant a CRT-P because of high RV pacing requirements pacing-induced cardiomyopathy. Given that the patient had cleared the bacteremia and chronic suppressive antibiotic therapy, the CIED infection risk should be lower.

Percutaneous lead extraction is preferred over open surgical extractions due to significantly reduced morbidity for patients.[2,8] Open extractions are favored in patients with high-risk transcutaneous extractions, large lead masses (> 2.5 cm), or who have open-heart surgery needs, such as severe valvular insufficiency or endocarditis-associated valvular dysfunction requiring surgical repair.[3] Our patient was not a candidate for open extraction due to prohibitive surgical risk. Percutaneous extraction was performed to reduce the infection burden with a plan for chronic suppressive antibiotic therapy.

SUMMARY POINTS

- Percutaneous lead extraction is preferred over open surgical extractions except in cases with indication for open heart surgery.
- Preprocedure CT angiography could help risk stratify patient and identify potential high-risk area during extraction (severe lead adhesion within the vessel).
- When encountering a trapped lead during extraction, it may be due to lead-to-lead binding. Switching your extraction to a different lead can often free up the lead-to-lead binding and facilitate extraction of other leads.
- Blunt dissection at the lead tip is critical to avoid vascular or myocardial tear.
- In case with complete IVC occlusion, placement of a Bridge occlusion balloon above the SVC from the subclavian or internal jugular vein can be attempted.

REFERENCES

1. Akowuah EF, Davies W, Oliver S, Stephens J, Riaz I, Zadik P, Cooper G. Prosthetic valve endocarditis: Early and late outcome following medical or surgical treatment. *Heart*. 2003;89:269–272.
2. Huang X-M, Fu H-X, Zhong L, et al. Outcomes of transvenous lead extraction for cardiovascular implantable electronic device infections in patients with prosthetic heart valves. *Circ Arrhythm Electrophysiol*. 2016;9.
3. Kusumoto FM, Schoenfeld MH, Wilkoff BL, et al. 2017 HRS expert consensus statement on cardiovascular implantable electronic device lead management and extraction. *Heart Rhythm*. 2017;14:e503–e551.
4. Svennberg E, Jacobs K, McVeigh E, Pretorius V, Birgersdotter-Green U. Computed tomography–guided risk assessment in percutaneous lead extraction. *J Am Coll Cardiol EP*. 2019;5: 1439–1446.

5. European Heart Rhythm Association (EHRA) international consensus document on how to prevent, diagnose, and treat cardiac implantable electronic device infections—endorsed by the Heart Rhythm Society (HRS), the Asia Pacific Heart Rhythm Society (APHRS), the Latin American Heart Rhythm Society (LAHRS), International Society for Cardiovascular Infectious Diseases (ISCVID) and the European Society of Clinical Microbiology and Infectious Diseases (ESCMID) in collaboration with the European Association for Cardio-Thoracic Surgery (EACTS). *EP Europace* 2020;22(4):515–549. Available from: https://academic.oup.com/europace/article/22/4/515/5614580
6. El-Chami MF, Soejima K, Piccini JP, et al. Incidence and outcomes of systemic infections in patients with leadless pacemakers: Data from the Micra IDE study. *Pacing Clin Electrophysiol.* 2019;42:1105–1110.
7. Beurskens NEG, Tjong FVY, Dasselaar KJ, Kuijt WJ, Wilde AAM, Knops RE. Leadless pacemaker implantation after explantation of infected conventional pacemaker systems: A viable solution? *Heart Rhythm*. 2019;16:66–71.
8. Patel D, Khan F, Shah H, Bhattacharya S, Adelstein E, Saba S. Cardiac implantable electronic device lead extraction in patients with underlying infection using open thoracotomy or percutaneous techniques. *Cardiol J.* 2015;22:68–74.

VIDEO LEGENDS

Video 22.1 CT angiography cine showing the brachiocephalic vein obstruction due to lead adhesion. [00:01]

Video 22.2 Left femoral venogram showing occlusion at the IVC with contrast filling of the hemiazygos system (arrow). The amputated epicardial lead was seen in this view. Left femoral venogram shows complete obstruction at the IVC. [00:09]

Video 22.3 Videos 22.3A and 22.3B show the CS lead removal allowed the passing of a stiff wire and the occlusion balloon through the brachiocephalic vein. The occlusion balloon was deployed in the SVC–RA junction through the brachiocephalic vein. [00:12] [00:01]

Video 22.4 Countertraction was applied on the RV lead at the lead tip-myocardium interface and freed the lead from the myocardium. [00:11]

23 | A Patient with Congenital Atrioventricular Block and Severe Tricuspid Valve Regurgitation

Roshan Karki, MD; Siva K. Mulpuru MD, MPH

CLINICAL VIGNETTE

A 28-year-old female with a permanent pacemaker and symptomatic severe tricuspid valve regurgitation (TR) was referred to our institution for lead extraction and tricuspid valve surgery.

Her cardiovascular history was significant for congenital complete atrioventricular (AV) block for which she underwent implantation of a pacing device at the age of 5 years. She has had multiple prior revisions, and the most recent device components (**Figure 23.1**) are summarized below.

She was first seen at our institution in the context of hemolytic uremic syndrome requiring hemodialysis in February 2018. She had biventricular failure with reduced left ventricular (LV) ejection fraction of 23% and moderate-to-severe right ventricular (RV) enlargement. In addition, she had severe TR (**Video 23.1**) with incomplete coaptation of the tricuspid valve leaflets and impingement of the RV pacemaker leads on the septal leaflet. With guideline-directed medical therapy, LV size and systolic function improved; however, severe TR remained unchanged. Over the next 2 years, she had progressive increase in fatigue and exertional dyspnea (NYHA class II-III). Therefore, the decision was made to extract the old leads, repair the incompetent tricuspid valve, and implant a new pacing system.

PREPROCEDURAL PLANNING

The patient had a multidisciplinary evaluation by cardiac electrophysiology, heart failure cardiology, cardiothoracic surgery, and anesthesia teams. The patient underwent routine laboratory tests, transthoracic echocardiography (TTE), chest radiography, and cardiac computed tomography (CT). The TTE showed calcific encapsulation of an RV lead on the tricuspid valve (**Video 23.2**) causing entrapment of the septal leaflet. CT of the chest showed significant calcification at different points along the course of the leads. (**Video 23.3**) There was significant calcification around the leads at the innominate vein–SVC junction. One RV lead had extensive calcified encapsulation in the right atrium, protruded slightly into the inferior vena cava (IVC) with increased calcification at the RA–IVC junction, and went up over the tricuspid valve annulus, where it is encapsulated with a large calcified mass (see Figure 23.1 and Video 23.3). The other RV lead had calcification at the level of right atrium as well. Given the need for tricuspid valve surgery, the decision was made to proceed with hybrid surgery-assisted percutaneous transvenous lead extraction (TLE) and tricuspid valve surgery. Since her underlying rhythm was complete heart block and junctional escape rhythm, the patient would also require a new

Device Details

Device and Leads	Manufacturer/Model	Date of Implant	Location
Pulse generator	St. Jude Medical 2240 Assurity	10/2017	Left upper chest
Right atrial (RA) lead	St. Jude Medical 1999 OptiSense	10/2017	Right atrial appendage
Right ventricular (RV) lead	Pacesetter 1358C AV Plus DX	08/2006	Right ventricular apex
Right ventricular (RV) lead	Pacesetter 1358C AV Plus DX	Unknown	High right ventricular septum
Epicardial RV lead × 2	Unknown	Unknown	Abandoned
Epicardial RA lead	Unknown	Unknown	Abandoned

 Cardiotext Publishing. ISBN: 978-1-942909-54-5

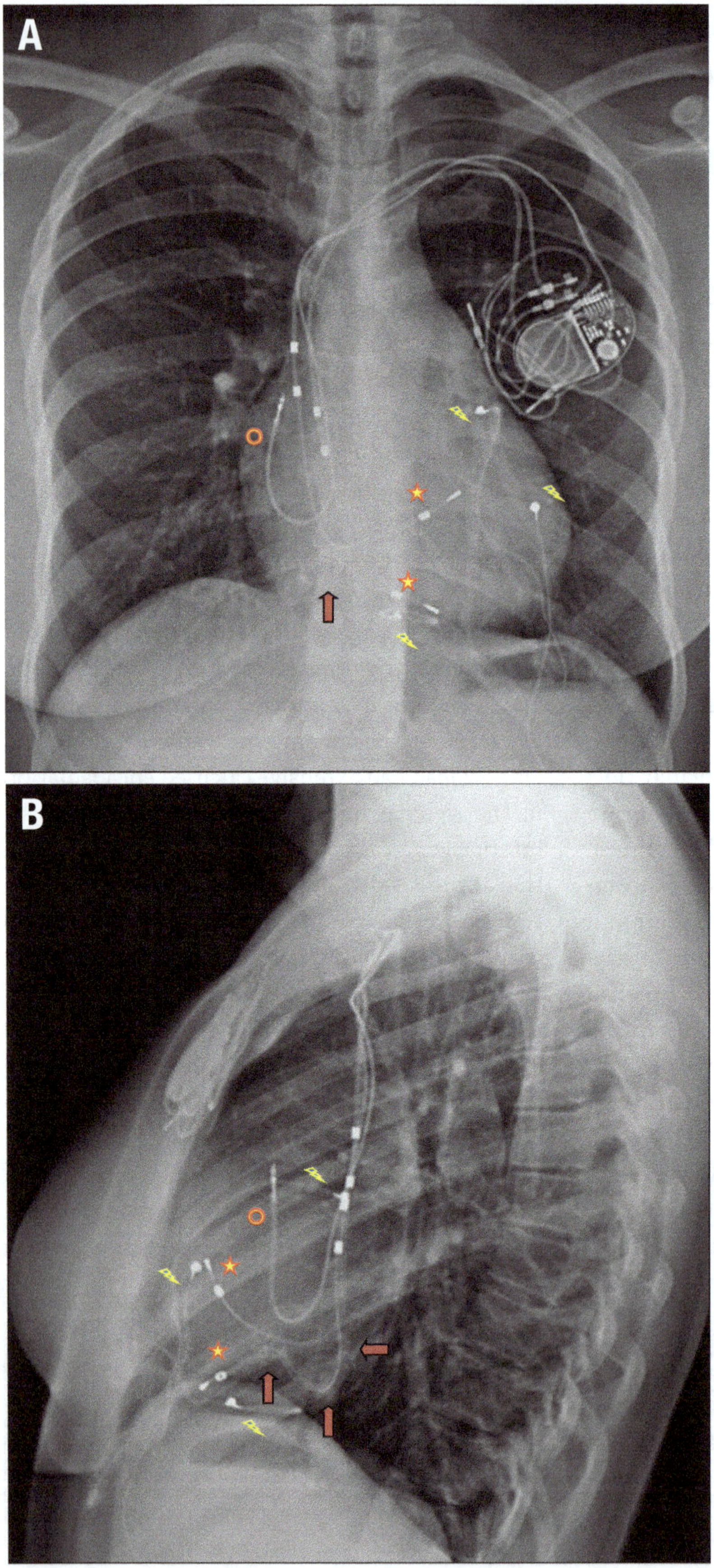

Figure 23.1 Preextraction CXR, postero-anterior view (**Panel A**) and lateral view (**Panel B**). There are 1 active fixation right atrial lead (**yellow donut with red border**), 2 passive fixation endocardial right ventricular leads (**yellow star with red border**), and 3 (1 atrial and 2 ventricular) abandoned epicardial leads (**blue flash with yellow border**). Note the course of the right ventricular lead that protrudes from the right atrium into the inferior vena cava (IVC) and turns over the tricuspid valve annulus to the inferior right ventricle. There are sizable calcifications encapsulating the lead at the tissue-lead interfaces (**red arrows with black border**). The right atrial and the second RV lead appears be on the lateral border of the superior vena cava (SVC). The pulse generator has two connector pins connector to the header. There are 3 connector pins abandoned in the pocket.

pacing system, for which an epicardial system was considered. The arrangement for 4 units of cross-matched, packed red blood cells was requested.

PROCEDURAL DETAILS

The patient underwent general anesthesia and was prepped and draped in the usual sterile fashion. A transesophageal echocardiography (TEE) probe was advanced and baseline images were obtained (▶ **Video 23.4**). After prophylactic intravenous cefazolin was administered, arterial and venous accesses were obtained under ultrasound guidance. The cardiothoracic surgical team began the procedure with sternotomy. The pleural cavities were opened on either side, and temporary epicardial right ventricular pacing wires were placed and connected to a backup pacing generator.

The cardiac electrophysiology team took over at this point. A skin incision was made in the left infraclavicular chest over the pacemaker pocket. The capsule was opened and the pulse generator was taken out. The leads were then disconnected from the pulse generator. Careful dissection was performed to free the leads with initial plan to salvage the RA lead. However, the decision was modified to extract all the transvenous leads because of disruption of the RA lead insulation.

A regular stylet was advanced into the RA lead as distal as possible, and the screw was successfully retracted. However, application of gentle traction did not free up the RA lead at the tip. The RA lead connector was cut off, a Liberator Beacon Tip locking stylet (Cook Medical) was advanced through the inner lumen as distally as possible, and the locking mechanism deployed. To avoid bunching of the insulation, a 2-0 Prolene suture (Ethicon Inc.) was tied distally at the cut end of the lead with lock stitch applied at the loop handle of the locking stylet. A 9-Fr TightRail rotating dilator sheath (Philips Medical) was slowly advanced over the RA lead down to left branchiocephalic–SVC junction. At that point, the lead was freed up, pulled into the sheath and removed in totality.

Then, we attempted extraction of the RV leads. The locking stylet could not be passed distally into the tip of the lead. Therefore, a Bulldog lead extender (Cook Medical) was used to crimp the insulation and conductor cables individually of both the RV leads. A gentle pull of the RV leads failed to release the tip of the passive fixation leads. An 11-Fr TightRail rotating dilator sheath was advanced over the RV lead. The mechanical sheath could not be advanced past the left clavicle (▶ **Video 23.5**). Instead, an 11-Fr Excimer laser sheath (Philips Medical) was advanced over the RV lead, short bursts of laser was applied to break the adhesions while traction-countertraction forces were applied, and the lead was eventually freed down to the right atrium (▶ **Video 23.6**). The second RV lead was also freed down to the right atrium (▶ **Video 23.7**) by a similar method to that described for the first RV lead.

After this, the cardiothoracic surgical team took over, cardiopulmonary bypass was initiated and right atriotomy was performed. The IVC was opened, but there was a large, hard mass at the RA–IVC junction interfering with IVC cannulation. The IVC cannula was eventually placed in a retrograde fashion via the right femoral vein cut-down. A portion of RV lead was protruding into the IVC, coming back to the right atrium and then crossing the tricuspid valve in the commissure between the septal and the posterior leaflet where there was a 1.5-cm to 2-cm circumferential mass of calcium (▶ **Video 23.8**). The atrial portion of the RV leads were surrounded by calcium and incorporated into the myocardial wall. In the right ventricle, one lead was attached to the septum and the other to the inferior wall. Attempt was made to break the calcified mass over the lead attachment. However, it was not safe to remove the entirety of the lead without potentially causing a significant risk of damage to tricuspid annulus, tricuspid valve, and the RV myocardium (▶ **Video 23.9**). Therefore, the RV leads were transected flush with the RV myocardium. The leads were divided, the distal end pulled through the SVC, and the proximal end pulled through the pacemaker pocket. The mechanism of the TR was felt to be a combination of tricuspid annular dilatation, mass of calcium in the commissure between the septal and posterior leaflets, and some prolapse of the anterior leaflet.

The tricuspid valve was initially repaired with a 26-mm Contour 3D annuloplasty ring (Medtronic), but optimal repair could not be achieved. Subsequent annuloplasty was successfully performed using a 28-mm CarboMedics band (CarboMedics Inc.), reducing the tricuspid regurgitation to only mild degree (**Video 23.10**). The right atriotomy and IVC were closed, and the patient weaned off from the bypass. Then, two bipolar suture-on drug-eluting epicardial leads (Medtronic 4968 CapSure Epi) were placed on the anterior wall of the right ventricle (**Figure 23.2**) and one bipolar suture-on drug-eluting epicardial lead (Medtronic 4968 CapSure Epi) over the right atrium. The leads were then tunneled across the anterior chest wall into the left infraclavicular subcutaneous pocket. Two leads (1 RA and 1 RV) were interfaced with a pulse generator (Boston Scientific L121 Essentio EL) and the second RV epicardial lead was capped. Primary closure of the both the sternotomy incision and the pacemaker pocket was then performed. The final device components are shown in the postoperative chest X-ray (CXR) in **Figure 23.3**.

POSTPROCEDURAL CLINICAL COURSE

The patient's postoperative course was uneventful. The TTE showed residual mild tricuspid regurgitation. She was discharged on the fifth postoperative day. Since discharge, she has been doing well with improvement of exertional dyspnea. She is currently undergoing cardiac rehabilitation.

DISCUSSION

TR has been increasingly recognized in a small proportion of patients who undergo implantation of transvenous RV pacing or defibrillator lead(s).[1] Lead-related TR can be associated with significant morbidity and increased mortality.[1] Lead-related TR can result acutely from leaflet perforation, laceration, or avulsion of papillary muscles. Other mechanism includes mechanical interference of the tricuspid valve leaflets mobility and coaptation by lead impingement or entrapment. In the long term, connective tissue sheath will form at the tissue–lead interface and may extend throughout the endovascular course of the lead. Such fibrotic encapsulation of the lead can be calcified over time in a significant proportion of the

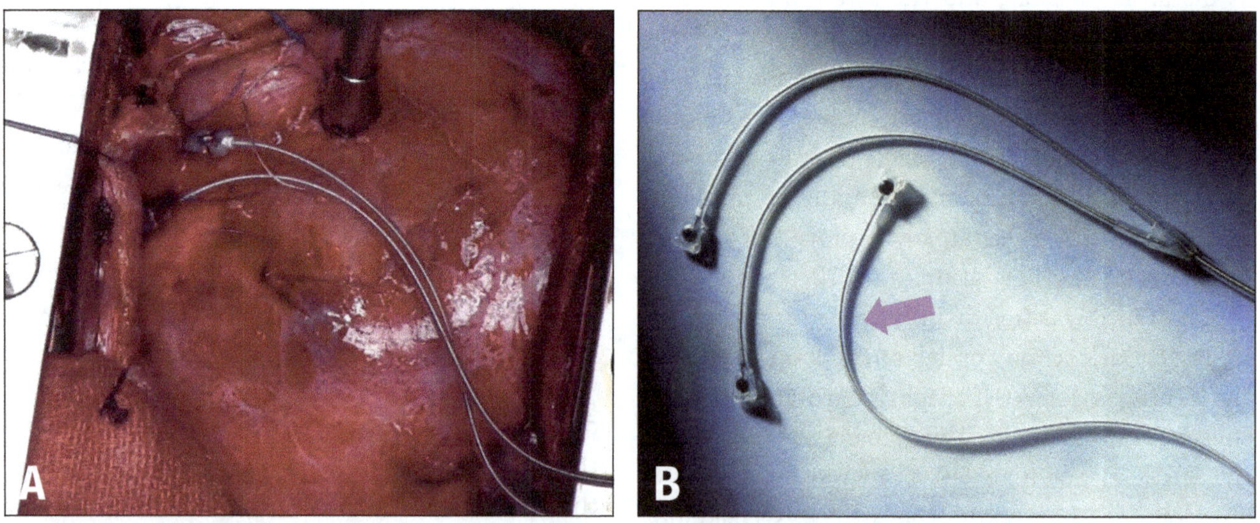

Figure 23.2 Epicardial lead implantation. **Panel A:** Intraoperative view of a bipolar suture-on steroid-eluting ventricular epicardial lead sutured on to the epicardium. **Panel B:** Medtronic Capsure 4968 bipolar (**pink arrow**) and unipolar suture-on pacing leads.

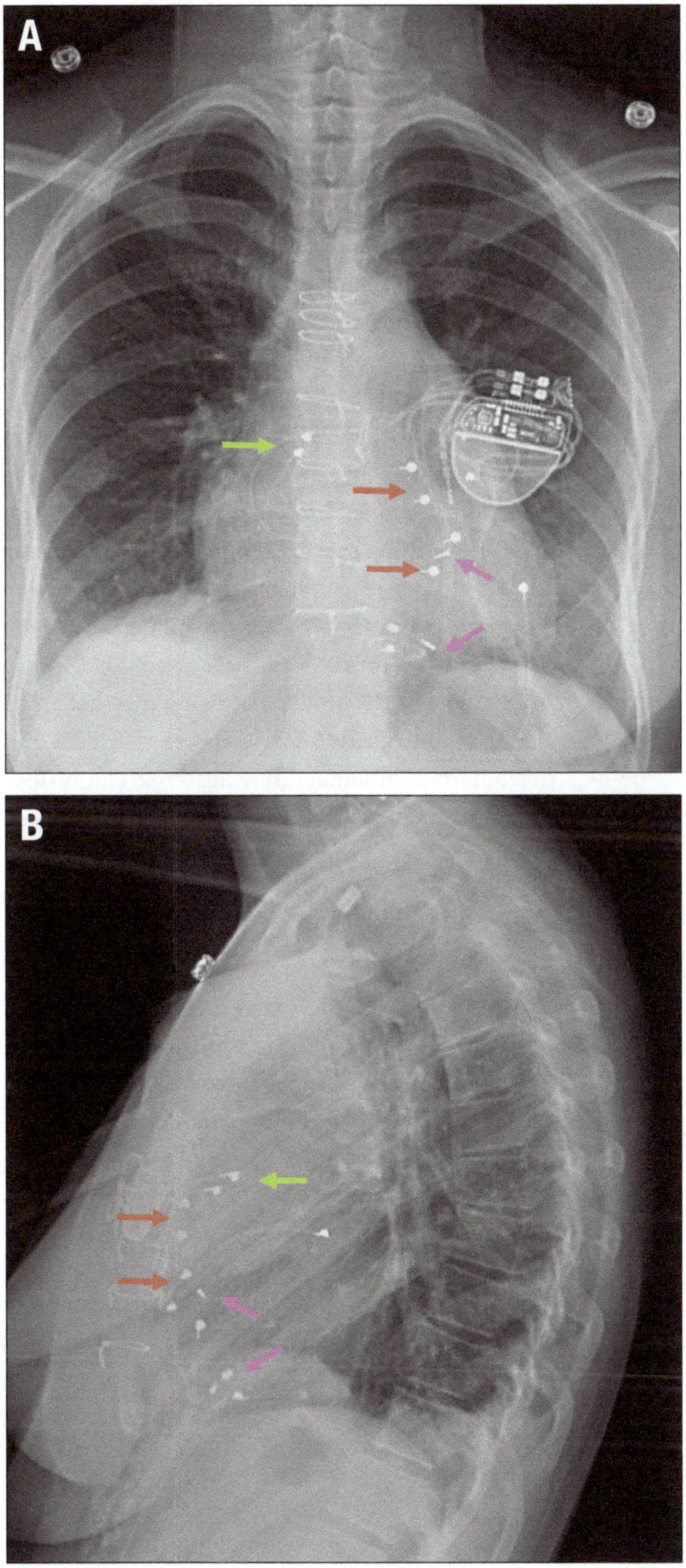

Figure 23.3 Postprocedure CXR, posteroanterior view (**Panel A**) and lateral view (**Panel B**). The **purple arrows** show abandoned tip of the RV lead that was cut flush with the myocardium. The **red arrows** indicate 2 newly implanted bipolar epicardial ventricular leads and the **green arrows** indicate one bipolar epicardial atrial lead. The previously abandoned epicardial leads are also seen but not labeled (see Figure 23.1).

patients.[2] The exact causes of calcification remain to be elucidated with certainty but putative mechanisms include (1) hypoxia of encapsulating tissue, leading to osseous differentiation, and (2) foreign body giant cell reaction to insulation (silicone or polyether polyurethane) breakdown.[2,3]

While right atriotomy routinely performed during tricuspid valve surgery provides reasonable access to RA and RV, fairly extensive surgery may be required to break fibrotic and calcific adhesions in the left subclavian vein, the innominate vein and the SVC. Percutaneous extraction using laser and/or mechanical sheaths can help avoid such extensive procedure. However, it may not be possible to break the calcified encapsulation of the lead on the tricuspid valve with percutaneous extraction techniques without causing significant damage to the valve. In addition, there are no tools currently available for safe percutaneous transection of the lead that would be theoretically tricuspid valve sparing. The resultant loss of structural integrity of the tricuspid valve would preclude tricuspid valve repair that would be preferred in a young patient to replacement with tissue valve or mechanical prosthesis. The solution to this complex problem would be a hybrid procedure with combined percutaneous transvenous extraction of the lead down to the RA and surgical extraction of rest of the lead, as demonstrated with our case.

Hybrid transvenous and surgical extraction techniques have been previously described.[4-6] The common reasons cited for hybrid extraction are (1) prevention of pulmonary embolism in patients with large lead thrombus or vegetation[5]; (2) complete removal of the fractured or abandoned leads[5]; (3) failed prior extraction[5]; and (4) extravascular lead (e.g. right atrial lead perforating into the pericardial space).[4] In patients with concomitant CIED infection and severe valvular endocarditis requiring surgery, hybrid extraction procedure has been reported.[6] In our institution, we usually perform extraction and valve surgery in a staged manner. The need for type of surgical approach minimally invasive right thoracotomy versus median sternotomy and need for cardiac bypass depends on case-by-case basis.

The hybrid procedure also offers additional benefit—an opportunity to implant an epicardial pacing system. Although an epicardial pacing system is an attractive option, it is not without issues. The epicardial leads tend to fail over time due to fibrosis at the lead tip causing progressive rise of pacing threshold and disruption of lead integrity due to mechanical trauma. The suture-on (Capsure 4968, Medtronic) epicardial leads have steroid-eluting tip to circumvent the problem of rising threshold. The screw-in (Myodex 1084T, Abbott) lead does not have steroid elution. A screw-in steroid elution lead is commercially available in Europe. Burger et al.[7] compared these lead designs and demonstrated similar performance and durability at 24 months after implantation. The alternative options of ventricular pacing in patients with a desire to avoid crossing the tricuspid valve include leadless AV pacemaker (Micra AV, Medtronic) and placing a lead through the coronary sinus.

If an epicardial system is not desired or feasible, alternatives for sparing the tricuspid valve include: (1) percutaneous implantation of a transvenous lead in the anterior interventricular or middle cardiac vein (CV) (**Figure 23.4**), and (2) surgical placement of transmyocardial leads (**Figure 23.5**).

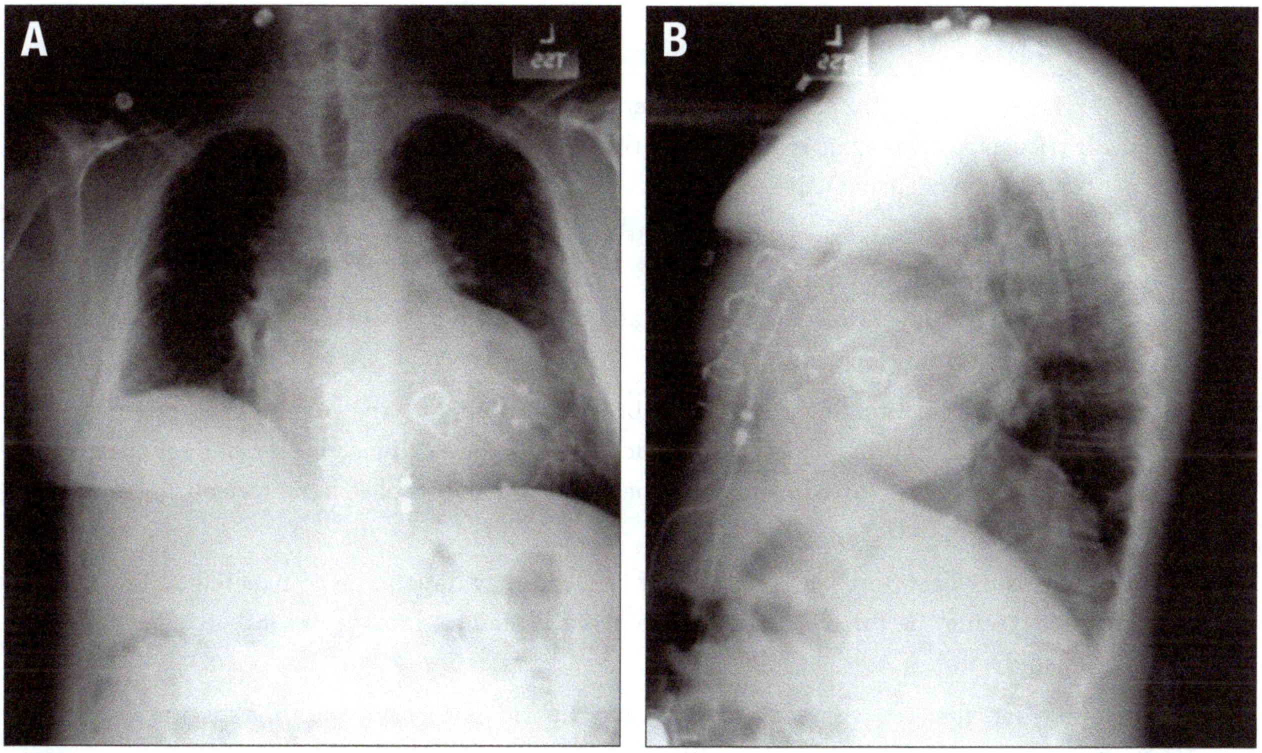

Figure 23.4 Images of CXRs (**Panels A** and **B**).

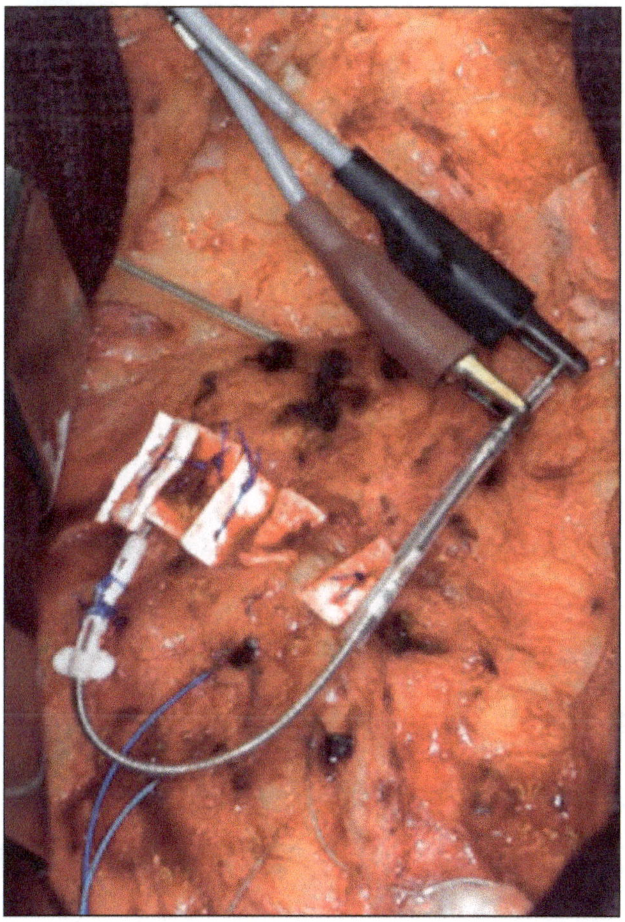

Figure 23.5 Intraoperative view of a trans-myocardial lead implanted in the right ventricle from a different case.

SUMMARY POINTS

- Lead-related TR needs tricuspid valve surgery (repair or replacement) if severe and symptomatic. If tricuspid valve repair is considered, the patient will require extraction of the RV lead(s) that traverse the tricuspid valve.
- Hybrid percutaneous and surgical approach to lead extraction should be considered in patients who undergo combined lead extraction and tricuspid valve surgery. The lead extractor can free up the leads using laser and mechanical sheaths down to the RA and surgeon removes rest of the leads.
- Percutaneous extraction of the leads may be complicated, and the current tools are not effective in cutting through significant calcification around the leads especially if encapsulated near a vital structure. In addition, there is no current tool to percutaneously transect a lead in a safe manner.
- Even with surgical approach, a portion of the lead may have to be transected and left behind if freeing the calcified lead can potentially lead to damage of vital structures such as tricuspid valve.
- In appropriate patients who undergo surgical or hybrid extraction, epicardial pacing system with steroid eluting leads should be considered.

REFERENCES

1. Al-Bawardy R, Krishnaswamy A, Rajeswaran J, et al. Tricuspid regurgitation and implantable devices. *Pacing Clin Electrophysiol.* 2015;38(2):259–266.
2. Kołodzińska A, Kutarski A, Koperski Ł, Grabowski M, Małecka B, Opolski G. Differences in encapsulating lead tissue in patients who underwent transvenous lead removal. *EP Europace.* 2012;14(7):994–1001.
3. Stokes K, Anderson J, McVenes R, McClay C. The encapsulation of polyurethane-insulated transvenous cardiac pacemaker leads. *Cardiovasc Pathol.* 1995;4(3):163–171.
4. Rizkallah J, Kent W, Kuriachan V, Burgess J, Exner D. Troubleshooting during a challenging high-risk pacemaker lead extraction: A case report and review of the literature. *BMC Res Notes.* 2015;8(1):94.
5. Goyal SK, Ellis CR, Ball SK, et al. High-risk lead removal by planned sequential transvenous laser extraction and minimally invasive right thoracotomy. *J Cardiovasc Electrophysiol.* 2014;25(6):617–621.
6. Yildirim Y, Petersen J, Tönnis T, Reichenspurner H, Pecha S. Hybrid transvenous lead extraction during cardiac surgery for valvular endocarditis. *J Cardiovasc Electrophysiol.* 2020;31(8):2101–2106.
7. Burger H, Kempfert J, van Linden A, et al. Endurance and performance of two different concepts for left ventricular stimulation with bipolar epicardial leads in long-term follow-up. *Thorac Cardiovasc Surg.* 2012;60(01):070–077.

VIDEO LEGENDS

Video 23.1 Color Doppler echocardiography of the tricuspid valve showing severe regurgitation. [00:05]

Video 23.2 2D echocardiography showing encapsulated calcification of the right ventricular pacing lead abutting the tricuspid valve causing leaflet entrapment. [00:05]

Video 23.3 Cine of chest CT (coronal view) showing the course of each lead and calcification around the leads. [00:06]

Video 23.4 Preoperative TEE showing impingement of the RV lead on the tricuspid valve and calcification (left) and severe tricuspid regurgitation (right). [00:02]

Video 23.5 Cine-fluoroscopy showing inability to pass the mechanical sheath beyond the junction of left clavicle and the first rib. [00:06]

Video 23.6 Cine-fluoroscopy showing freeing of the first RV lead down to the RA with the laser sheath. [00:14]

Video 23.7 Cine-fluoroscopy showing freeing of the second RV lead down to the RA with the laser sheath. [00:05]

Video 23.8 Intraoperative view of the calcified encapsulation of the RV lead at the tricuspid valve. Please note the calcification is being crushed. [02:15]

Video 23.9 Intraoperative view showing the RV lead embedded with the tricuspid valve leaflet and papillary muscles. [02:15]

Video 23.10 Postrepair TEE showing tricuspid valve ring (left) and trace-to-mild residual tricuspid regurgitation. [00:02]

24 | Management of Epicardial Leads in Device Infections

Erik A. Green, MD, MPH; Travis Pollema, DO

CLINICAL VIGNETTE

A patient is a 72-year-old male with a history of diabetes mellitus and coronary artery disease who previously underwent coronary artery bypass grafting (CABG) 6 years ago at an outside facility. During his admission for CABG, a biventricular implantable cardioverter-defibrillator (ICD) was placed. A left ventricle (LV) epicardial pacing lead was placed due to inadequate coronary sinus target branches. He subsequently presented to our emergency department with fever, leukocytosis, and cardiac implantable electrical device (CIED) pocket infection with an externalized epicardial pacemaker lead. Three months prior to his current presentation, he had undergone a generator replacement. Following the replacement, he developed erythema and purulent discharge from his CIED pocket. The generator and 2 transvenous leads had been removed, but the epicardial LV lead remained in place, which had become externalized (**Figure 24.1**).

PREPROCEDURAL PLANNING

The patient was seen by a multidisciplinary team, including cardiac electrophysiology, cardiothoracic surgery, and infectious disease. He was started on antibiotics, and preprocedure imaging was obtained. This included a chest X-ray (CXR), computed tomography (CT) scan of the chest, echocardiogram, and a coronary CT for his CABG history. The chest film confirmed the presence of only one remaining epicardial lead (**Figure 24.2**). Lab work showed a leukocytosis peak at 15,200, and blood cultures drawn were negative. A baseline ECG demonstrated normal sinus rhythm with a narrow QRS. Transthoracic echocardiogram (TTE) showed a moderately reduced ejection fraction of 40% and did not reveal any valvular vegetations.

PROCEDURE DETAILS

The patient was taken to the operating room and underwent an open lead extraction procedure via an exploration of his previous deltopectoral pocket

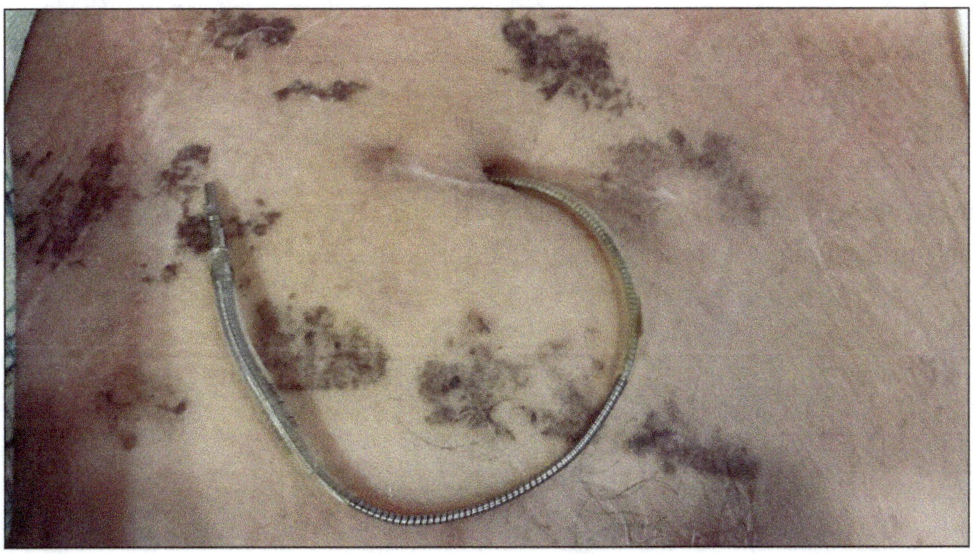

Figure 24.1 Externalized epicardial lead in a patient with CIED infection.

CASE 24

 Cardiotext Publishing. ISBN: 978-1-942909-54-5

at the site of lead exteriorization and excision of the third costal cartilage to mobilize the lead. The subcutaneous and muscular tissues appeared to be free of infection. Significant adhesions of the distal lead to surrounding structures ultimately led to amputating the lead but still allowing for removal of the entire exposed proximal portion of the lead. As the distal portion of the lead was not infected and no mediastinitis was suggested by CT scan, the risk of injury to the lung or previous patent bypass grafts outweighed the potential benefit of complete lead removal. A PET scan can often give a better indication of ongoing infection but was not done. The incision was closed in layers, but the skin around the lead's exit site was excised and loosely closed with interrupted sutures to allow for drainage at the externalization site.

FOLLOW-UP

The patient recovered well and was discharged from the hospital without complications. He was continued on oral doxycycline for 2 weeks after discharge. At 3 months follow-up, he had no further signs or symptoms of infection, and his wounds were well healed. The patient had no CRT requirements and did not receive a new CIED system as per discussions with him and his family.

DISCUSSION

Clinical Indications for Epicardial Leads

Indications for placement of epicardial pacing leads include the need for pacing in the pediatric patient population, adult patients with congenital heart disease, and patients in whom transvenous lead placement is either not possible or not preferable. Dependability for epicardial leads is mostly acceptable long-term.[1–3] In patients requiring CRT, as in this patient, placement of an epicardial LV lead is a viable alternative to transvenous LV leads; they account for up to 12% of all LV leads placed, based on national registry data[4] and have similar outcomes.[5] While they are often used after transvenous placement failure, epicardial LV leads offer a greater variability and placement location specificity. Therefore, they can be particularly helpful in patients with anomalous or difficult venous and coronary sinus anatomy or when the lead must be targeted to a specific site in the LV.[5]

Surgical Implantation

Epicardial leads (**Figure 24.3**) may be placed by sternotomy, video-assisted thoracotomy, mini-thoracotomy (**Figure 24.4**), or a subxiphoid approach, depending on patient characteristics, history, or concomitant procedures performed. Placement of an epicardial pacing system can also be considered when continued pacing is required to remove an infected transvenous system.[6]

Practitioners should be familiar with the type of epicardial leads and the common locations of epicardial lead placement. **Table 24.1** shows the most commonly used epicardial leads currently available.

Epicardial patches (**Figure 24.5**) are no longer routinely used, as modern transvenous ICD leads replaced them. Epicardial patches require more invasive placement approaches and are associated with complications such as restrictive pericarditis. However, they may still be seen in various populations, especially in patients, adults, or children with congenital heart disease. Transvenous

Table 24.1 Epicardial lead models

Lead Model	Manufacturer	Type	Fixation Method	Steroid-Eluting
4965	Medtronic	Unipolar	Suture-on	Yes
4968	Medtronic	Bipolar	Suture-on	Yes
5071	Medtronic	Unipolar	Screw-in	No
Myopore (511211)	Greatbatch	Unipolar/Bipolar	Screw-in	No

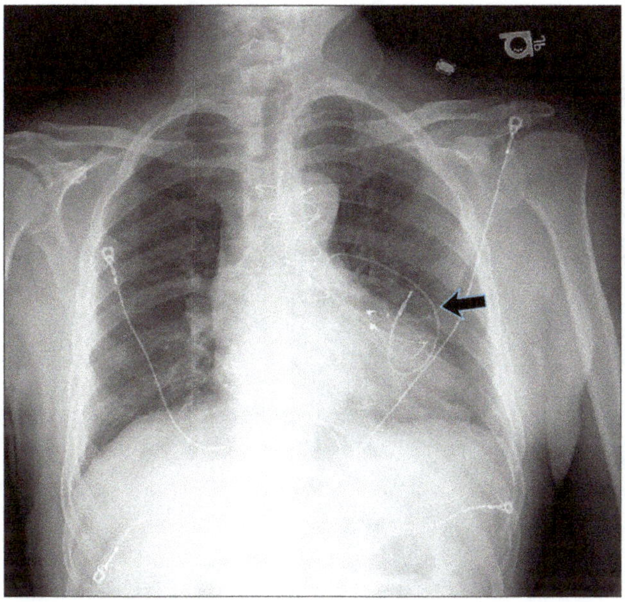

Figure 24.2 The patient's CXR showing the externalized lead (**black arrow**).

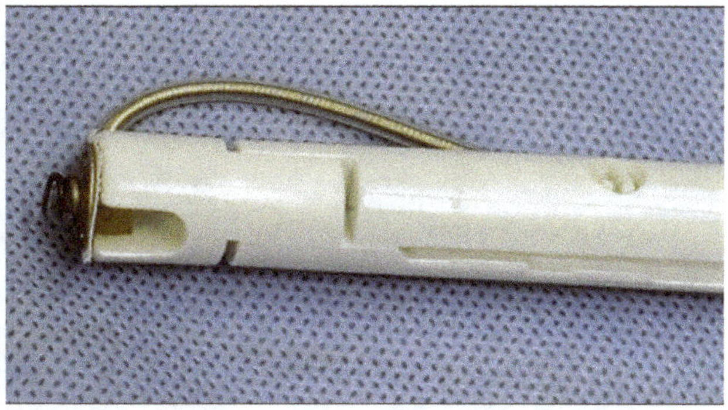

Figure 24.3 Myopore (Greatbatch Medical) epicardial lead on an insertion device.

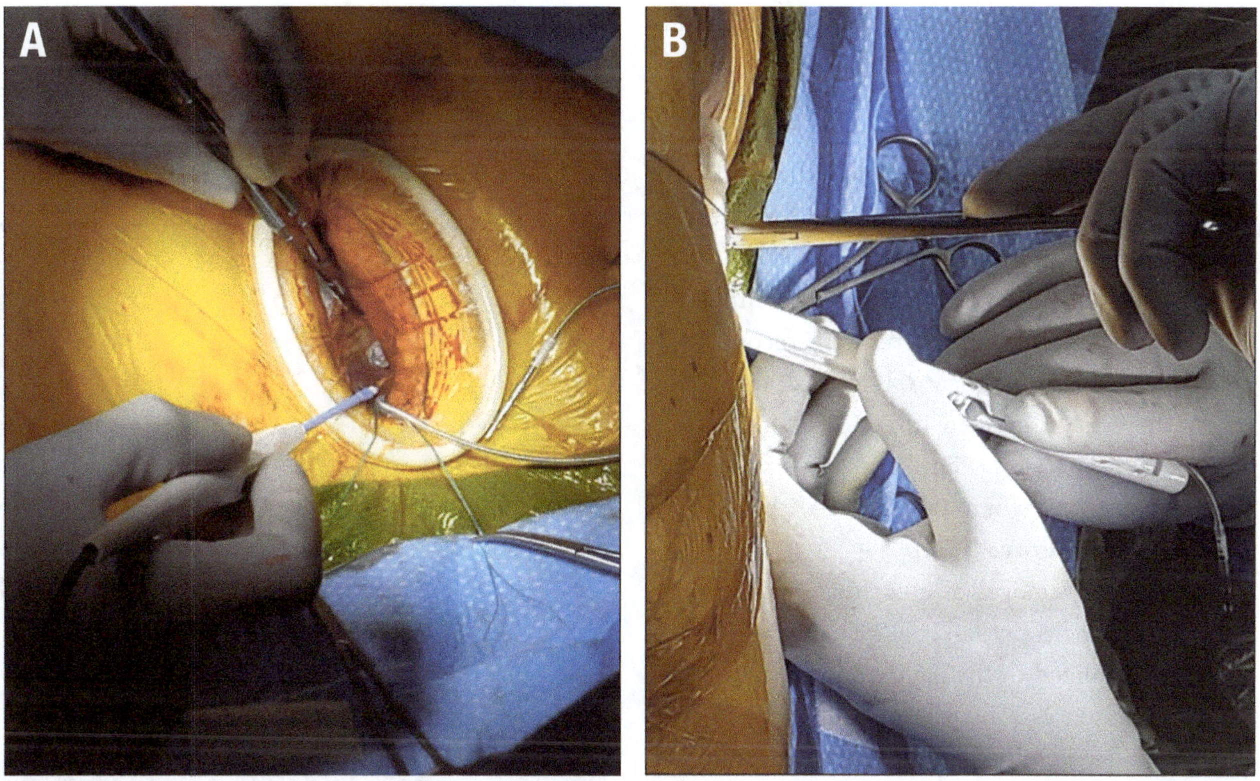

Figure 24.4 Insertion of epicardial lead, via anterior mini-thoracotomy approach. **Panel A** shows a rib spreader (Alexis retractor, Applied Medical), and **Panel B** shows lead fixation using the insertion tool.

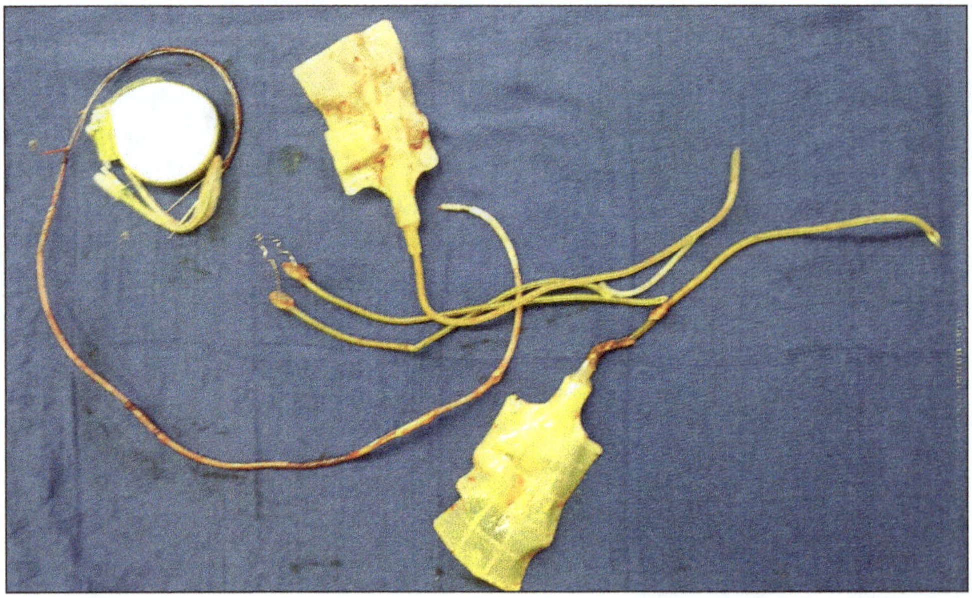

Figure 24.5 Epicardial patches removed due to infection.

lead placement is limited due to venous and cardiac anatomy or patient size.[7] Therefore, clinicians should be familiar with epicardial patches, as patients may present with patch-related complications from old CIED systems.

Epicardial Lead Removal

There is limited data regarding indications for epicardial lead removal. Indications for removal are often infection and lead fracture.[8] The 2017 Heart Rhythm Society consensus guidelines on lead management and extraction recommend complete removal of epicardial leads and patches when there is confirmed infection of the lead's intrathoracic portion.[9] Similarly, leads should be removed entirely when associated with ongoing mediastinitis (**Figure 24.6**).

Incomplete removal of epicardial leads can be considered in select cases. In patients who have an infection localized to the device pocket, an incomplete extraction may be performed by amputating the lead under traction and extracting the proximal portion of the lead via a separate incision, away from the thoracic entry site.[9] Access for lead removal can be through the generator pocket or lead entry sites via mini-thoracotomy. In complicated lead infections, or those involving epicardial patches, more aggressive surgical access may be required, including subxiphoid, thoracotomy with rib or costal cartilage resection, mini-sternotomy, or full sternotomy approaches.[8] The type and degree of surgical approach should be based upon the severity of infection present and lead involvement.

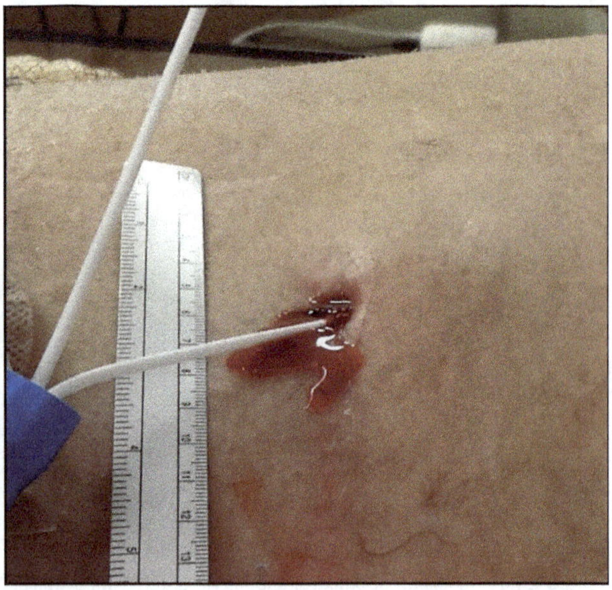

Figure 24.6 CIED and epicardial leads with associated infection. An infected sinus tract from the skin and pocket down to the mediastinum resulting in overt mediastinitis.

SUMMARY POINTS

- Epicardial leads and patches with clear lead infection should be completely removed.
- Epicardial leads with pocket infection but without infection of the intrathoracic portion should ideally be completely removed but may be amputated under traction.
- Minimally invasive approaches are feasible for epicardial lead and patch removal and should be considered when possible to avoid sternotomy.

REFERENCES

1. Lau KC, Gaynor JW, Fuller SM, Smoots KA, Shah MJ. Long-term atrial and ventricular epicardial pacemaker lead survival after cardiac operations in pediatric patients with congenital heart disease. *Heart Rhythm.* 2015;12(3):566–573.
2. Kubus P, Materna O, Gebauer RA, Matejka T, Gebauer R, Tláskal T, Janousek J. Permanent epicardial pacing in children: Long-term results and factors modifying outcome. *Europace.* 2012;14(4):509–514.
3. 3. Burger H, Pecha S, Hakmi S, Opalka B, Schoenburg M, Ziegelhoeffer T. Five-year follow-up of transvenous and epicardial left ventricular leads: Experience with more than 1000 leads. *Interact Cardiovasc Thorac Surg.* 2020;30(1):74–80.
4. 4. Kremers MS, Hammill SC, Berul CI, et al. The National ICD Registry Report: Version 2.1 including leads and pediatrics for years 2010 and 2011. *Heart Rhythm.* 2013;10(4):e59–e65.
5. 5. Chen L, Fu H, Pretorius VG, et al. Clinical outcomes of cardiac resynchronization with epicardial left ventricular lead. *Pacing Clin Electrophysiol.* 2015;38(10):1201–1029.
6. 6. Amraoui S, Sohal M, Li A, et al. Comparison of delayed transvenous reimplantation and immediate surgical epicardial approach in pacing-dependent patients undergoing extraction of infected permanent pacemakers. *Heart Rhythm.* 2015;12(6):1209–1215.
7. Stephenson EA, Batra AS, Knilans TK, et al. A multicenter experience with novel implantable cardioverter defibrillator configurations in the pediatric and congenital heart disease population. *J Cardiovasc Electrophysiol.* 2006;17(1): 41–46.
8. Rusanov A, Spotnitz HM. A 15-year experience with permanent pacemaker and defibrillator lead and patch extractions. *Ann Thorac Surg.* 2010;89(1):44–50.
9. Kusumoto FM, Schoenfeld MH, Wilkoff BL, et al. 2017 HRS expert consensus statement on cardiovascular implantable electronic device lead management and extraction. *Heart Rhythm.* 2017;14(12):e503–e551.

25 | Pacemaker Infection Treated with Chronic Suppressive Antibiotic Therapy

Fatima A. Ali-Ahmed, MD; Siva K. Mulpuru, MD, MPH

CLINICAL VIGNETTE

A 72-year-old female presented to the clinic with an erosion of her pacemaker pocket associated with purulent drainage and exposed leads. Her past medical history included antiphospholipid antibody syndrome with deep venous thrombosis, underwent inferior vena cava (IVC) filter placement, hypertension, type 2 diabetes, morbid obesity (BMI, 50.3 kg/m^2), and permanent atrial fibrillation. In 1996, during treatment for deep venous thrombosis, she developed heart block, and she underwent implantation of a temporary pacemaker from the left subclavian system. A left-sided superior vena cava (SVC) was identified at that time, and she subsequently underwent implantation of a right-sided dual-chamber permanent pacemaker. In 2012, her RV lead demonstrated high impedance. Her RV lead was abandoned, and a new RV lead was implanted. In 2019, the pulse generator was changed as the device reached elective replacement. Her device details are as follows.

Device Details

Device Component	Manufacturer/ Model	Date of Implant
Pulse generator	St. Jude Allure RF	09/2019
Right atrial lead	Medtronic 4068	11/1996
Right ventricular lead	St. Jude 2088TC	11/2012

A few months after the device surgery, partial erosion of the pocket was noted. She was treated with antibiotics and local wound care, but the erosion persisted.

On physical examination, she was afebrile; her right-sided pocket showed erosion with purulent drainage and exposed leads. A chest X-ray (CXR) showed the presence of 3 intracardiac leads: 1 atrial and 2 ventricular leads. Her leads from 1996 were implanted from the right internal jugular vein and were tunneled over the right clavicle. Her echocardiogram revealed an ejection fraction of 50%, moderate to severe tricuspid valve insufficiency, and suggested the presence of a left SVC. There was no overt evidence of endocarditis. A chest CT showed the presence of a left SVC without a communicating innominate vein, extensive coronary calcification, and an IVC filter located transversely with the tip pointed into the renal vein. Device interrogation revealed atrial flutter with complete heart block.

PREPROCEDURAL PLANNING

Device erosion or CIED infection is a class I indication for extraction. The defined extraction approach and goals are tailored toward the patient's risk factors and procedure complexity. The risks can be divided into patient factors and device factors. Patient risk factors for a complication during lead removal include: advanced age over 65 years old, female gender, and renal dysfunction/ESRD, while device risk factors include the presence of multiple leads, lead dwell time more than 10 years, and dual-coil ICD lead.

In our case, the option of complete system extraction in the operating room was discussed by a team of electrophysiology, infectious disease, general surgery, and cardiothoracic surgery. Multiple factors such as female gender, multiple leads, more than 20-year-old passive fixation leads, and other comorbidities (morbid obesity, and diabetes mellitus) placed her at a high risk for complications. Additionally, the cardiothoracic

Cardiac Lead Extraction: A Case-Based Contemporary Approach.
 Cardiotext Publishing. ISBN: 978-1-942909-54-5

surgery team felt she was high risk for surgical resuscitation in the event of a vascular tear. The patient understood the risks of chronic antibiotic suppression and did not feel the surgical risks of lead extraction were acceptable for her. Due to her high risk for complications, a shared decision was made to remove the generator, amputate the leads as distally as possible, and debride the right chest pocket. A transesophageal echocardiogram (TEE) was done to confirm there was no valve or lead vegetation. Since she is pacemaker dependent, the plan was first to establish a safe pacing system, after which debridement would be carried on and plan for chronic antibiotic suppression. The decision was made to implant a leadless pacemaker. If there is difficulty traversing the IVC filter, an alternative would be a left-sided permanent pacemaker via the left subclavian through the left-sided SVC into the right ventricle. General surgery evaluated the patient and discussed wound management of the pocket, including initial washout, debridement, and application of a wound VAC device. They suggested returning to the OR every 48 hours for washout until the pocket appears amenable to delayed primary skin closure with a drain.

PROCEDURAL DETAILS

Consent and appropriate preoperative testing and evaluation were performed. The patient was taken to the hybrid operating room. She was intubated and an arterial line placed for continuous blood pressure monitoring during the procedure. The chest and bilateral thighs were prepped and draped in a sterile fashion. Wound cultures were collected, and then IV cefazolin, IV vancomycin, and IV clindamycin were administered. Venous accesses were obtained using ultrasound guidance and modified Seldinger's technique. An 8-Fr sheath was placed in the right femoral vein and 6-Fr in the left femoral vein. Through the right-sided 8-Fr sheath, an Amplatzer stiff guidewire (Boston Scientific) crossed the IVC filter and was advanced to the SVC. The 8-Fr sheath was then removed and was serially dilated to accommodate the guiding catheter for the leadless pacemaker leadless. The 27-Fr leadless pacemaker delivery sheath was advanced through the right femoral vein up to the IVC filter level. The IVC filter was malpositioned (**Figure 25.1**), and the leadless pacemaker delivery sheath would not advance across the IVC filter. Therefore, this approach was abandoned. The sheath was removed, and hemostasis was achieved with a figure-eight suture.

The alternative option was a left-sided permanent pacemaker. The patient had a known left SVC without a communicating innominate vein. A contrast injection in the left arm confirmed the patent left SVC (**Figure 25.2**). The sheath was placed, and the pacemaker lead was negotiated to the right atrium. With curved stylet and manipulation, the lead was passed across the tricuspid valve into the region of the right ventricular outflow tract (RVOT). There were no spontaneous R waves available for sensing. The pacing threshold was 0.4 V at 0.5 ms and impedance 794 ohms. With 10 V output, there was no extracardiac stimulation. The stylet was removed, and the lead was sewn in place. A recheck of pacing and sensing showed stable values. A left-sided pocket was created for the pulse generator with electrocautery and blunt dissection. The pocket was then irrigated with saline solution. The lead was attached to a new Medtronic single-chamber pacemaker pulse generator. The pulse generator and leads were placed in the pocket, and the pulse generator was sutured loosely to the posterior aspect of the wound. The pocket was then closed with three running layers of 2-0 PDS Stratafix suture and one running layer of 4-0 Monocryl Stratafix suture (Johnson & Johnson Medical). The wound was dressed in a sterile manner.

After re-gloving, attention was turned to the right upper chest pacemaker pocket. There were four open wounds: superior lateral (5 × 6 × 2 cm), inferior lateral (7 × 10 × 3 cm), superior medial

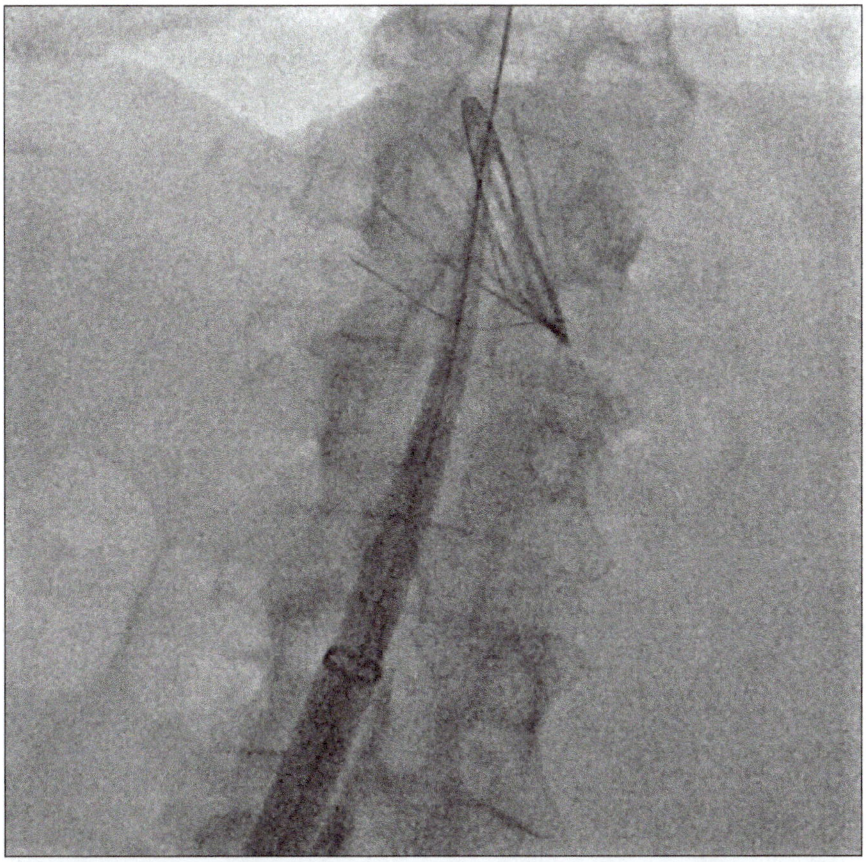

Figure 25.1 The malpositioned IVC filter was obliquely oriented, and leadless pacemaker delivery sheath could not be advanced through the splines.

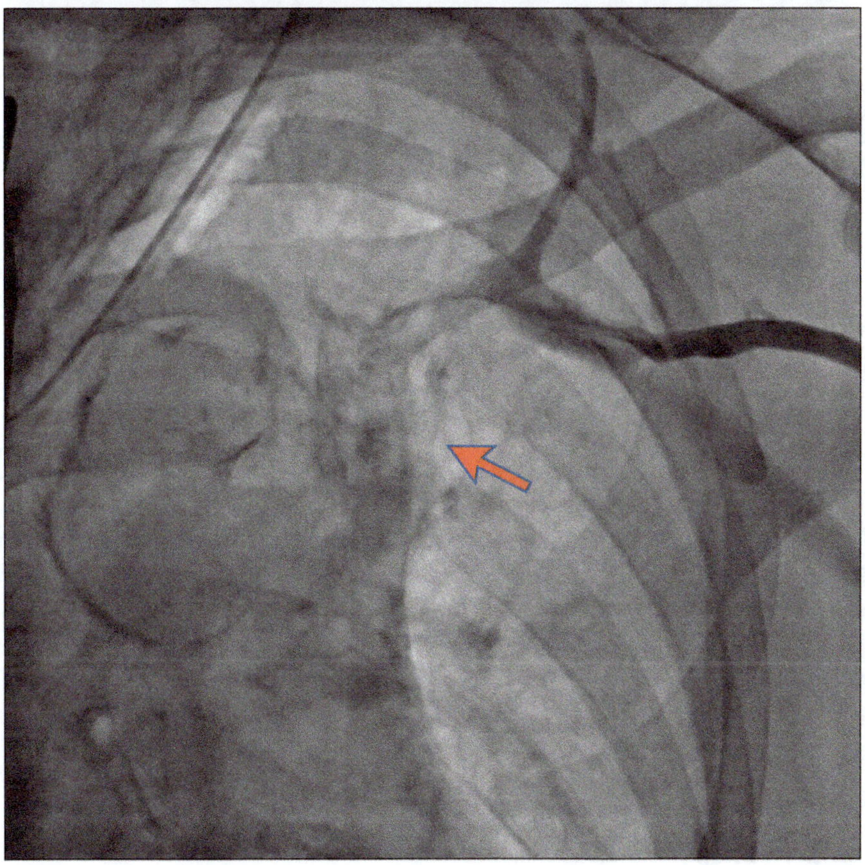

Figure 25.2 A contrast injection through a peripheral IV, demonstrating a known left SVC without a communicating innominate vein (**red arrow**).

(2 × 2 × 1 cm), and the inferior medial (5 × 6 × 3 cm). The leads were pulled through after clipping of the pins, and the leads were retracted. At the medial-most incision of the site of the erosion, there was obvious purulence and coagulum. Cultures had been taken earlier in the procedure before the administration of antibiotics. The leads were pulled through to this site and then at another counter-incision site near the clavicle (**Figure 25.3**). Then a general surgery team joined the procedure for initial washout, debridement, and wound VAC.

POSTPROCEDURAL COURSE

The patient was transferred to the ICU and extubated. Postoperatively she continued IV vancomycin and was started on doxycycline. Postprocedure CXR identified no abnormalities (**Figure 25.4**). On postoperative day #2, the patient returned to the OR for a wound VAC removal. A 10-Fr drain was placed in the inferior lateral wound. The wound was then quilted with interrupted 3-0 PDS (P-dioxane) to obliterate the dead space. The superior lateral wound, inferior lateral wound, and superior medial wound were closed with a 4-0 vertical mattress nylon suture. The inferior medial wound (**Figure 25.5**) was packed with moist Kerlix (Cardinal Health). The drain was placed to suction. A sterile dressing was applied. Forty-eight hours later, the drain demonstrated low output and was removed. Dressing changes on the inferior medial wound were done 3 times daily, and the wound was allowed to heal by secondary intention. Final wound cultures grew *Staphylococcus epidermidis* and *Corynebacterium amycolatum*. The patient was discharged to receive 6 weeks of IV Vancomycin, followed by lifelong suppression with oral doxycycline 100 mg bid.

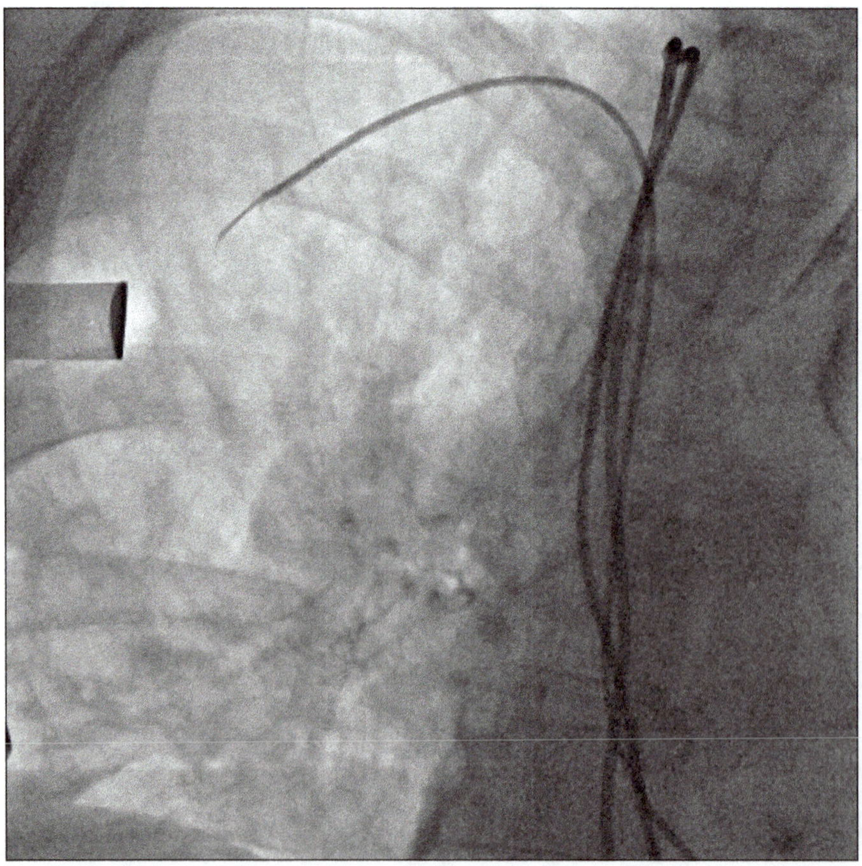

Figure 25.3 Amputation of the leads was performed as distally (towards the lead tip and away from the pin) as possible.

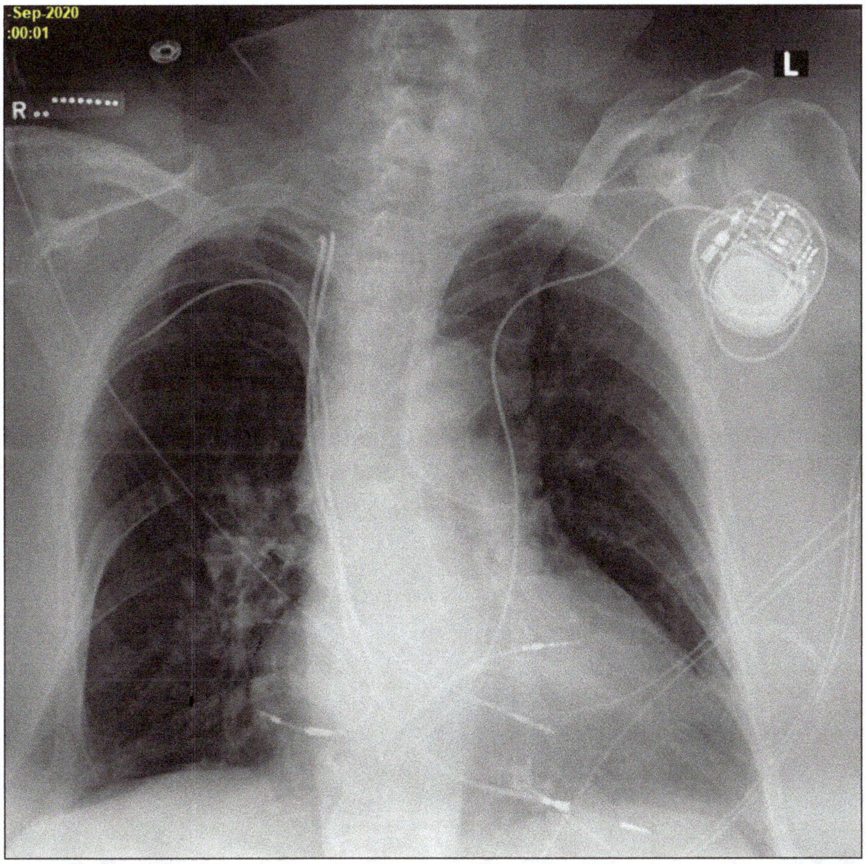

Figure 25.4 Postprocedure CXR demonstrating the amputated leads and a new left-sided, single-chamber pacemaker.

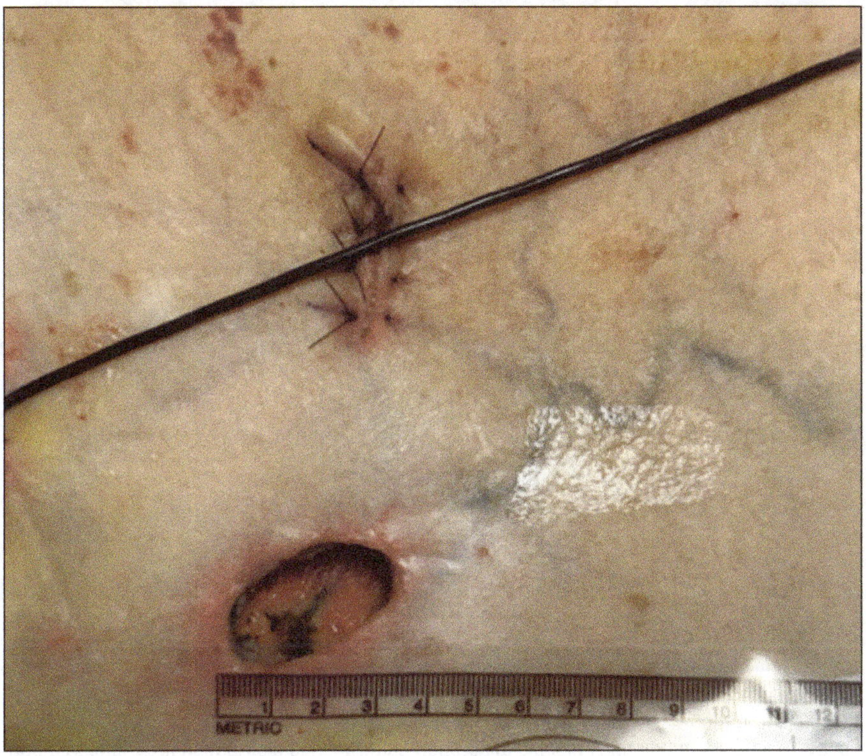

Figure 25.5 An open inferior medial wound after removal of the drains on the right upper chest. The wound was allowed to heal by secondary intention.

DISCUSSION

As cardiovascular implantable electronic devices (CIED) implantation increases, CIED infections become increasingly prevalent. CIED infections are grouped into pocket or systemic infections and are managed appropriately.[1] Typically, the course of antibiotics can range from 2–6 weeks. It is a class I recommendation for CIED removal when there is valve vegetation, lead vegetation, or pocket infection/erosion.[1] However, in selected patients with CIED infections who are high-risk candidates for a complete system removal, chronic antibiotic suppression, similar to our patient, is an option. Given the limited data, the choice of antibiotic therapy and its dosing is empirical. One study by Tan et al.,[2] demonstrated that device retention in patients with CIED infection was associated with a high rate of mortality and an increased rate of relapse at follow-up one year later. Another conservative approach described by Puri et al.,[3] is 5 days of povidone-iodine closed irrigation, followed by reimplantation of a new ICD on the contralateral side. A recent small study evaluating the continuous, in-situ targeted, ultra-high concentration of antibiotics (CITA) showed salvage of 86% of the device infections confined to the pocket without bacteremia.[4] The serum antibiotic levels were adjusted by adjusting the concentration and flow of the pocket irrigation (**Figure 25.6**). However, long-term outcomes are unknown. Therefore, these approaches are only considered when the patient declines extraction, or the risk of conventional

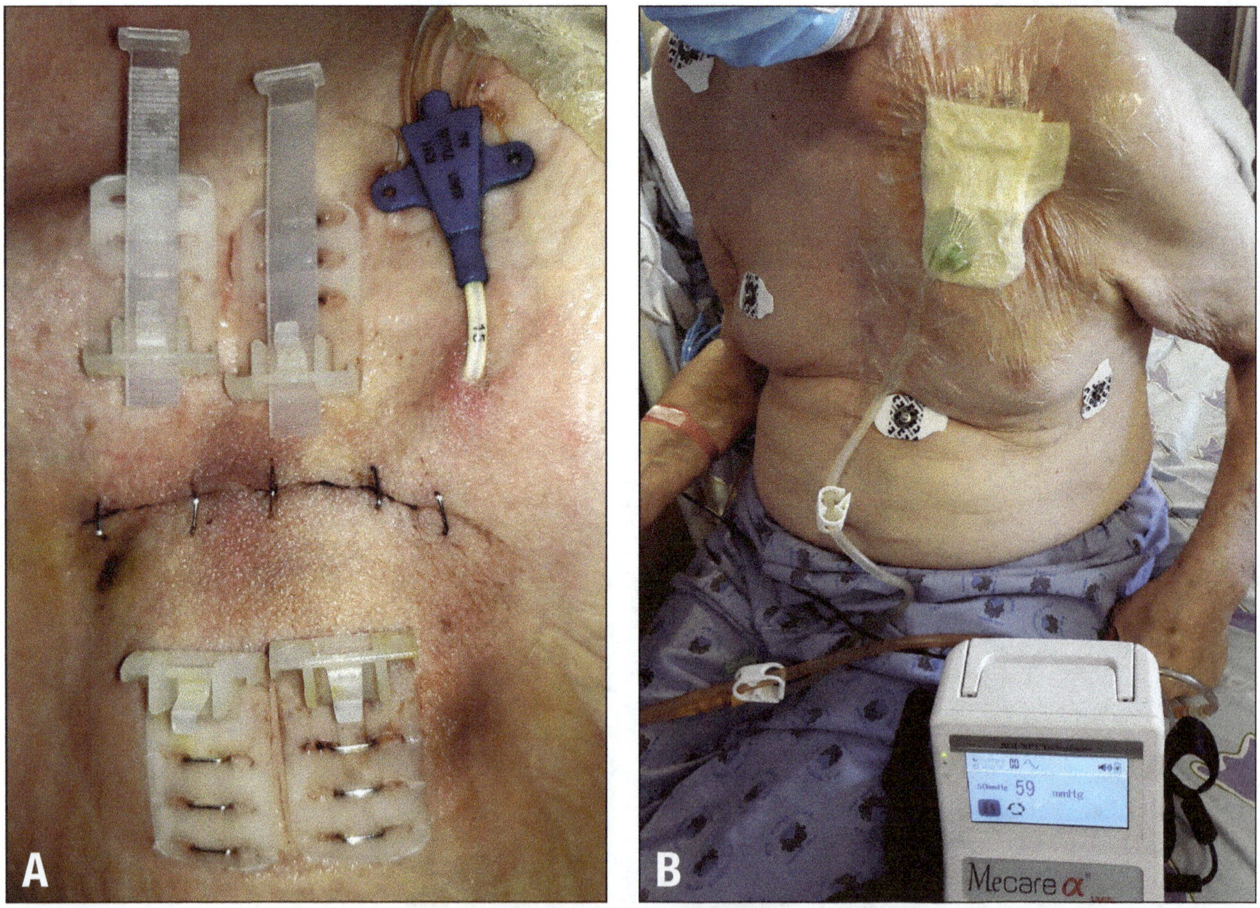

Figure 25.6 Continuous in-situ targeted, ultra-high concentration of antibiotics (CITA) treatment. The Topaz procedure was designed for conservative salvage of infected CIED's by wound irrigation with CITA provided continuously to the infected pocket (**Panel A**). CITA provides antibiotics that spread to the entire body by diffusion gradient. Antibiotic absorption and systemic distribution are monitored and confirmed by serum level assays. The total antibiotic dose correlated with the daily recommended dose. The Top Closure tension release system allows for wound edge approximation (**Panel A**) and the wouwnd is isolated by regulated negative pressure therapy (**Panel B**). (Figures courtesy of Moris Topaz MD, PhD, Israel.)

management outweighs the benefit in individuals who are at high risk for procedural complications. The current guidelines only recommend long-term antimicrobial suppression therapy as a palliative approach and is the last option compared with the recommended curative lead extraction approach.[1] The options are summarized below.

- Local debridement and removal of hardware to the extent possible. Chronic antibiotic suppression is often prescribed. If infection flares up, the lead extraction option should be reconsidered.
- Local infusion of antiseptics or antibiotics through a closed infusion pump.
- Hybrid extraction procedures. During these procedures, a portion of the lead is freed up by percuatenous techniques, and the remainder of the lead is taken out by minimally invasive surgical techniques.

When deciding the appropriate approach for an individual patient with a CIED infection, their overall risk needs to be taken into account, and a shared decision-making process between the patient and the treating physicians should take place. The 6 elements of good decision aid are listed in **Figure 25.7**. The 2017 Heart Rhythm Society expert consensus[1] recommends the following information be discussed with the patient during the shared-decision making encounter: (1) the annual lead extraction volume at that center; (2) the lead extraction clinical success rate; and (3) major procedure-related complication/death rates during hospitalization. Lastly, if extraction is planned, cardiothoracic surgery backup is imperative. If there is no cardiothoracic surgery backup, a referral to an experienced, high-volume extraction center with cardiothoracic surgery backup will facilitate the best patient care outcomes.

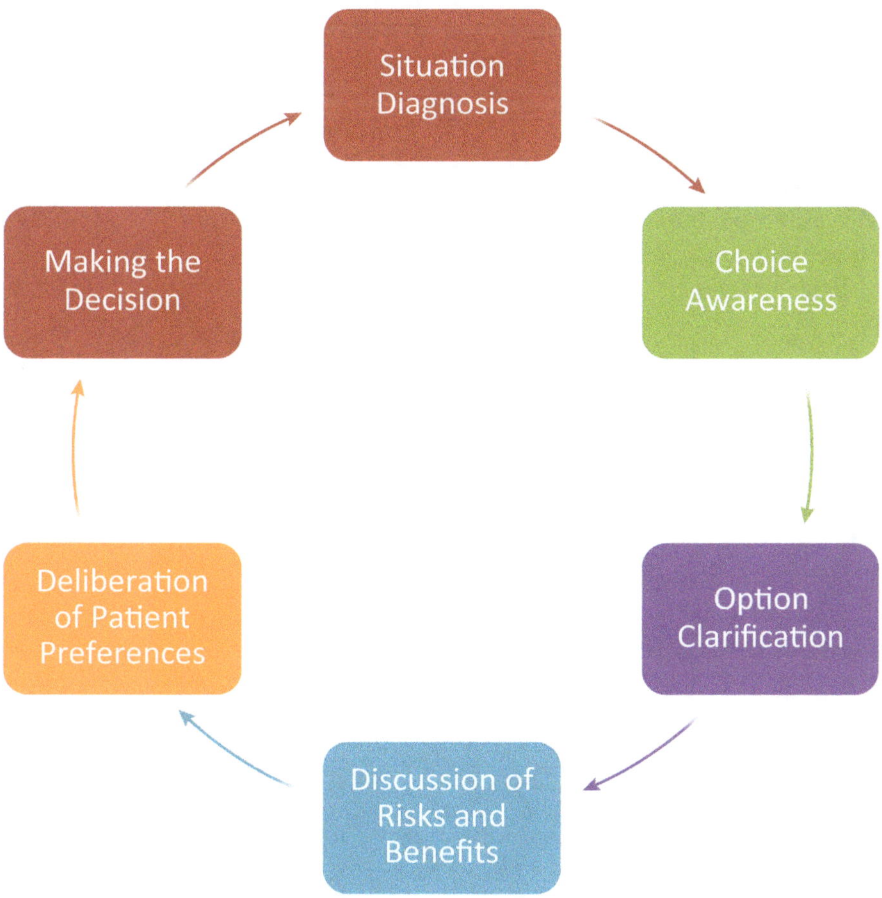

Figure 25.7 The 6 important elements of a decision aid used for shared decision making. The shared decision making starts with the patient's problem at hand (situational diagnosis) that requires management. The patient is made aware of the importance of his/her preferences when multiple options are available for management (choice awareness). Subsequently, the provider and the patient deliberate decision making after clarifying options (option clarification), discussion of risks and benefits (discussion of risks and benefits) associated with each choice with the incorporation of patient preferences (deliberation of patient preferences). The patient makes a final decision with the team members.

SUMMARY POINTS

- Some patients with CIED infection may be at high risk for management of surgical complications or may not prefer to undergo lead extraction procedures due to their individual preferences.
- Shared decision making involving a decision aid should be used to make such complex medical decisions. The decision aid should have the following components: (1) situational diagnosis; (2) choice awareness; (3) option clarification; (4) discussion of risks and benefits; (5) deliberation of patient preferences; and (6) making the decision.
- Antiseptic/antibiotic infusion through a closed circuit has been described among patients with CIED infection who were not candidates for extraction procedures.
- Chronic antibiotic suppressive therapy can be considered in patients with CIED infection who are not candidates for extraction procedures. If the patient develops a flare of infection on appropriate antibiotic treatment, the option of lead extraction should be revisited.

REFERENCES

1. Kusumoto FM, Schoenfeld MH, Wilkoff BL, et al. 2017 HRS expert consensus statement on cardiovascular implantable electronic device lead management and extraction. *Heart Rhythm.* 2017;14(12):e503–e551.
2. Tan EM, DeSimone DC, Sohail MR, Baddour LM, Wilson WR, Steckelberg JM, Virk A. Outcomes in patients with cardiovascular implantable electronic device infection managed with chronic antibiotic suppression. *Clin Infect Dis.* 2017 Jun 1;64(11):1516–1521.
3. Puri R, Psaltis PJ, Nelson AJ, Sanders P, Young GD. Povidone-iodine irrigation-a possible alternative to lead extraction. *Indian Pacing Electrophysiol J.* 2011;11(4):115–119.
4. Topaz M, Kazatsker M, Ashkenazi I, et al. A novel antibiotic delivery approach enhances salvage of infected cardiovascular-implantable electronic devices. *Circulation.* 2020;142(Suppl 3):A15682.

26 | Lead Extraction Using Single Sheath Mechanical Dilatation

Luca Segreti, MD; Mario Giannotti Santoro, MD; Stefano Viani, MD; Andrea Di Cori, MD; Antonio Maria Canu, MD; Giulio Zucchelli, PhD, MD

CLINICAL VIGNETTE

A 48-year-old male patient was referred to our center for the management of a defibrillator lead malfunction. The patient had a dilated cardiomyopathy with severe systolic dysfunction (ejection fraction [EF], 22%). In 2012, a single-lead implantable cardioverter-defibrillator (ICD) system with atrial sensing electrodes (VDD-ICD) had been implanted at another Italian center. The successive follow-ups revealed clinical stability with the persistence of reduced systolic function. In 2021, 9 years after the VDD-ICD implantation, a routine interrogation of the device revealed nonsustained noise oversensing on the ventricular ICD channel, marked in the ventricular fibrillation (VF) zone (**Figure 26.1**). Capture threshold, sensing, and lead impedance values were in the normal range. The decision was made to perform lead extraction and the ICD was programmed a longer tachycardia detection interval to avoid inappropriate therapy (VT zone: 171–222 bpm, 40 cycles, onset 20%, stability 12 ms; VF zone: > 222 bpm, 24/30 cycles).

Device Details

Device Component	Manufacturer/Model	Date of Implant
Generator	Biotronik Lumax 740 VR-T DX	10/24/2012
Defibrillator lead	Biotronik Linox Smart ProMRI S DX 65/15	10/24/2012

The defibrillator lead was a single-coil lead with an atrial dipole and an active fixation mechanism. The patient was in sinus rhythm with a complete left bundle block with a wide QRS (160 ms) (**Figure 26.2**) and a New York Heart Association (NYHA) class II. There were no clinical signs of infection.

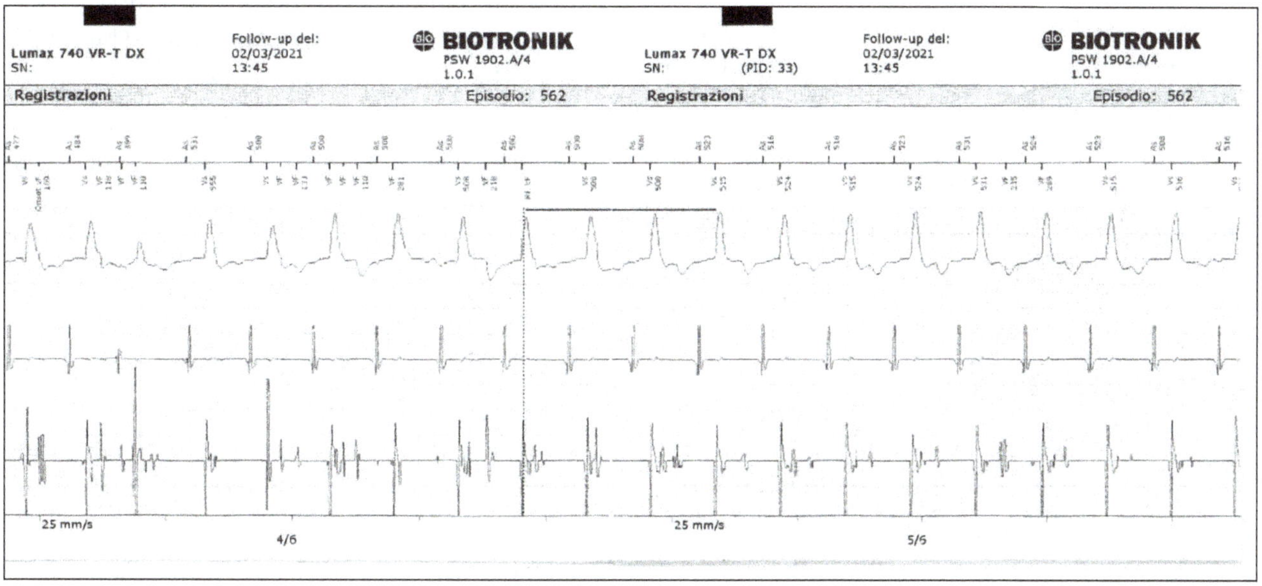

Figure 26.1 Atrial and right ventricular electrogram recordings. There are make-or-break signals consistent with noise and suggestive of lead integrity failure.

CASE 26

 ISBN: 978-1-942909-54-5

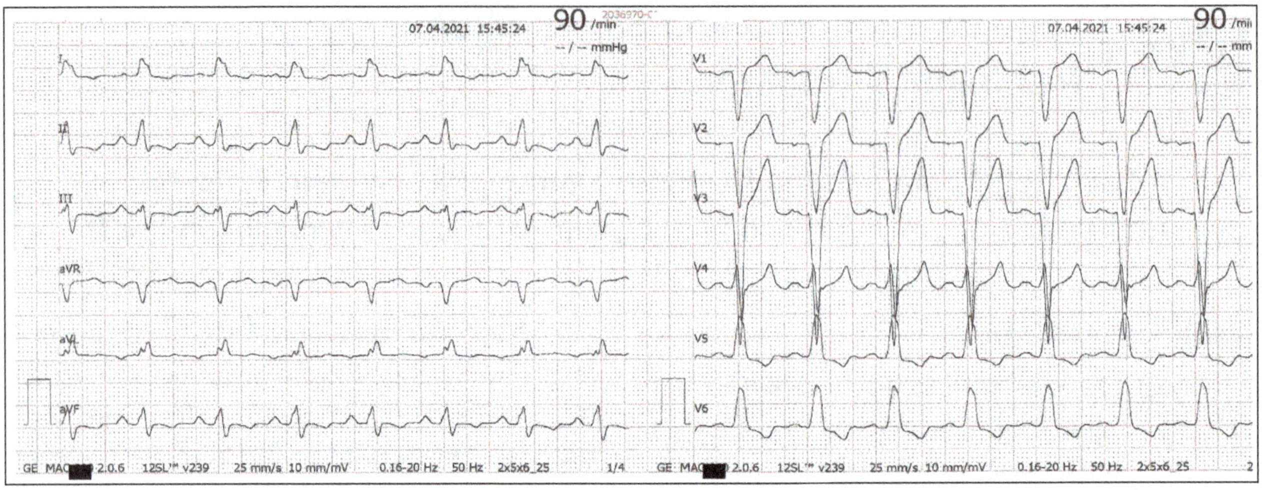

Figure 26.2 A 12-lead electrocardiogram showing sinus rhythm, with a complete left bundle block with a wide QRS (160 ms).

PREPROCEDURAL PLANNING

Chest X-ray (CXR) revealed the regular position of the lead without signs of fracture or insulator defects (**Figure 26.3**, Panels A and B). A new interrogation of the device showed reproducible noise during extreme abduction of the left arm. Venous angiography performed from a left antecubital peripheral access revealed a patent subclavian and central venous system, with signs of adherences at the innominate tract (**Video 26.1**). There was an excessive lead loop before entering the tricuspid valve, suggesting the possible location of the damage and presence of binding sites (**Video 26.2**).

We opted for transvenous lead extraction (TLE) of the malfunctioning lead, and ipsilateral cardiac resynchronization therapy and defibrillator (CRT-D) reimplantation during the same procedure.

PROCEDURAL DETAILS

The procedure was performed in the cardiac electrophysiology laboratory after obtaining informed consent. A cardiothoracic surgery stand-by was available. General anesthesia was administered, and the patient was intubated. The patient was prepared with the application of cutaneous pads for defibrillation, transvenous temporary pacing from femoral venous access, invasive arterial blood pressure from the femoral artery, and pulse oximetry monitoring. The pulse generator pocket was opened, and the lead was freed by electrocautery from their adhesions down to the venous insertion site. A new extrathoracic subclavian venous access was obtained, and we advanced a wire in the inferior vena cava. We cut the lead 10 cm out of the venous entry site. A stiff normal stylet (6293–85 cm, Medtronic) was introduced into the lead body, but its tip could not advance in the ventricle tract since it stopped at the tricuspid level. The retraction of the helix was ineffective. A special tie of non-absorbable silk suture material (Ethibond Excel 0, Ethicon, Johnson & Johnson Medical) was secured around the insulation of the lead. A modified Fisherman's knot was performed: it is a compact knot, does not increase the lead diameter, jams when tightened, and the working ends can be cropped very close to the knot. We performed dilatation using polypropylene sheaths. Dilatation was started by using a single sheath with the inner diameter as close as possible to the lead body diameter (8.5-Fr Byrd Dilator Sheath Set (A) Polipropylene, Cook Vandergrift Inc.). Traction was maintained on the silk ties while the sheath was advanced under fluoroscopy following the lead

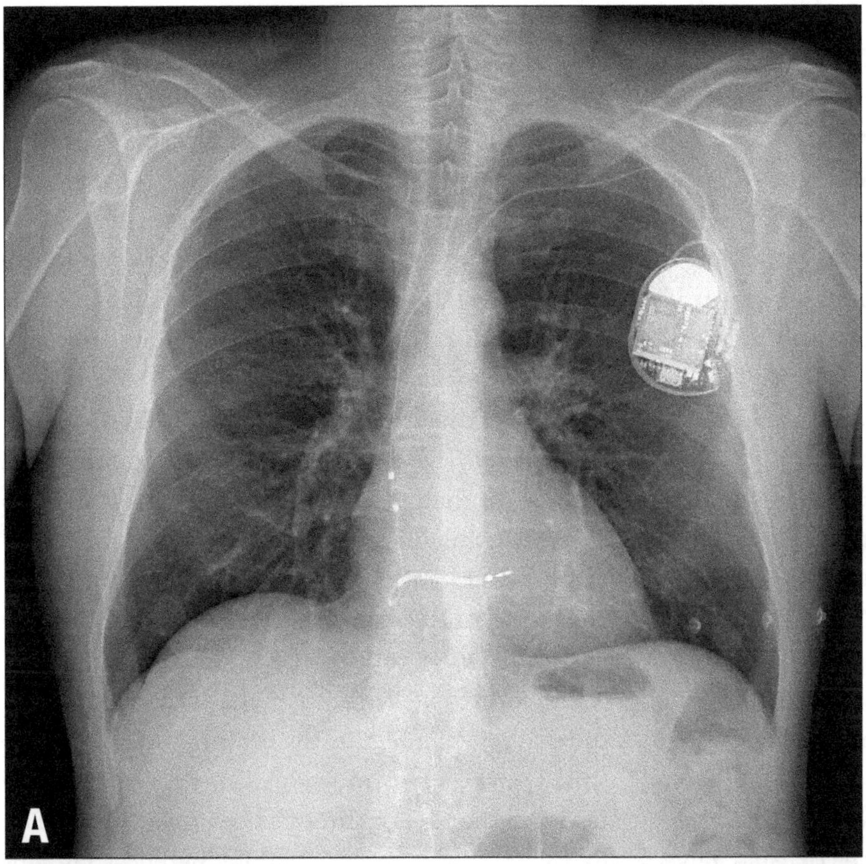

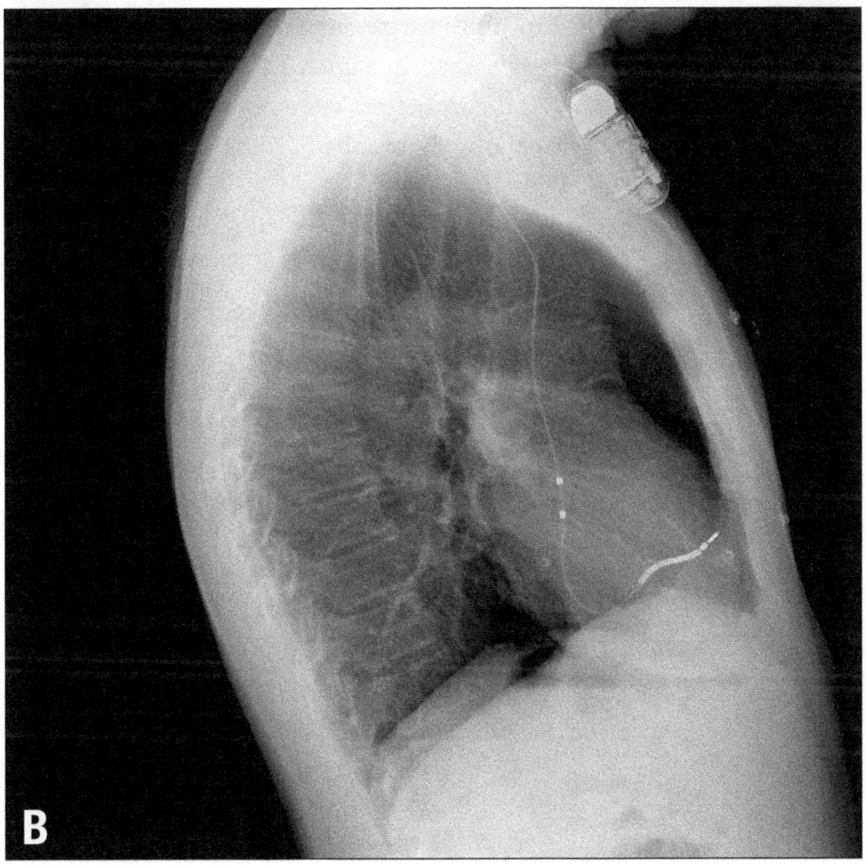

Figure 26.3 Posteroanterior and lateral chest radiography. The lead has a regular location for a VDD lead, with a septal fixation. There are no signs of fracture or of insulator defects.

course and avoiding any angle (**Video 26.3**). The advancement of the sheath was performed by rotating it alternatively clockwise and counterclockwise with 2 or 3 turns, using a dedicated handle around the sheath (My Good Block, accessory for percutaneous dilatator sheaths, Fiab). While dilating, we performed smooth traction to keep the lead in tension but avoiding myocardial wall invagination or coil lengthening and lead damage. When the advancement of the sheath was difficult, it was retrieved for a few millimeters, and dilatation restarted. The advancement in the subclavian and innominate vein was challenging for a strong adherence, so the dilatator was changed to a new one of larger diameter (10.0-Fr Byrd Dilator Sheath Set (B) Polipropylene, Cook Vandergrift Inc.), also used in a telescopic manner (**Video 26.4**). Another tough adherence was present in the proximity of the atrial dipole, and we overcame it with a larger dilatator (11.5-Fr Byrd Dilator Sheath Set (C) Polipropylene, Cook Vandergrift Inc.) (**Video 26.5**). At the level of the tricuspid valve, the lead presented a large and strong adherence, requiring sheath upsizing (**Video 26.6**, **Video 26.7**, and **Video 26.8**). At this point, the lead showed a defect of the insulator with externalization of a wire, so we needed additional sheath oversize to incorporate it (**Video 26.9**). The possibility of grasping the lead proximally to the site of adherence and making it free-floating was checked to evaluate the possibility of crossover to the internal jugular approach in case we were unsuccessful with the standard venous entry site approach (**Video 26.10**, and discussion for other technical details). After many attempts from the venous entry site, we overcame the adherence with the largest dilatator available (13.0-Fr Byrd Dilator Sheath Set (D) Polipropylene, Cook Vandergrift Inc.). After that, the tip was reached; the stylet was inserted while exerting mild traction and maintaining it; dilatation was performed by continuous clockwise and counterclockwise rotation of the sheath in order to dissect the distal binding site; and fluoroscopy was used to check that the sheath did not overcome the tip of the lead (**Video 26.11**). Once the tip was freed, we removed the lead and the sheath through the implant vein. The extracted lead showed 3 main adherences (at subclavian-innominate, atrial, and tricuspid valve level) as shown in **Figures 26.4**, **26.5**, and **26.6**. The vital parameters were normal, and transthoracic echocardiography (TTE) showed an absence

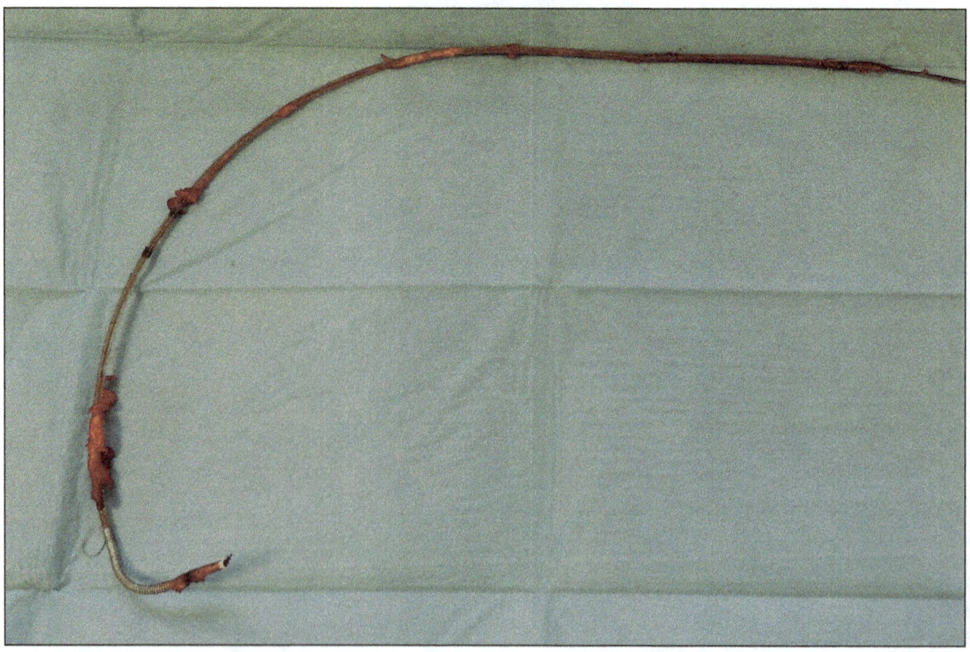

Figure 26.4 Examination of the extracted lead. There are 3 visible adherences corresponding with the tracts where there were difficulties and the need to use larger sheaths (subclavian and innominate tract, just proximally to the atrial dipole and in proximity of the ICD coil).

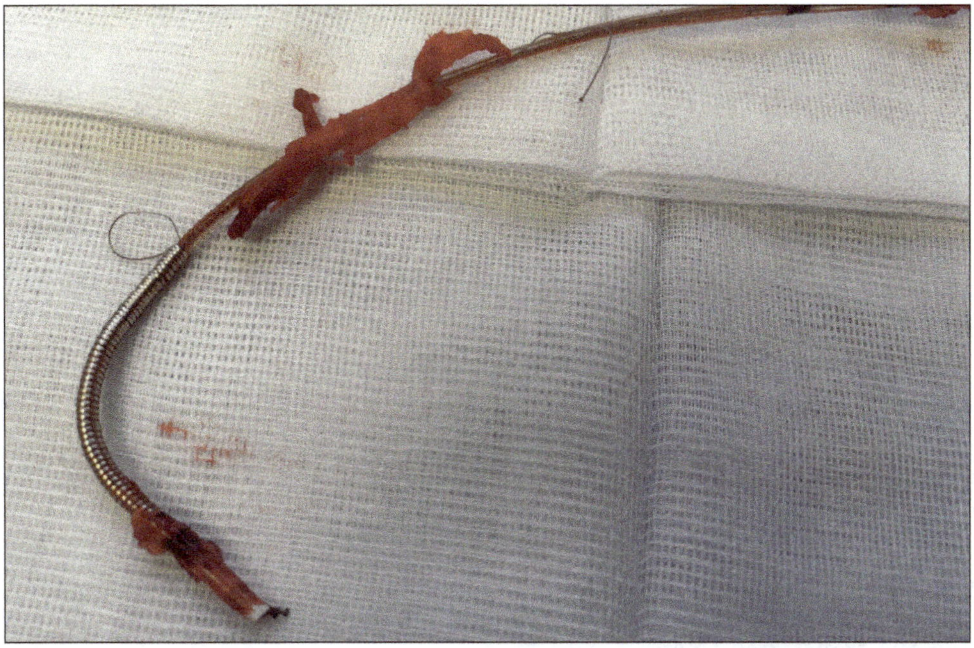

Figure 26.5 A detail of the main adherence in proximity of the coil. Note the exposed and deformed helix and the externalization of the wire in the corresponding tract where the stylet cannot be advanced.

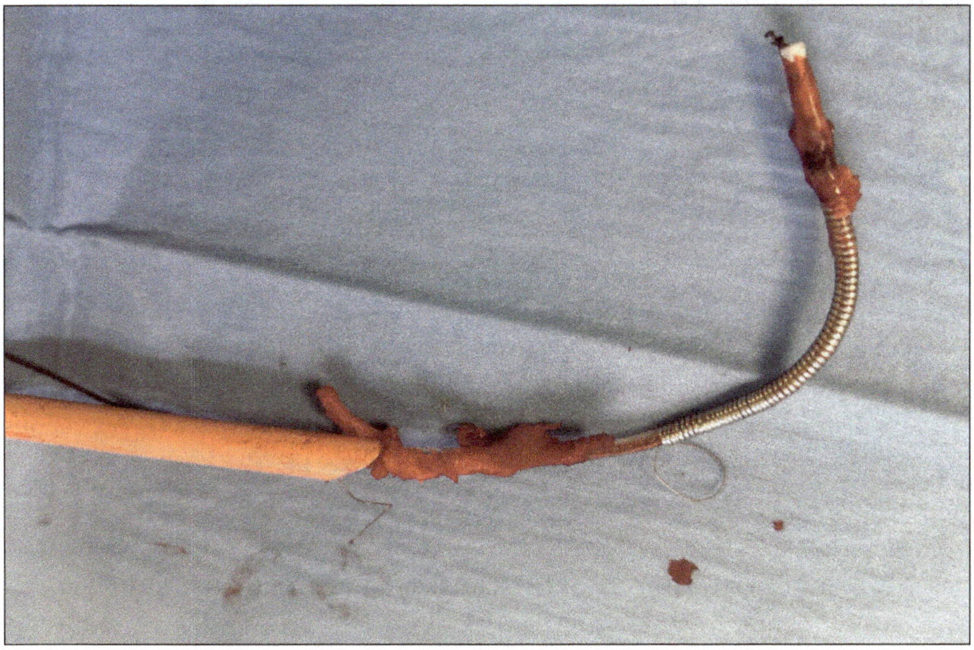

Figure 26.6 A detail of the largest used sheath to overcome the strong adherence in proximity of the coil.

of pericardial effusion. Finally, it was contextually performed as a new ipsilateral CRT-D reimplantation, using the venous access previously obtained and 2 new extrathoracic subclavian venous accesses (Device: Neutrino NxT HF; atrial lead: Tendril STS 2088TC; defibrillator single-coil active fixation lead: Durata 7122; coronary sinus lead: Quartet 1456Q; Abbott). (**Video 26.12**, A and B; **Video 26.13**, A, B, and C). At the end of the procedure, we programmed the device and enabled antitachycardia therapies, and temporary cardiac pacing was removed. The final ECG documented atrial-synchronous biventricular paced rhythm, with a narrow QRS (**Figure 26.7**).

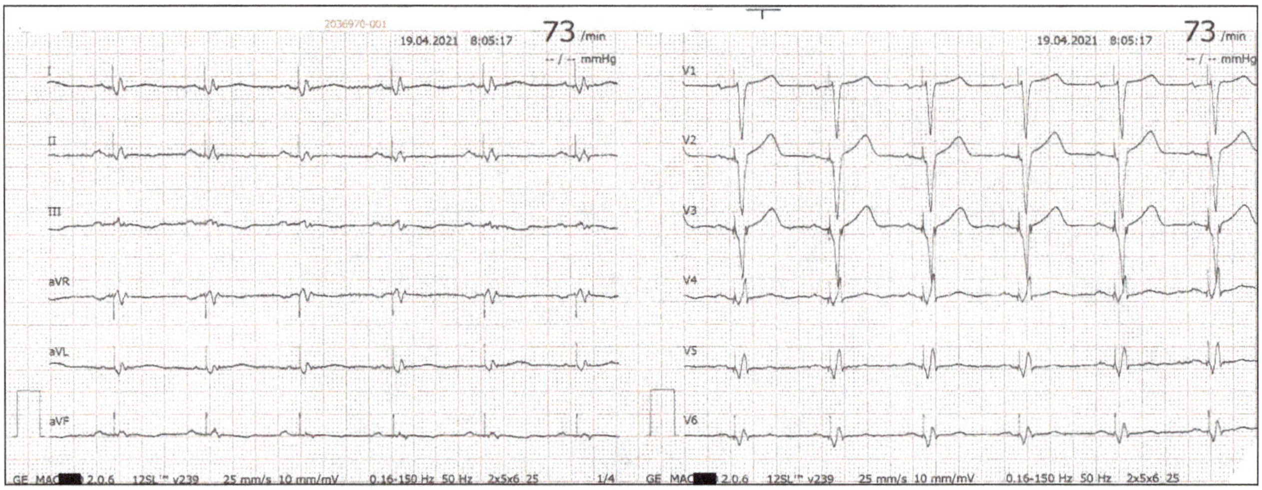

Figure 26.7 12-lead ECG: atrial-synchronous biventricular paced rhythm.

POSTPROCEDURAL COURSE

The patient was extubated and transferred to an intensive cardiologic unit for a 24-hour observation. During the first postoperative day, femoral introducers were removed, and the patient was mobilized. A CXR and the electronic interrogation of the device resulted in range. The patient was discharged from the hospital 3 days after the procedure in good clinical conditions and the first follow-up is scheduled after one month.

PERSONAL EXPERIENCE IN LEAD EXTRACTION AND INTERNAL JUGULAR APPROACH

From January 1997 to December 2020, we treated 2839 patients (75.9% males, mean age 65.2 years), with 5210 leads (4090 pacemakers, 1120 ICDs, mean pacing period 73.6 months).[1–4] Indications to removal were infective in 78% (systemic infection 27% and local infection 51%) and noninfective in 22%.

In our center, we perform all extraction procedures with mechanical dilatation, with a high rate of clinical success (97.4%) and low rates of major complications (0.77%) or death (0.18%). We never experienced superior vena cava tears.

In the reported case, we described a lead extraction procedure using mechanical sheaths from the venous entry site. In our experience, we consider the crossover to the internal jugular approach when dilation is stopped at any binding site for more than 5 minutes, despite the use of larger sheaths, or when dilation is judged too risky. The internal jugular approach increased the mechanical dilation success rate from 89.7% (when performed through the venous entry-site approach) to 97.4%.

Indications to the internal jugular approach were: the presence of tight binding sites (40%), intravascular leads (16%), lead damaged during dilatation (13%), incomplete stylet advancement (10%), narrow costoclavicular space (10%), venous thrombosis (9%), and other (2%).

In brief, a grasping tool (pigtail catheter, deflectable electrophysiological catheter, or tip-deflecting wire) is advanced via the femoral vein and the lead is grasped at the level of the right atrium or SVC, distally to the site where dilatation is stopped. We apply slight traction in order to assess the possibility of slipping the lead and making it free-floating (see Video 26.10). When the lead could not be slipped through, the possibility of grasping it proximal to the site of adherence and making it free-floating is checked. After removal of the stylet and the suture, we make the lead free-floating by applying traction from the femoral vein through the tip-deflecting wire. The right internal jugular vein is then percutaneously cannulated with an 11-Fr introducer. A Lasso (Osypka GmbH) is advanced through the jugular vein, the proximal end of the lead is captured as close as possible to its end, and the lead is retrieved through the jugular vein and exposed. The exposed lead is then extracted with a percutaneous procedure that uses the previously described mechanical dilators (**Figure 26.8**; **Video 26.14**).

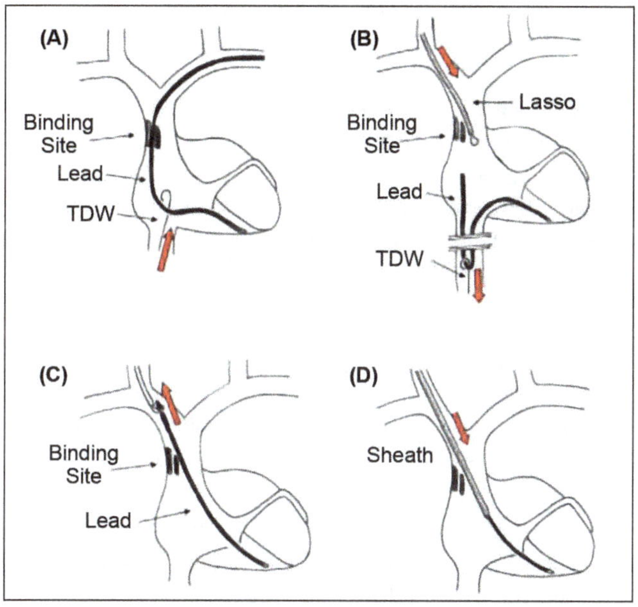

Figure 26.8 Consecutive steps of the internal transjugular approach in case of free-floating leads with anchored tips. **Panel A:** A tip deflecting wire is advanced via the femoral vein in order to assess the possibility to grasp the lead and to move it. **Panel B:** Once the lead has been grasped, it is pulled down in the inferior vena cava; a Lasso, introduced through the internal jugular vein, is advanced near the proximal end of the lead. **Panel C:** The lead is caught by the Lasso and then pulled up and exposed through the jugular vein. **Panel D:** Dilatation using a dilating sheath is performed.

SUMMARY POINTS

- A young patient with a malfunctioning lead should be considered for lead extraction to avoid abandoned leads.
- A preprocedural venography and fluoroscopy predict the complexity of the procedure, showing the location of adherences and the venous system patency.
- The standard stylet provides a good track for the dilator, without the stiffness of the locking stylet, and allows easy removal and re-insertion in case of crossover to a different venous approach.
- The ligature of the lead makes the lead a single body, preventing the development of the insulator. A correct technique application prevents the "snowplowing" effect.
- Bigger adherences need larger dilators, also used in telescopic mode.
- Excess lead loops may be at risk for malfunction and for difficulties during the extraction, for the development of strong adherences.
- Mechanical dilatation must always be performed with gentle, rotational sheath advancements up to the tip, avoiding excessive lead traction and angulations between sheaths and leads (rail effect).
- In absence of infective indications, contextual homolateral reimplantation is workable.
- Jugular approach may be considered in challenging procedures.

ACKNOWLEDGMENT

I would like to address a special thanks to Dr. Maria Grazia Bongiorni, our leader and mentor, who has made the development and the spread of this wonderful lead extraction technique possible. Working with the team, led by Dr. Bongiorni, has given me the opportunity to learn from her about the field of lead extraction and arrhythmology. Every day and every procedure with Dr. Bongiorni is a growth opportunity: simple things and little details make the difference! I am sure it is her pleasure to share with you this instructive case.

—*Luca Segreti, MD*

REFERENCES

1. Bongiorni MG. *Transvenous Lead Extraction: From Simple Traction to the Internal Transjugular Approach*. Springer-Verlag Italia; 2011.
2. Bongiorni MG, Soldati E, Zucchelli G, et al. Transvenous removal of pacing and implantable cardiac defibrillating leads using single sheath mechanical dilatation and multiple venous approaches: High success rate and safety in more than 2000 leads. *Eur Heart J*. 2008;29(23): 2886–2893.
3. Bongiorni MG, Segreti L, Di Cori A, et al. Safety and efficacy of internal transjugular approach for transvenous extraction of implantable cardioverter defibrillator leads. *Europace*. 2014; 16(9):1356–1362.
4. Segreti L, Giannotti Santoro M, Di Cori A, et al. Safety and efficacy of transvenous mechanical lead extraction in patients with abandoned leads. *Europace*. 2020;22(9):1401–1408.

VIDEO LEGENDS

Video 26.1 Angiography performed from a left antecubital peripheral access. Patency of the central venous system is demonstrated, with the presence of adherence in the subclavian and innominate vein tract. [00:06]

Video 26.2 A fluoroscopy zoom on the coil shows no insulator defects. There is an excess lead loop before the tricuspid valve, suggesting it as the possible location of the damage. [00:10]

Video 26.3 The sheath is inserted, taking care to be coaxial with vein entrance. [00:19]

Video 26.4 The adherence in the subclavian and innominate tract, predicted by the venography, was overcome using a larger dilator (10.0-Fr Byrd Dilator Sheath Set (B) Polypropylene, Cook Vandergrift Inc.). [00:48]

Video 26.5 Another adherence, just before the atrial dipole, was overcome with larger size dilator (11.5-Fr Byrd Dilator Sheath Set (C) Polypropylene, Cook Vandergrift Inc.). The transition zone, with small caliper differences, is usually at risk for the development of adherences. [00:56]

Video 26.6 The subsequent adherences present in the atrium were easily overcome with the same dilator. [00:31]

Video 26.7 A larger dilator was repositioned to engage the strong adherence before the tricuspid valve (13.0-Fr Byrd Dilator Sheath Set (D) Polypropylene, Cook Vandergrift Inc.). [00:17]

Video 26.8 It was challenging to engage this adherence. Moreover, the lack of advancement of the stylet over the tricuspid valve added difficulties in this passage. [00:56]

Video 26.9 The externalization of a wire from the lead is visible, with a loop conformation. The wire was engaged with the oversize sheath. [00:53]

Video 26.10 The possibility of grasping the lead proximal to the site of adherence and making it free-floating was checked, in order to evaluate a cross-over to jugular approach in case subclavian access was unsuccessful. [00:17]

Video 26.11 The strong and large adherence localized just before the tricuspid valve, was overcome with the largest dilator available (13.0-Fr Byrd Dilator Sheath Set (D) Polipropylene, Cook Vandergrift Inc.). The dilator was advanced up to the tip, so the lead was totally removed only after all the lead was covered by the sheath. [00:56]

Video 26.12 Videos 26.12A and 26.12B show that after the cannulation of coronary sinus, an angiography with a Swan Ganz catheter was performed, revealing a posterior-lateral branch with a good caliper. [00:17]

Video 26.13 Videos 26.13A–C feature the final fluoroscopy showing the ipsilateral CRT-D reimplantation. [00:04]

Video 26.14 A case of despiralized dual-coil ICD removed with the internal jugular approach. [00:47]

Author Disclosures

Fatima A. Ali-Ahmed—None

Samuel J. Asirvatham—None

Walid M. Barake—None

Ulrika Birgersdotter-Green—No relevant conflicts of interest

Antonio Maria Canu—No disclosures

Yong-Mei Cha MD—None

Gregory A. Cogert—Consulting for Medtronic reviewing ICD electrograms

Freddy Del-Carpio Munoz—None

Andrea Di Cori—No disclosures

Paul A. Friedman—Global PI on the Medtronic Extravascular ICD study and has served as an advisor, with all funds going to Mayo Clinic

Bradley Genovese—No disclosures

Mario Giannotti Santoro—No disclosures

Shane M. Gillespie -None

Erik A. Green—No disclosures

Akbar H. Khan—No conflicts of interest

Klitos Konstantinidis—None

Gurukripa N. Kowlgi—None

Fred M. Kusumoto—No conflicts

Adetola Ladejobi—No relevant disclosures

Chin Lee—No disclosures

Justin Z. Lee—None

Charles J. Love—Abbott Medical, Boston Scientific, Convatec, Medtronic, Philips Medical

William J. Mauermann—None

Olurotimi Mesubi—None

Kevin J. Mulligan—No disclosures

Siva K. Mulpuru—No conflicts

Travis Pollema—No disclosures

Luca Segreti—No disclosures

Samuel A. Shabtaie—None

Imran S. Syed—No conflicts to disclose

Martin van Zyl—None

Pierce J. Vatterott—Paid consultant for Boston Scientific, Cook Medical, Medtronic, Philips Medical

Stefano Viani—No disclosures

Giulio Zucchelli—No disclosures

Index

S

T

V

W

www.ingramcontent.com/pod-product-compliance
Lightning Source LLC
LaVergne TN
LVHW080645011026
849160LV00014B/1324
9781942909545